PENGUIN CANADA

LIVING WELL WITH ARTHRITIS

DR. DIANNE MOSHER is professor of medicine at Dalhousie University and past president of the Canadian Rheumatology Association. She has practised rheumatology at the QEII hospital in Halifax for the past sixteen years.

DR. HOWARD STEIN has been a practicing rheumatologist for more than twenty-five years. Based in Vancouver, Dr. Stein has been on staff at St. Paul's Hospital, the Arthritis Centre, and at the G. F. Strong Rehabilitation Centre. He is honorary professor of medicine at the University of British Columbia.

DR. GUNNAR KRAAG is chief of the Division of Rheumatology at the Ottawa Hospital and professor of medicine at the University of Ottawa. He is past chair of the Canadian Council of Academic Rheumatologists and vice president of the Canadian Rheumatology Association.

Living well *with* arthritis

A SOURCEBOOK FOR UNDERSTANDING AND MANAGING YOUR ARTHRITIS

Dianne Mosher, MD

Howard Stein, MD

Gunnar Kraag, MD

PENGUIN
CANADA

PENGUIN CANADA

Published by the Penguin Group

Penguin Group (Canada), 90 Eglinton Avenue East, Suite 700, Toronto, Ontario, Canada M4P 2Y3
(a division of Pearson Penguin Canada Inc.)

Penguin Group (USA) Inc., 375 Hudson Street, New York, New York 10014, U.S.A.
Penguin Books Ltd, 80 Strand, London WC2R 0RL, England
Penguin Ireland, 25 St Stephen's Green, Dublin 2, Ireland (a division of Penguin Books Ltd)
Penguin Group (Australia), 250 Camberwell Road, Camberwell, Victoria 3124, Australia
(a division of Pearson Australia Group Pty Ltd)
Penguin Books India Pvt Ltd, 11 Community Centre, Panchsheel Park, New Delhi – 110 017, India
Penguin Group (NZ), cnr Airborne and Rosedale Roads, Albany, Auckland 1310, New Zealand
(a division of Pearson New Zealand Ltd)
Penguin Books (South Africa) (Pty) Ltd, 24 Sturdee Avenue, Rosebank, Johannesburg 2196, South Africa

Penguin Books Ltd, Registered Offices: 80 Strand, London WC2R 0RL, England

First published in a Viking Canada paperback by Penguin Group (Canada),
a division of Pearson Penguin Canada Inc., 2002
Published in this edition, 2006

(WEB) 10 9 8 7 6 5 4 3 2

This publication contains the opinions and ideas of its authors and is designed to provide useful advice in regard to the subject matter covered. The authors and publisher are not engaged in rendering health or other professional services in this publication. This publication is not intended to provide a basis for action in particular circumstances without consideration by a competent professional. The authors and publisher expressly disclaim any responsibility for any liability, loss or risk, personal or otherwise, that is incurred as a consequence, directly or indirectly, of the use and application of any of the contents of this book.

Manufactured in Canada.

LIBRARY AND ARCHIVES CANADA CATALOGUING IN PUBLICATION

Mosher, Dianne
Living well with arthritis : a sourcebook for understanding and managing your arthritis / Dianne Mosher, Howard Stein, Gunnar Kraag.

Includes bibliographical references and index.

ISBN 0-14-305558-5

1. Arthritis—Popular works. I. Kraag, Gunnar II. Stein, Howard III. Title.

RC933.M68 2005 616.7'22 C2005-905930-3

Visit the Penguin Group (Canada) website at **www.penguin.ca**

This book is dedicated to my two sons, Christopher and Jeffrey, my father, Eric, and to the memory of my mother, Carol Cole Mosher.

– Dianne Mosher

To my family for their patience and support: Sunni, Jaime, Jordan, Rhoda, Anne, and Morris, and to my brother Steven for encouraging me to write a book.

– Howard Stein

To my loving wife, Marilyn, for her enduring patience and support.

– Gunnar Kraag

Contents

Foreword

As president of the Arthritis Society, I'm thrilled to introduce you to *Living Well with Arthritis*. I salute the team of dedicated arthritis specialists who have contributed, chapter by chapter, piece by piece, to put the arthritis "puzzle" into perspective through this book.

In many ways, arthritis is still a mystery to all of us—laypeople and physicians alike—but we have made great headway in developing new treatments for the more than 100 kinds of arthritis.

The Arthritis Society and other members of the arthritis community have also worked to develop programs and services to help those living with this painful and often disabling disease. One of these initiatives is the Canadian Arthritis Bill of Rights, a document that describes arthritis patients' rights and responsibilities, provides some facts and figures about arthritis, and suggests action that can be taken by Canadian citizens and our governments at all levels to improve the lives of people with arthritis, both now and in the future.

Patients are also taking on the challenge of battling the disease. Together, they are working with their doctors, health care professionals, and decision makers to make life better for those with arthritis, and are now sitting at the table to ensure that health policies are developed that deal with arthritis.

Not only does this book serve as a guide for information about how the disease works, but it also takes on issues that until recently haven't been discussed in an open forum, such as COXIBs, biological agents, anesthesia for arthritis surgery, complementary therapies, sexuality, research and the patient, and the workplace and insurance.

I know the struggle only too well, as I talk with so many patients who ask, "Why me?" or "Why my child?" and "What can I do?" I hope you take the time to read this book page by page so that you, your family, and those in your life who have been hit hard by this disease can better deal with the challenges you face.

—Denis Morrice, president of the Arthritis Society

Acknowledgements

First and foremost, we would like to thank Ms. Jennifer McTaggart (previously of Prentice Hall Publishing) for convincing us to take this project on, and Ms. Nicole de Montbrun (our editor at Penguin Books) for her invaluable support. We are very grateful to Ms. Laurel Sparrow for turning our written ideas into readable prose. We would also like to acknowledge the work of Dr. Faith Dodd, who developed the outline for this book while working as a medical student.

Many people have made significant contributions along the way. We would like to acknowledge the professional input, review of chapters, and support of our friends and colleagues: Dr. Gillian Graves (gynecologist); Mr. David Farrar (lawyer); Dr. Mary Lynch (psychiatrist and pain specialist); Dr. Lee Kirby (physiatrist); Ms. Karen Van Mahltzen (occupational therapist); Mr. Ed Dubois (friend and patient); Ms. Wendy Turner (physiotherapist); Dr. Michael Gross (orthopedic surgeon); and Ms. Sherrie Lynch (of the Mary Pack Arthritis Centre).

Mr. Lance Woolaver's book, *The Illuminated Life of Maud Lewis* (published by Nimbus Publishing Limited), was an excellent source of information about Maud Lewis's life. We would also like to acknowledge Mrs. Anne Kitz and Ms. Laurie Hamilton of the Art Gallery of Nova Scotia for their assistance in obtaining information on Maud Lewis. We thank Ms. Beth Brooks for kindly agreeing to allow us to use her father's photograph of Maud Lewis. (Mr. Bob Brooks was a well-known photojournalist who did the photos of Maud for *Star Weekly* magazine in 1965.)

We would also like to acknowledge Ms. Jill Babcock, our illustrator and a patient with arthritis, for her beautiful drawings that bring our book to life.

The support of peers is also necessary for a publication such as this. The Division of Rheumatology and the Department of Medicine at Dalhousie University have graciously supported Dr. Mosher's sabbatical leave to write a portion of this book. We would also like to thank Mr. Denis Morrice and Ms. Norma Kent, both of the Arthritis Society.

Last, but certainly not least, we wish to acknowledge our patients, who continually inspire and educate us.

Introduction

Our heroes are the many people who walk through life with crippled joints, daily pain, and profound fatigue, but despite this, do not have a disabled spirit. Maud Lewis was one of these people. She was not our patient; in fact, she never saw a rheumatologist. Her story is a portrait of a hero, however, and also illustrates the natural progression of inflammatory arthritis without treatment.

A Portrait of a Hero

Maud Lewis was a folk artist born in South Ohio, Yarmouth County, Nova Scotia, in 1903. She has been likened to a Canadian Grandma Moses and in 1999, a major exhibition of her work crossed Canada in a tour sponsored by Scotia Bank.

Maud's biographer, Lance Woolaver, states that "Maud suffered from multiple birth defects that left her shoulders unnaturally sloped and her chin resting on her chest." A 1967 article in the *Atlantic Advocate* by Doris McCoy stated that "Maud had been stricken with polio, which left her arms and legs crippled." Mr. Woolaver doubted that this was the case, and again described her hand, chin, and spinal deformities as part of her birth defects. It was generally acknowledged that in later years she suffered from arthritis. We also learn from Mr. Woolaver that Maud missed many days of school and that children made fun of her flat chin. If you examine pictures of Maud as a child, you will note that her chin is small. Also, her neck is bent sideways, a deformity that worsens with age. She has flexion contractures (bend) in her right elbow and right knee. Maud had juvenile onset rheumatoid arthritis.

Maud's father was a reasonably prosperous harness maker. At school, Maud went only as far as Grade 4, but her mother had taught her to paint and they sold Christmas cards door to door. She lived under the comfort and protection of her parents until their deaths in 1935 and 1937. Her brother, Charlie, did not want Maud living with him, and so she was shipped off to an aunt in Digby. Any inheritance from the family went to Charlie.

Unwilling to be completely dependent upon her aunt, Maud answered an ad from a local fishmonger looking for a live-in housekeeper. Maud walked seven kilometres to Marshalltown to meet Everett Lewis, and agreed to move in only on the condition that they marry. Two weeks later they were married, and Maud moved into Everett's 14-square-metre house, where she spent the rest of her life.

Maud Lewis

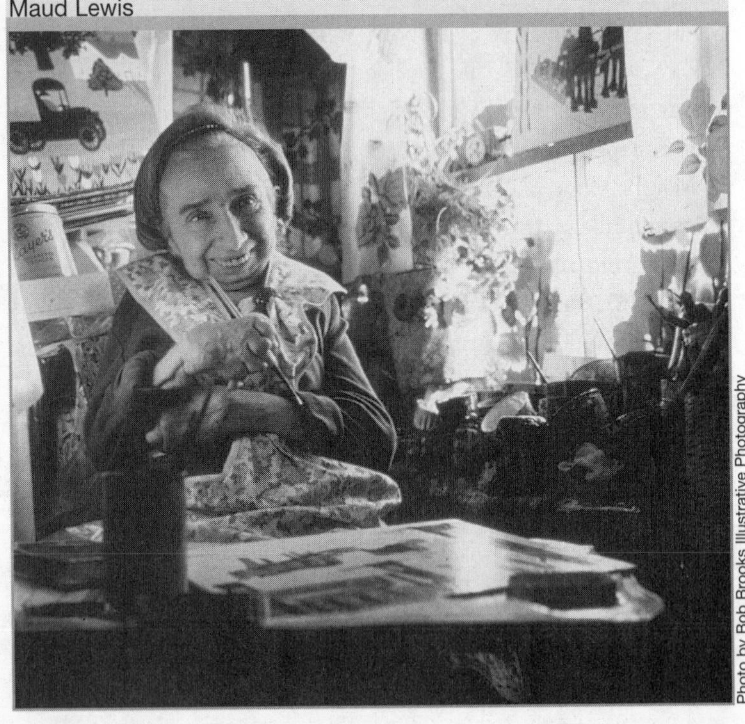

Photo by Bob Brooks Illustrative Photography

There was no running water, no bathroom, and the only bed was in a loft into which she was surely unable to climb.

She began by painting the small cabin, and later sold paintings at the roadside. Maud painted on a TV table with whatever paints Everett could find. Later, when she became famous, artists would visit her and give her supplies. She was given an easel but never used it; this was attributed to the fact that she was content with the pure simplicities of life, but it was more likely because of her arthritis. She had fixed flexion deformities of her wrists and elbows and no movement of her shoulders. She painted at the TV table by holding the brush in her hand and moving back and forth at her waist. It would have been impossible to use an easel.

When then-president of the United States Richard Nixon requested two of her paintings, her reply was, "Upon receipt of your $14, I will forward the two paintings." Eventually, enough money was coming into the household that Everett quit his job. He was described as a miser and would not allow Maud to spend any of the money she earned. There were never any improvements on the house that would have made Maud's life more comfortable.

In 1968, Maud fell and fractured her hip. The fracture was likely as a result of osteoporosis due to her arthritis, subsequent inactivity, and poor nutrition. She was a chronic smoker and died in 1970 of pneumonia.

Everett sold her belongings, and got $1 apiece for the sympathy cards (including one from Richard Nixon). It was rumoured that Everett kept all the money in the house, perhaps under the floorboards. In 1979, a young man broke in, looking for the cash box. In the ensuing battle, Everett was killed.

It is sad to think of Maud's life and how she was treated in her marriage. Maud would have lived every day in pain. With the extent of her arthritis, mobility would have been difficult, and she was deprived of any physical comforts even when she could well afford them. Yet despite this, she asserted her independence by marrying Everett Lewis. She accepted responsibility and even when ill was worried about her commissioned artworks. She forged a life for herself despite the odds, and painted beautiful, cheerful pictures. She was a hero.

Maud's story makes us realize what life must have been like for people with severe arthritis at that time: not only did they have to deal with the disease, but with social isolation and poverty as well. Arthritis is still affecting people today (four million in Canada), but in the past five years, there have been many new developments in the treatment and management of arthritis. Now, more than at any time in the past, patients who suffer with arthritis can expect improvement in joint swelling, pain, mobility, and quality of life.

As most forms of arthritis are chronic in nature, it is crucial that people with arthritis understand their condition and what options for therapy are available to them. Each type of arthritis affects patients differently. People also have different ideas about what they consider to be important achievements for themselves: for some, a signficant accomplishment may be to move without help from a wheelchair to a bed, while for others, it is to run a marathon. Some people are by nature willing to take greater risks and may want to participate in clinical studies; others prefer the conservative approach. All of this together means that each person's management of arthritis must be individualized: there is no cookbook recipe, and there is no magic.

A purpose of this book is to provide you with information about arthritis and how it can be managed in the long term. It is also a resource to direct you to more information about the disease. However, its most important reason for being is to give you the knowledge and confidence to take control of the care of your arthritis, so that you too can live well with arthritis.

How to Use This Book

This book deals with the various common forms of arthritis, as well as soft tissue rheumatism and chronic pain syndromes, which are frequently confused with arthritis. It discusses the common forms of arthritis, musculoskeletal pain that is not arthritis, and childhood arthritis, pregnancy and delivery, medications and therapies, surgery, complementary medicine, exercise, diet and nutrition, assistive devices, pain and fatigue and their management. Very importantly, we have included a section on health care providers and what their role should be. This book also deals with sex and relationships, the workplace and disability, and research and the patient.

Appendix I contains more detailed information on the hereditary and environmental components of arthritis. Appendix II contains a list of resources that can provide you with more detailed and specific information about your type of arthritis. Dr. Stein has been answering "Ask a rheumatologist" questions for the Arthritis Society of Canada's website and has collected an excellent dossier of frequently asked questions.

We have recognized the need for an informative, practical book on arthritis that is oriented to Canadians. Because of our many years of experience in practice we have chosen areas that we feel need to be covered. This book stems from the questions patients ask us, and what we think they ought to know.

1 Not all arthritis is created equal

In my years in practice as a rheumatologist, I have noted that among patients and the medical community alike, there are some major misconceptions about arthritis.

The most common misconception may have come from the slogan "Arthritis: there is no cure." Many equate the slogan to "Arthritis: there is no *treatment*." Time and again, I have seen patients who have been told, "It's arthritis and nothing can be done, so go home and live with it."

The most dangerous misconception is that arthritis is not a serious disease. In fact, arthritis is the number one cause of disability in North America and affects people of all ages: it is not only a disease of the old.

It is also not true that all arthritis is the same: there are approximately 100 forms of arthritis. The most common form is osteoarthritis, which affects approximately 55 percent of us by age 65. Rheumatoid arthritis is less common, but does affect approximately 1 percent of the population; most of these people begin to be affected between the ages of 30 and 50.

What Is Arthritis?

Arthritis is derived from the Greek *arthron* (joint) and *itis* (inflammation). Therefore, arthritis by this definition would mean inflammation within a joint.

A joint is the structure that connects two bones. The joint is held together by ligaments and tendons and a capsule. The ends of the bones are covered with cartilage and the capsule is lined by a synovial membrane (see illustration below).

Cartilage is the white glistening stuff you have probably seen at the end of a chicken bone. It allows bones to glide smoothly over each other, with synovial fluid acting as a lubricant, and also absorbs the forces that impact on the joints. Cartilage is made up of collagen (protein fibres), water, chondrocyctes (the cartilage cells), and proteoglycans. Normal cartilage is essential to a well-functioning joint.

In arthritis, the cartilage may have become damaged. It may have thinned and eventually disappeared, leading to bone rubbing on

A joint

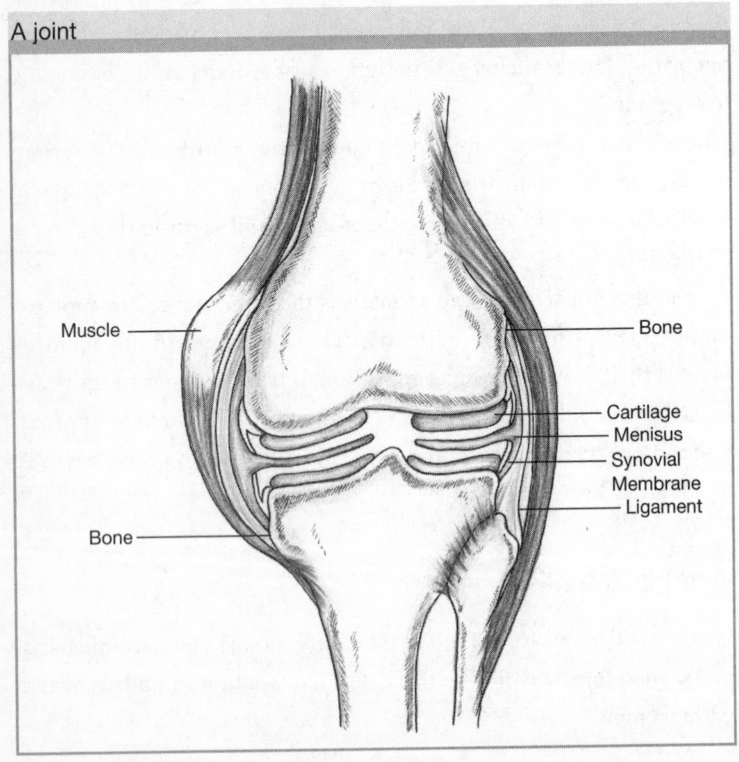

bone. The damage to cartilage can occur in different ways, and this is why we have different forms of arthritis. The two major types of arthritis are degenerative (wear and tear) and inflammatory.

Degenerative arthritis is known as osteoarthritis. In this form of arthritis, the primary problem occurs in the cartilage. The cartilage may be damaged by a previous injury to the joint, or by a chronic stress on the joint (as in osteoarthritis in the knees of obese females). The cartilage itself may be abnormal because of a genetic defect that can lead to premature osteoarthritis in whole families. Degenerative arthritis used to be referred to as "non-inflammatory arthritis," however, researchers have become increasingly aware that inflammation is an important factor in the progression of osteoarthritis.

In inflammatory arthritis, the inflammation in the joint causes the damage. The signs of inflammation are redness, heat, swelling, and pain. In the joint, this leads to loss of function. An example of an inflammatory arthritis is rheumatoid arthritis, in which the immune system is overactive, leading to inflammation mainly (but not always) in the synovium and the joint fluid. The inflammation itself causes pain and a poorly functioning joint, but ultimately, the cartilage is damaged and the joint is finished. Rheumatologists want to treat the inflammation before this happens.

Other conditions such as bursitis or tendonitis are not arthritis. They do not occur in the joint. They are referred to as soft tissue rheumatism, and are discussed in Chapter 2, "Not All Musculoskeletal Pain Is Arthritis."

Osteoarthritis

Osteoarthritis is a common disease characterized by pain in the joint, stiffness, and loss of movement. It is also referred to as degenerative joint disease and osteoarthrosis. It is a slowly evolving disease that is part of the aging process. Autopsy studies have shown that by age 40, 90 percent of all persons have changes in the weight bearing joints (knees, hips) although, of course, all of these people did not have symptoms. By age 65, approximately 60 percent of us will have symptoms of osteoarthritis.

Not only is osteoarthritis common, but it has been around for a long time: dinosaur bones and Egyptian mummies all show evidence of osteoarthritis. Yet we still understand very little about this disease and specific treatment has eluded us.

Osteoarthritis is classified as a non-inflammatory arthritis. This implies that there is no inflammation, but recent research shows that this is not true. The factors that cause the disease (which starts in the cartilage) are not completely known. It is known that early on, although there is no inflammation yet, the cartilage starts to wear away and fragment, and the bone under the cartilage thickens. Loose pieces of cartilage cause an immune response and inflammation, which is known to be responsible for some of the progression of the disease. As the disease evolves, the cartilage thins and disappears. As well, new bone is formed at the joint edges (this is referred to as an osteophyte) and the bone under the cartilage continues to thicken.

Dr. Stein discusses in detail some of the causes of osteoarthritis in Appendix I, "Heredity and Environment," but we will summarize some of the causes here:

- Trauma may lead to osteoarthritis (whether this is sudden, severe trauma, or a repetitive strain such as seen in obese females and osteoarthritis of the knees).
- The tendency to develop osteoarthritis can also be passed from parent to child in the genes, as we see with congenital hip dysplasia or erosive osteoarthritis of the hands (which seems to be passed from mother to daughter most commonly).

Classification of Osteoarthritis

Generally, osteoarthritis is divided into primary and secondary forms: primary osteoarthritis has no underlying cause; secondary

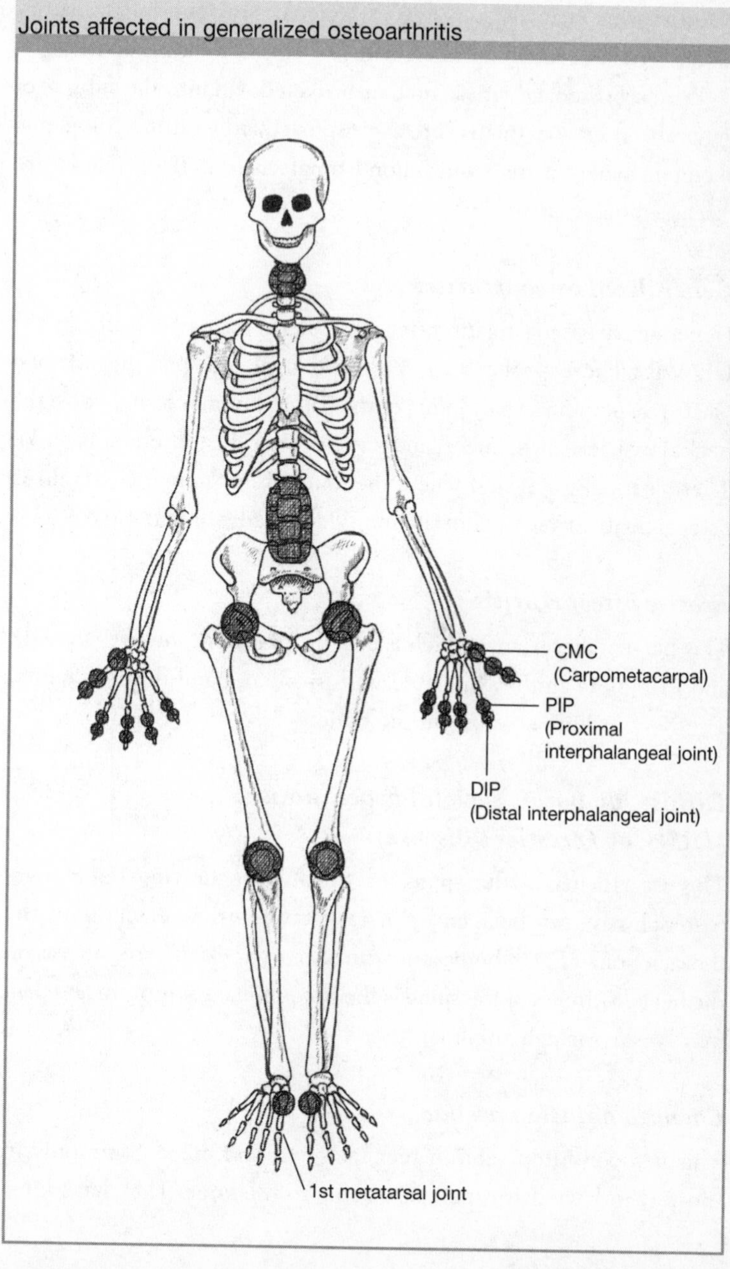
Joints affected in generalized osteoarthritis
CMC
(Carpometacarpal)
PIP
(Proximal
interphalangeal joint)
DIP
(Distal interphalangeal joint)
1st metatarsal joint

osteoarthritis may be a result of trauma, previous inflammatory diseases such as rheumatoid arthritis, or crystal induced diseases.

Primary osteoarthritis is further broken down into the subsets of generalized osteoarthritis, erosive osteoarthritis, diffuse idiopathic skeletal hyperostosis, and chondromalacia patellae. These are discussed below.

Generalized osteoarthritis

Generalized osteoarthritis refers to osteoarthritis that affects the DIP (distal interphalangeal), PIP (proximal interphalangeal), and CMC (carpometacarpal) joints of the hands, but may also involve the neck, low back, hips, knees, and big toes (see illustration on page 5). There is usually a period where the joints are inflamed. Generalized osteoarthritis occurs primarily in middle-aged women.

Erosive osteoarthritis

This particular variant, which is usually inherited, involves the DIP and PIP joints and is associated with swollen, painful finger joints. The X-rays show erosions in the bone.

Diffuse idiopathic skeletal hyperostosis (DISH, or Forestier's disease)

This is arthritis in the spine, in which huge flowing bone spurs (osteophytes) can be seen on X-ray between the vertebrae of the thoracic spine. Large bony spurs can also occur elsewhere, such as on the heels. Stiffness of the spine is the predominant symptom and pain may be surprisingly minimal.

Chondromalacia patellae

This is a condition seen in teenage girls, and more commonly in those who have had repeated trauma to the knee. They have knee pain that is made worse with squatting, kneeling, and going down stairs. What has happened is that the cartilage behind the kneecap has softened and split into fibres, and the kneecap has been allowed too much sideways movement because of looseness in its supporting muscles and tendons. What is needed is an exercise program to strengthen the muscles, after which the cartilage can go back to normal.

Symptoms

The joints that are commonly affected by osteoarthritis include the DIP, PIP, and CMC joints of the hands, the neck, lower back, hips, knees, and the big toes (or first metatarsal phalangeal joint). (See again the illustration on page 5.) If other joints are involved, it is usually as a result of trauma to that joint or an inflammatory arthritis (which will be discussed on page 15 of this chapter).

Pain

Pain is a predominant feature of osteoarthritis. Early in the disease, the pain accompanies movement, is aggravated by prolonged activity, and is made better with rest. When the condition is more severe, there is pain at rest and it will also awaken you at night.

The pain in osteoarthritis is not coming from the cartilage, which does not have nerve endings. The pain may be from the joint capsule, or from tendons around the joint that are being stretched because of the swelling or deformity of the joint. The pain may also be caused by stretching of the lining of the bone (periosteum) at the sites of new bone growth. If the bone spurs protrude into the space where the nerves travel (as in the neck or back) then the pain is from the nerve irritation or compression. Such a pain would travel down your arm or leg and would be a burning type of pain; there may be weakness or loss of feeling in the affected limb.

Stiffness

People with osteoarthritis often experience morning stiffness that usually lasts for less than 30 minutes.

Swelling

Once the cartilage has been damaged, bits of it actually cause an immune response and associated swelling, heat, redness, and pain (inflammation). Another cause of an acutely inflamed joint in osteoarthritis is the presence of calcium crystals in the joint space. Sometimes, the joint may appear to be swollen but it is actually enlarged as a result of the new bone growth. This is referred to as bony enlargement.

Crepitus

Crepitus is the grinding and creaking of the joint as it is being moved. This is common in osteoarthritis.

Deformity

The bony enlargement of the DIP joint of the finger is called a Heberden's node. The enlargement of the PIP joint is called a Bouchard's node. These can begin as a swelling like a cyst filled with jelly-like material. At times they become inflamed and painful. Once the inflammation has settled, they stop hurting and become hard and bony.

At the base of the thumb is the CMC joint, which can be involved with osteoarthritis. The joint can be very painful, like a boil, and becomes enlarged and bony. Often physicians refer to this as squaring of the joint.

There are two common deformities of the knees. The first, *genu valgus* or knock knees, occurs with loss of the lateral joint space of the knee and is more common in women. The second, *genu varus* or bow legs, is due to loss of the medial joint space of the knee and is more common in men.

The other common deformity of osteoarthritis is a *hallux valgus* deformity of the big toe: this is your common bunion.

Investigations

There are no specific laboratory tests for osteoarthritis: the diagnosis is based on the clinical findings and X-rays. This disease stays in the joints and the tests for inflammation (such as the ESR or the CRP) are usually normal.

The typical changes we see on X-ray include loss of cartilage, thickening of the bone under the cartilage, and bony spurs. You do not usually need more sophisticated X-rays, such as a CAT scan (computerized axial tomography) or MRI (magnetic resonance imaging). The MRI does show the cartilage changes better, however, and so would probably be used in clinical studies where it would be important to determine whether new therapies have an effect on the cartilage.

Management

The management of osteoarthritis includes treating the pain, maintaining the range of motion of the joints, and preventing disability. To do this, patients use medications, exercise, supportive devices, modification of daily activities, and surgery. To date, the most significant improvement in the management of osteoarthritis has been the replacement surgery for the knee and hip.

Medications

Medications are discussed much more fully and in more detail in Chapter 7, "Medications." This section is intended to be an overview of medications available for treating osteoarthritis in particular.

No medication is currently available that repairs the cartilage, although considerable research is being done into the development of what are termed the "disease modifying osteoarthritic drugs."

There is no harm in trying acetaminophen first. It should be taken on a regular basis, up to 650 mg (or two regular-strength pills) four times a day. If this is not working, then an NSAID (non-steroidal anti-inflammatory drug) can be tried, provided there is not a contraindication to its use. If you have had a previous bleed from a stomach ulcer, then you should be on something to protect your stomach (such as misoprostil or a proton pump inhibitor) or you could take a COX-2 selective drug, which is easier on the stomach. If you have high blood pressure, kidney problems, or congestive heart failure, then check with your physician before using an NSAID.

There are several topical agents used in osteoarthritis for pain control. Most of these contain capsaicin, which is derived from cayenne pepper. These products are rubbed over the skin three to four times a day, and may provide moderate relief of pain. There are also topical non-steroidal preparations, but the difficulty with these is that we don't know how much is absorbed, and they have the potential for the same side effects as NSAIDs that you take by mouth.

There are several products that are labelled as viscosupplements (including Synvisc and Orthovisc). These are derivatives of hyaluronic acid, which is a naturally occurring part of the joint fluid, and they are given to supplement or add to what the body already makes. These drugs are given as a weekly joint injection (usually into the knee) for three weeks. They help with pain and improve mobility in 50–60 percent of cases. This effect lasts approximately six months to one year. Viscosupplementation works best in patients who have mild to moderate osteoarthritis of the knee.

Low doses of amitriptyline or other tricyclic antidepressant medications are very useful for pain control. They are used at night in small doses and they help you with sleep, have a direct effect on pain, and help relax your muscles.

Narcotics are occasionally recommended for the control of chronic pain and are sometimes necessary to control the pain of osteoarthritis.

As mentioned, disease modifying osteoarthritis drugs are not available yet, but glucosamine and chondroitin sulfate have been used to treat osteoarthritis. These are available in pharmacies and natural food and supplement stores. These products have been studied in Europe more than in North America, but the results to date suggest that both have an effect on pain, although the better designed studies showed them to have less of a benefit than placebo. Both are well tolerated; some people reported stomach upset, but this was mild. There may be an increase in blood sugar levels in diabetics on glucosamine, so this should be monitored. These products are not regulated, and it is therefore advisable to buy from a reputable manufacturer to ensure that you have purchased the advertised compound. There is a website (www.drtheo.com) that reports on the independent laboratory analysis of products from the nutriceutical industry, and you might do well to check the website to get unbiased information about a product that you're thinking about taking.

Corticosteroids are only used to treat osteoarthritis by injection into the joint, which provides short-term relief (usually in the range of four weeks).

Tetracycline and minocycline are antibiotics that may actually help prevent cartilage loss in osteoarthritis, and clinical studies are now underway to investigate this.

Therapies

A physiotherapist can help to settle an acute flare of osteoarthritis, and can also provide an appropriate exercise regime, which is essential for patients with osteoarthritis. Acupuncture and massage are often very beneficial in the control of arthritis pain.

This next section will cover specific therapies that rheumatologists have found helpful for the management of osteoarthritis in specific joints.

Osteoarthritis of the hands usually affects the DIP, PIP, and CMC joints. As these joints can frequently be inflamed, it is useful to use an NSAID when the joint is swollen, red, and tender. Some people find that they need these drugs only periodically, while others need them on a regular basis. If you are using them as an anti-inflammatory, then they need to be taken for at least two weeks on a regular basis to have their full effect. If one or two joints are particularly inflamed, then an injection of corticosteroids into the joint is helpful (particularly for the CMC joint).

Hot wax therapy makes the joints feel good. If this is not possible, you might get a similar effect by rubbing mineral oil into your hands, putting on tight rubber gloves, and putting your gloved hands into hot water.

It is important to exercise your hands regularly so that you prevent loss of range of motion.

Occasionally, surgery is necessary if you are experiencing pain that is not otherwise controlled or if there is progressive deformity. The CMC joint can be replaced or fused; the surgery works well. The DIP joint can be fused. The PIP joint can be replaced or fused.

Osteoarthritis in the cervical spine occurs in the small joints and is usually associated with degeneration of the discs and bone spur formation. Arthritis of the cervical spine leads to a stiff and painful neck and limited range of movement. The muscles may also be in spasm, and patients tend to sleep poorly.

Management first involves avoiding activities that might aggravate the pain. For example, if your job requires you to talk on the phone a long time, you should use a headset. If you are working on a computer, make sure that it is at a proper height and that you have a comfortable chair. This is not to say that you should cease all activity, however, because exercise is important for maintaining range of movement and strength. Even a few simple stretches in the shower are helpful.

It is important to get a good sleep. Cervical pillows are helpful, and the water-filled pillows seem to work best for most people. Sometimes a low dose of a tricyclic antidepressant is very useful as it relieves the pain, gets you to sleep, and also relieves the muscle spasm. NSAIDs are useful to try, and some people find it helpful to take regular Tylenol or Tylenol with codeine at bedtime.

A soft collar is helpful if you are having a lot of pain. It should not be worn for more than a few hours a day, however, as wearing it too long leads to muscle weakness and worsening of the problem.

Surgery is an option if the nerve root is irritated or compressed to the point that pain is running down the arm and there is numbness or loss of strength in the hand. These types of symptoms are referred to as radiculopathy. The symptoms will sometimes settle on their own, however if they are persistent or severe, then surgery may be needed.

Osteoarthritis in the lumbosacral spine occurs at the back of the spine at the facet joints and the discs. The treatment includes NSAIDs, painkillers (narcotics), physiotherapy, exercise, and supportive devices.

In the condition called spinal stenosis, the spinal cord and nerves coming from the cord are being crowded or pinched by the bone spurs or protruding discs. The pain occurs when walking, is improved with leaning forward, and is relieved with a few minutes' rest. This condition, if severe, requires surgery.

Patients with pain from osteoarthritis in the facet joints often experience pain in the buttock region. Many refer to this as hip pain, although it is not from the hip but from the lower back. This pain may radiate down the back of the leg to just above the knee, and is made worse by arching the back. The best treatment is an exercise program to strengthen the muscles. Physiotherapy can be helpful for some to settle the pain, but an exercise program is needed to prevent the pain from recurring. A girdle or a lumbosacral corset can be helpful if you have to stand for any length of time. Do not use the corset too much, however, as this can lead to muscle weakness.

Lower back pain that is originating with the discs is usually across the mid-lower back. If a nerve is being pinched, then the pain will radiate down the whole leg and there may be numbness or loss of strength in the leg. This is, again, a radiculopathy. The treatment includes an exercise program and pain medication. If the pain is persistent and severe, surgery may be needed.

The symptoms of **osteoarthritis of the hip** are pain, stiffness, and loss of range of movement. Hip pain is usually felt in the groin and down the thigh, and may sometimes be felt in the knee (this is a referred pain pattern for the hip). One of the first symptoms may be difficulty in putting on your socks or pantyhose.

Continuing to walk is important, as are range-of-motion exercises. Impact sports (such as running, basketball, or squash) should be avoided. If you are experiencing a lot of pain on walking, then it is important to use a cane. (If your left hip is involved, you carry the cane in your right hand and put your left foot forward as the cane moves forward on the right side.) This will take 40 percent of your weight off the bad hip, which can make a huge difference.

The use of NSAIDs and acetaminophen can be helpful. Once the pain and loss of movement are significantly interfering with your lifestyle and/or you are waking at night with pain, you might consider a hip replacement. Because the artificial hips do not last forever and each repeated surgery is more difficult, surgeons ask their younger patients to delay the surgery as long as possible.

Osteoarthritis of the knees causes pain, stiffness, and loss of mobility. An exercise program is essential to maintain strength and range of motion. If the knee pain occurs mainly with kneeling, squatting, or walking downstairs, then the pain may be caused by the kneecap scraping against the knee. This is best managed with physiotherapy and an exercise program for patellofemoral disease.

Using a cane can be very beneficial with knee osteoarthritis, as it removes 40 percent of your weight from the knee. A support bandage or brace may sometimes provide stability and comfort.

Swelling is often associated with osteoarthritis of the knees, and NSAIDs can be beneficial. If these do not settle the swelling, an injection of corticosteroids can help.

Patients with mild to moderate osteoarthritis and those for whom surgery is contraindicated may wish to try viscosupplementation (see Chapter 7, "Medications") for some relief of the pain on walking.

Arthroscopic surgery to clean out the joint may temporarily help with the symptoms of osteoarthritis of the knee, and a high tibial osteotomy for osteoarthritis of the medial joint space can buy time before a knee replacement. If the above have failed, however, and you are experiencing significant pain, loss of function, and night pain, a knee replacement needs to be considered. (Please see Chapter 10, "Surgery.")

Osteoarthritis of the first MTP joint (also known as a bunion joint) is a very common problem. The initial treatment is to buy shoes, with or without orthotics, that are comfortable and accommodate your foot. If the pain is interfering with activities, then surgery can be considered, but this surgery is not minor: recovery takes from six weeks to three months. (Again, please see Chapter 10, "Surgery.")

Rheumatoid Arthritis

Rheumatoid arthritis is the most common form of chronic inflammatory arthritis. It affects 1 in 100 people, and roughly 300 000

Canadians have the disease. Three times as many females as males are affected, and it can occur at any age, although the most common age of onset is between 30 and 50 years.

Rheumatoid arthritis causes swelling, pain, and stiffness of the small joints of the hands, wrists, elbows, knees, and feet. It can, in fact, affect almost any joint, but usually spares the lower back and thoracic spine. Rheumatoid arthritis is also a systemic disorder, meaning that more is affected than the joints: the eyes, lungs, small blood vessels, and other organs can all be involved. People with rheumatoid arthritis experience fatigue, anemia, and a general feeling of being unwell. They are usually stiff in the mornings for more than an hour, and the more severe the arthritis, the longer the morning stiffness will last.

In autoimmune disorders in general, the immune system is revved up and attacks one's own tissues, cells, or molecules. In the case of rheumatoid arthritis in particular, most of the action is at the joint, although other tissues are involved. Other examples of autoimmune diseases include diabetes, thyroid disease, systemic lupus, erythematosus, and Crohn's disease.

This immune response in rheumatoid arthritis causes inflammation and thickening of the lining of the joint (the synovium), and causes fluid to move into the joint space (see the illustration of a rheumatoid joint below). This leads to a swollen, hot, painful joint. The immune cells release hormones called cytokines, which control the release of enzymes that damage the cartilage, bone, ligaments, and tendons. New therapies for rheumatoid arthritis inhibit the bad cytokines or promote the good ones. The cytokines that have become the targets of therapies are tumor necrosis factor alpha (TNFα) and interleukin-1 (Il-1).

Please see Appendix I, "Heredity and Environment," for further information on the causes of rheumatoid arthritis.

A rheumatoid joint

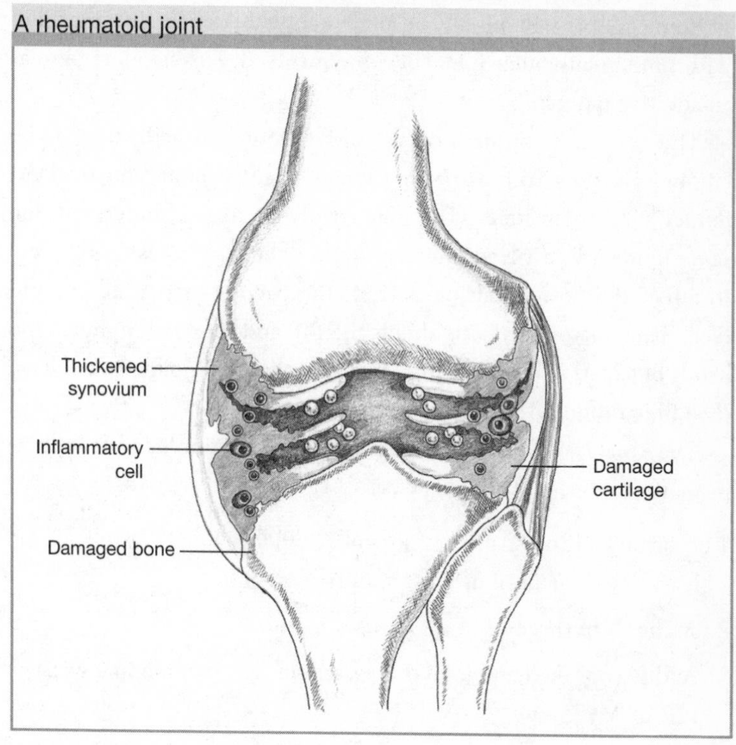

Symptoms

Rheumatoid arthritis begins differently in different people. Some awaken in the morning with diffuse swelling in the hands, wrists, ankles, and feet.

Others have swelling in a joint for 48 hours and then the swelling disappears, but soon recurs in another joint. The arthritis migrates from joint to joint. This is called palindromic rheumatism, and approximately one-third of the time it settles into rheumatoid arthritis.

In elderly patients, the arthritis may start with severe stiffness and discomfort in the shoulders and hips, mimicking a condition called polymyalgia rheumatica. However, the development of swelling in the hands or feet makes rheumatoid arthritis a more likely diagnosis.

Some people will initially be affected only in one or two joints but with time, many other joints become involved. This is referred to as an additive pattern.

The general symptoms or signs of rheumatoid arthritis may be fatigue, morning stiffness lasting longer than an hour, and swollen, tender, and warm joints. The joint involvement is symmetrical: the same joints are involved on both sides of the body. It is more likely to affect the peripheral joints (i.e., the hands, wrists, ankles, and feet). Rheumatoid arthritis affects the PIP and the MCP joints in the hands but spares the DIP joints. It affects the MTP joints of the feet. (See illustration on page 19.)

The American College of Rheumatology has identified the following seven criteria for the diagnosis of rheumatoid arthritis:

1. Morning stiffness: stiffness in and around the joints lasting at least one hour until maximal improvement
2. Arthritis of three or more joints
3. Arthritis of the hand joints: at least one area swollen in a wrist, PIP, or MCP joint
4. Symmetric arthritis
5. Rheumatoid nodules
6. Serum rheumatoid factor
7. Radiographic changes typical for rheumatoid arthritis

A patient must have four out of the seven to satisfy criteria, and the first four conditions in the list above must have been present for at least six weeks. A patient may not meet criteria but still have rheumatoid arthritis.

Investigations

Early diagnosis and treatment of rheumatoid arthritis is important because damage can occur within the first three months of disease. Once damage has occurred, it is permanent. You should therefore see your family physician if you have joint pain, swelling, and stiffness. If rheumatoid arthritis is suspected, the physician should order the following tests and refer you to a rheumatologist.

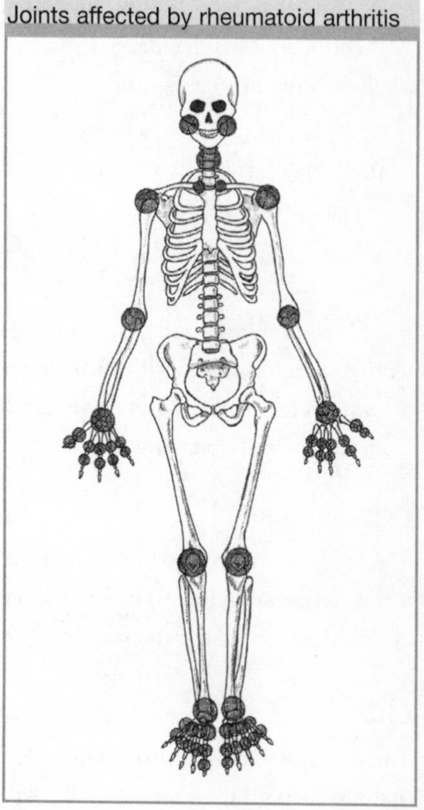

Joints affected by rheumatoid arthritis

Rheumatoid factor test

Also called a latex fixation test, this blood test measures for an IgM antibody to IgG; this antbody is called the rheumatoid factor. Of patients with definite rheumatoid arthritis, 90 percent have a positive rheumatoid factor. It can usually be positive in patients with the rheumatoid factor, but can also be positive with Sjogren's syndrome (see page 35 of this chapter), with age, and with other chronic diseases (but usually at low levels). The rheumatoid factor test is useful but not essential in making a diagnosis in a patient with joint pain, stiffness, and swelling. High levels of the rheumatoid factor predict a more severe disease.

CBC

The CBC, or complete blood count, is a routine test for many conditions. The abnormalities that might be seen in rheumatoid arthritis are as follows:

- Anemia (low hemoglobin, low numbers of red blood cells) may be noticed. In active disease, patients may have what is called anemia of chronic disease.
- The platelet count may be increased if there is a lot of inflammation. Platelets help with blood clotting, and an increased count is usually not dangerous. In Felty's syndrome, the platelet count can be low. (See the discussion of Felty's syndrome on page 22, in the section on complications of rheumatoid arthritis.)
- The white blood cell count (WBC) is generally normal in rheumatoid arthritis. It can be low from medications or Felty's syndrome, or with lupus. (See the discussion of lupus on page 29 in the section on connective tissue diseases.)

ESR

ESR, sed. rate, erythrocyte sedimentation rate: these are all different terms for the same thing. The ESR is an indirect measure of the amount of inflammation. The higher the level, the more inflammation there is.

CRP

The CRP, or C-reactive protein test, is another measure of inflammation. As with the ESR, the CRP test may be one of several things that would help your doctor decide if treatment is working.

ANA

The ANA, or antinuclear antibody test, is more commonly positive in lupus. Approximately 10 percent of patients with rheumatoid arthritis will have a positive ANA.

X-rays or radiographs

These are usually normal in early disease. The X-ray only shows changes when damage has occurred. In rheumatoid arthritis, changes occur first in the feet and hands.

Other Disease Manifestations and Complications of Rheumatoid Arthritis

Rheumatoid arthritis is a systemic disease, meaning that it affects more than the joints. Its most common effect on the body at large is fatigue, which is worse when the disease is more active and can be more bothersome than the pain or swelling. Controlling the underlying disease will improve the fatigue.

Nodules

Rheumatoid nodules are rubbery, firm, rounded lumps found under the skin in approximately 20 percent of patients who have rheumatoid factor positive disease. They are sometimes stuck to the bone and at other times are mobile, but they usually occur in places where you put pressure, such as where you lean on your elbows. Rheumatoid nodules can also occur in the lungs, and are not harmful.

There is no specific treatment for the nodules. If the disease gets better with treatment, they will sometimes recede. If they are surgically removed, they will return. Methotrexate can make them worse, and can cause more small nodules to appear on the fingers.

Eye effects

The most common effect on the eyes is that they become dry. Dryness of the eye is treated with lubricant drops or gel. The combination of dry eyes and dry mouth is referred to as sicca syndrome.

Inflammation of the sclera (the white covering of the eyeball) is called episcleritis. It can occur from the eye dryness or as a result of inflammation in the small blood vessels of the sclera. If the inflammation goes deeper, it is referred to as scleritis. If it is severe and left untreated, the eyeball can perforate. If you have a red and/or painful eye, you should see your doctor.

Lung effects

Lung involvement occurs in up to 28 percent of people with rheumatoid arthritis. The most common effect—thickening of the lung's lining (the pleura)—does not usually cause any symptoms.

Sometimes people will develop pleuritis, in which the lining of the lung becomes inflamed (causing pain when breathing in) and the pleural space may become full of a fluid (pleural effusion). This sometimes will improve on its own, or may require treatment with a drug such as prednisone.

The lungs may become scarred as a result of chronic inflammation. This is called interstitial fibrosis, and is associated with more severe rheumatoid disease.

An extremely rare but very serious complication is called bronchiolitis obliterans. It is uncertain if this is due to the disease itself or if it is a complication of drug therapy (specifically gold or penicillamine). I have only seen one case in 12 years.

Felty's syndrome

In this syndrome seen in rheumatoid arthritis, patients have an enlarged spleen and a low white blood cell count. They may also have a low platelet count, and bacterial infections are more common. It usually improves with DMARDs (disease modifying anti-rheumatic drugs) but sometimes the spleen has to be surgically removed.

Vasculitis

In rheumatoid vasculitis, inflammation in the small blood vessels causes them to become damaged and plugged off, cutting off the blood supply to the tissue that the vessel was supplying. Resultant damage can include leg ulcers, nerve damage that usually affects sensation in the arms or legs, loss of strength and ability to move, and gangrene in the feet or hands.

This condition is seen in severe rheumatoid arthritis in people with a high rheumatoid factor, and is rare. The treatment is high doses of corticosteroids and immunosuppressant drugs.

Ruptured popliteal cyst

This can occur with any condition that causes the knee to swell. The fluid in the swollen knee leaks back behind the knee through a one-way valve into a pouch (bursa). Since the fluid gets in but can't get out, the bursa or cyst gets bigger and bigger until it bursts. This causes the lower leg to become swollen, very painful, red, and hot.

The management is first to make sure that the problem is not a blood clot. This is done using a Doppler machine (a type of ultrasound), which looks at blood flow. If it is not a blood clot, then the management is to keep the leg elevated and to put ice on it. Analgesia is given for pain control, and narcotics may be required. Usually a shot of corticosteroids in the knee helps.

Neck effects

Because rheumatoid arthritis also affects ligaments and tendons, it can damage many of the supportive tissues in the neck, leading to unstable movement of the neck. Sometimes your rheumatologist or surgeon may ask for special X-rays of the neck to be sure there is not too much unstable movement, especially when bending the neck. This is an important complication because if it is not detected, it can lead to damage of the spinal cord. If it is severe, then treatment is to perform surgery in which the neck is fused.

Chronic deformities

The chronic deformities of rheumatoid arthritis include, in the hand, ulnar drift of the MCP joints and Boutonniere's or swan neck deformity of the fingers (see the illustrations on page 25). The wrist may rotate or drift towards the thumb. The elbow can become permanently bent. The shoulders usually are not deformed but they lose their range of motion. In the lower limbs, the legs may become bent at the knees and hips, and the ankles can roll inward. The big toe often drifts outward and the remaining toes bend upwards.

Control of the disease is the best way to prevent deformity. Splints may be used to prevent flexion contractions or bends in the joints. Wrist splints may be worn when working or at rest and may help prevent deformities of the wrist. Sterling silver ring splints can help prevent progression of the swan neck or Boutonniere's deformity.

The deformities of the foot are best accommodated with orthotics and supportive shoes.

Prognosis

Rheumatoid arthritis is a chronic disease that causes erosions in the bone and cartilage of the joints, which can be detected by X-rays. The degree of erosion development predicts the severity of disability. At the time of diagnosis, up to 30 percent of people will already have developed erosions. Early aggressive treatment is necessary to prevent erosions and hence disability.

Rheumatoid arthritis affects individuals differently. Approximately 15 percent of patients will have a benign course and therefore have very little damage, if any. (In elderly patients, particularly if their disease begins with stiffness in the shoulders and hips, the disease is often benign.) For approximately 50–60 percent of patients, the disease runs a moderate course. However, 25–35 percent of patients will have serious disease that is difficult to manage with traditional therapies. Predictors of more severe disease include: a strongly positive rheumatoid factor; HLA DR4; young age of onset and female; extra-articular features (disease outside the joint, in lungs, eyes, etc.); uncontrolled polyarthritis; structural damage and deformity; and functional disability.

Deformities in rheumatoid arthritis

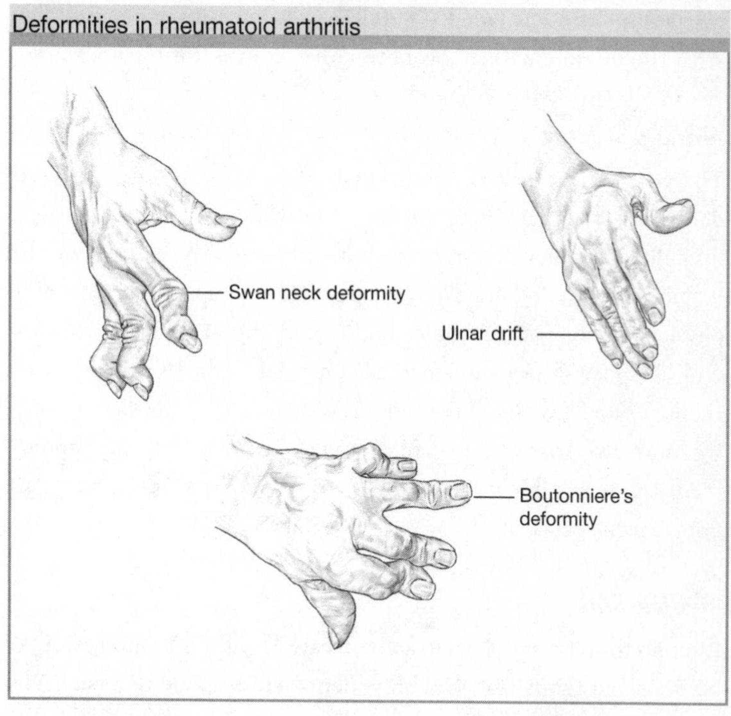

The ability to remain in the workforce is often determined by the physical demands in the workplace, the pace of work, and the amount of flexibility in the work schedule. Some studies have suggested that up to 50 percent of people with rheumatoid arthritis will be disabled and unable to work within five years of diagnosis.

A recent study suggests that the life expectancy of someone with rheumatoid arthritis is reduced by three years, on average. Those patients with more severe disease have a higher mortality rate.

Clearly, it is important to recognize the disease early and begin to treat it. For 20 years, we did not have any new therapies to offer patients. In the last five years, we have seen the introduction of the biological therapies and of a new drug called leflunomide, and have seen patients dramatically improve on these therapies when everything else has failed. Therefore, the future for people living with rheumatoid arthritis is better than ever before.

Management

The goal of therapy is to stop inflammation, control pain, prevent deformity, maintain function and, ultimately, prevent long-term disability. To achieve this requires a coordinated health care team that includes a physiotherapist, occupational therapist, nurse, family physician, orthopedic surgeon, and rheumatologist. Ideally, a patient with suspected or confirmed rheumatoid arthritis should see a rheumatologist within three months of the onset of the disease, since we know that irreversible damage can occur early. An early appointment is not possible in many parts of Canada, however, as there are not enough specialists.

Medications

Rheumatoid arthritis is usually treated with a combination of NSAIDs and DMARDs. Not all patients will respond to a particular medication. Often, a medication will work for a while and then become less effective. Most rheumatoid arthritis patients will, over the course of their disease, have been on a number of different NSAIDs and DMARDs. Some medications will have done nothing, some will have worked for a while, and some may have had to be stopped due to adverse effects.

The NSAIDs help with pain, swelling, and stiffness; however they alone do not control the disease process. Chapter 7, "Medications," will deal with the benefits and side effects of all the medications.

As soon as the diagnosis of rheumatoid arthritis is made, a disease modifying antirheumatic drug (DMARD) should be started to control the disease process. Clinical studies have shown that starting any DMARD early in the course of the disease will decrease the rate of formation of erosions, whereas someone who begins a DMARD later in the course of the disease can never catch up. Some people believe there is a window of opportunity for treating RA early on before the inflammation process becomes too well established.

Methotrexate is the most commonly used DMARD to treat rheumatoid arthritis. All new drugs are compared to it in studies. It can be used alone or in combination with other DMARDs. Other DMARDs include sulfasalazine, hydroxychloroquine, minocycline, gold, penicillamine, azathioprine, and cyclosporine. Several studies have shown that the combination of methotrexate, sulfasalazine, and hydroxychloroquine is more effective than methotrexate alone or the combination of sulfasalazine and hydroxychoroquine, particularly in early disease. Leflunomide (Arava) is a newer DMARD with efficacy similar to methotrexate. It can be used alone or in combination with methotrexate. Please see Chapter 7 "Medications" for a further description of these drugs.

The biologic response modifiers have been introduced in the past five years. This group of drugs includes the TNF inhibitors such as adalimumab (Humira), etanercept (Enbrel), and infliximab (Remicade). They are more effective when combined with methotrexate and represent a major advance in the treatment of rheumatoid arthritis. These drugs benefit 60 to 70 percent of cases.

Corticosteroids are very useful drugs for patients with rheumatoid arthritis. They are very effective when injected into an inflamed joint, and if a patient has several joints that just will not settle, this approach is used. They are sometimes given as an injection into the muscle during an acute flare of disease. They are also at times given orally as a steady daily dose or in tapering doses, but we try to avoid using them over the long term because of their adverse effects. Remember that if you are on corticosteroids (prednisone) and you have been on them for awhile, do not stop them on your own. Consult your physician on how to wean yourself from them. You can become very ill if you stop them suddenly.

Self-help

It is always important to maintain a positive attitude, and to remember that you are in control. It is essential that you understand the goals of therapy, the potential adverse effects, and the expected outcomes; this applies to drugs, exercise, and surgery—really, to any therapeutic intervention. It is important to find a physician who is knowledgeable about rheumatoid arthritis, and whose advice you trust. At times you may receive conflicting information on how to proceed, and sometimes must trust your doctor's clinical experience in having seen the same problem many times before.

You need to maintain as normal a lifestyle as possible, incorporating an appropriate exercise program and getting adequate rest, since fatigue is a huge problem for many patients. Exercise, splinting, pain control, lifestyle adjustments, and other forms of management will be dealt with in other chapters of the book.

So in summary, what can you do for yourself? Be informed, surround yourself with a heath care team whose opinions you trust, exercise, get enough sleep, eat well, don't smoke, don't waste your money on miracle cures, and stay in control.

The Connective Tissue Diseases

The connective tissue diseases are a group of autoimmune diseases that includes systemic lupus erythematosus (lupus), scleroderma, Sjogren's syndrome, polymyositis and dermatomyositis, and vasculitis. These diseases have many clinical manifestations and a book could be written about each of them, but one of their common features is arthritis that does not usually damage the joints. We will discuss the conditions and management in a broad sense and refer you to more detailed resources if you wish to investigate these diseases further.

In all of these connective tissue diseases, the body's immune system has an abnormal response to something foreign to the body (an antigen), and ends up producing antibodies against itself (autoantibodies). Some of the antibodies mediate the disease, but others do not.

Systemic Lupus Erythematosus

There are three classifications of lupus: discoid lupus, subacute cutaneous lupus erythematosus, and systemic lupus erythematosus.

Discoid lupus refers to a rash that occurs on sun-exposed areas. This rash is red, raised, and can cause scarring. It is uncommon for it to progress to systemic lupus erythematosus.

Subacute cutaneous lupus erythematosus refers to a recurring rash that is sun-sensitive. The rash can form rings or scaly patches. There can be arthritis, fatigue, and general malaise, but it is unusual to have serious organ involvement. This form of lupus is associated with the antinuclear autoantibody (ANA) directed against Ro and La. In a pregnant woman the Ro autoantibody can cross the placenta and cause the baby to have neonatal lupus. (Please see Chapter 4, "Pregnancy, Delivery, and Arthritis.")

The arthritis associated with systemic lupus erythematosus is symmetrical and mainly involves the joints of the fingers, wrists, elbows, shoulders, knees, and feet. It can range from joint pains, with or without tenderness, to tender swollen joints. It can be mistaken for rheumatoid arthritis. The joints do not get damaged, but some patients develop swan neck deformities and ulnar drift.

Systemic lupus erythematosus (SLE) is more serious. It is associated with rashes (such as the butterfly rash on the face), reactions to sun exposure, hair loss, mouth sores, Raynaud's phenomenon (where your fingers turn white and purple in the cold), inflammation around the lining of the lungs and heart, anemia, low white blood cell and platelet counts, and kidney disease with the potential for kidney failure. It may also affect the neurological system, causing seizures, depression, or numbness and tingling in the face or a limb.

The disease is characterized by cycles of getting better and then worse, but the outlook for people with lupus has improved because of better treatments. Although lupus can be a serious disease, 90 percent of patients do well. It affects women more commonly than men, and often starts in young women. There is an increased risk of cardiovascular disease in patients with longstanding disease, and it is therefore important to screen these people for other risk factors of cardiovascular disease.

The diagnosis is sometimes difficult to make in the early stages or with milder disease, but laboratory tests can help.

Investigations

The blood work abnormalities that can be found include a low white cell count, a low platelet count, and/or a low red cell count (anemia).

The autoantibodies that can be detected in lupus include antinuclear antibodies (ANA), such as those directed against DNA, Sm, Ro, and La.

The ANA is an antibody to the antigens in the nucleus of the cell. They are seen in many conditions but it would be most unusual to have systemic lupus reythematosus and negative antinuclear antibodies. The dsDNA and Sm are specific antibodies for systemic lupus reythematosus. The DNA is seen at high levels in active disease and is associated with kidney disease. The antibodies to Ro and La are associated with milder forms of lupus, arthritis, rash, and fatigue. These antibodies are seen in Sjogren's syndrome and neonatal lupus. Please see Chapter 4, "Pregnancy, Delivery, and Arthritis."

Antibodies to phospholipids are seen in a subgroup of lupus patients who have a tendency to form blood clots in arteries and veins and to have frequent miscarriages. There are three types of antiphospholipid antibodies: anticardiolipin, lupus anticoagulant, and a false positive test for syphilis.

Complement levels are used to follow disease activity: if they are low, it may mean that the disease is more active.

The analysis of the urine can be abnormal with protein and red cells and white cells. Such a result suggests that the kidneys are affected by lupus.

Treatment

The treatment of systemic lupus erythematosus depends upon which organs are involved and the severity of the disease. Although there is no cure, the disease can be controlled or it can spontaneously settle.

Hydroxychloroquine (Plaquenil) is helpful for the fatigue, arthritis, and rash associated with systemic lupus erythematosus, and probably prevents flares of the disease. Corticosteroids are used to treat fluid around the lungs or heart, kidney disease, more severe rash, arthritis, low blood counts, and neurological disease. Methotrexate is helpful in controlling moderately severe arthritis and rash. Azathioprine (Imuran) is used to treat moderately severe kidney disease. Cyclophosphamide is given as a large, slow injection of medication into a vein every four to twelve weeks to treat diffuse proliferative glomerulonephritis (a severe form of kidney inflammation) and neurological disease. Mycophenolate mofetil is a new immunosuppressant drug to treat kidney disease; at the present time, it is used when cyclophosphamide has failed or has not been tolerated.

Antiphospholipid Antibody Syndrome

This syndrome may occur in association with lupus or on its own. The main signs of this syndrome are blood clots in the veins and arteries, and recurrent miscarriages. The clots can be deep in the veins of the leg (causing phlebitis), lodged in the lung (known as a pulmonary embolism), or lodged in the brain (causing strokes). The syndrome can also be associated with low platelet counts, a rash called *livedo reticularis*, and heart murmurs. The syndrome in a pregnant woman can cause miscarriages and stillbirths, especially in the second third of the pregnancy.

The blood tests would reveal the anticardiolipin autoantibody, lupus anticoagulant (in a prolonged clotting test called a PTT), and a false positive result for syphilis.

The treatment is warfarin (Coumadin) to thin the blood and prevent further clots. If you have a positive blood test for this syndrome but have never had any symptoms, no treatment is required.

Scleroderma

Scleroderma is, fortunately, uncommon. It is estimated that a family physician would see one case in his or her entire career. It is three times more common in women, and usually occurs between ages 34 and 65. Scleroderma can be classified into three categories: cutaneous, limited, or diffuse.

In cutaneous scleroderma, only the skin is involved. There may be isolated patches of thickened skin (called morphea), or widespread skin thickening (called generalized morphea). Long strips of thickened skin are called linear scleroderma, and represent another type of cutaneous scleroderma; they soften with time.

Limited scleroderma was previously called CREST syndrome. Compared with diffuse scleroderma, it is milder and has a better prognosis. Its symptoms include thickening of the skin of the hands and feet (but not of the forearms or legs), and the skin on the face can sometimes be involved. In addition, there is Raynaud's phenomenon, difficulty swallowing and heartburn (as a result of involvement of the esophagus), and the presence of tiny dilated blood vessels in the skin appearing as tiny red dots (telangectasia) and tiny calcium deposits under the skin (calcinosis). High blood pressure in the blood vessels of the lungs (pulmonary hypertension) is more common with this form of scleroderma.

Diffuse scleroderma (or progressive systemic sclerosis) is the most severe form of the disease. It causes widespread thickening of the skin that begins in the hands and the feet and spreads to the arms, legs, face, and trunk. The appearance of the face may change, as the skin thickening can cause pursing of the lips and loss of wrinkles. When there is rapid progression of the skin thickening in the early phases of the disease, it is a sign that the disease is serious and there is the potential for severe kidney problems. The leading cause of death with this disease used to be kidney failure: the blood pressure suddenly rose and the kidney function deteriorated. The development of the family of blood pressure pills (called ACE inhibitors) has dramatically improved the outcome of this complication. The leading cause of death from scleroderma now is progressive scarring of the lungs (interstitial fibrosis), which shows up as shortness of breath and a dry cough.

When scleroderma affects the esophagus, people experience heartburn, difficulty swallowing, and difficulty with food sticking in the throat. The speed of food passing through the bowel is slowed so that constipation and bowel obstruction can be a problem. The intestinal bacteria may become too numerous because of the slow bowel speed, and this will likely cause diarrhea that would be followed by malnutrition due to the inability to absorb all the nutrients.

Raynaud's phenomenon, where the fingers and toes become white and then purple, results from the reduced blood flow to the extremities that is caused by narrowing and spasm of the blood vessels. It is brought on by cold temperatures and by anxiety. If severe, it can lead to ulcers and gangrene in the fingers and toes. Smoking makes this condition much worse.

The heart muscle can become scarred. Problems with the rhythm of the heart and heart failure can result.

Investigations

There may be a low hemoglobin (anemia), and an elevated serum creatinine (showing reduced kidney function). The specific antibody abnormalities are as shown in the table below.

A chest X-ray, a CT scan of the lung, and pulmonary function testing are used to evaluate scleroderma involvement in the lung.

Treatment

There is no good treatment for the skin disease, but there is evidence that penicillamine, cyclosporine, and methotrexate might be of minor benefit.

The heartburn (or acid reflux) is treated by decreasing the acid in the stomach with drugs that are proton pump inhibitors (e.g., Losec). The problems of moving food through the esophagus are treated with metaclopramide. Antibiotics are used to treat the diarrhea that results from the bacterial overgrowth.

A renal crisis, which includes deterioration of the kidney function and high blood pressure, is treated with ACE inhibitors (e.g., Captopril). There is some evidence that corticosteroids might cause a kidney crisis in someone with diffuse scleroderma, so these must be used with some care.

The lung involvement has been treated with cyclophosphamide, cyclosporine, and azathioprine.

Specific Antibody Abnormalities

Type of scleroderma	Autoantibody
Cutaneous scleroderma	No specific antibody
Limited scleroderma	+ANA, anticentromere antibody found 90% of the time
Diffuse scleroderma	+ANA, antiScl 70 found 30% of the time

Sjogren's Syndrome

This condition can be associated with other connective tissue diseases or it can occur on its own. It causes dryness of the mouth, eyes, skin, and vagina, and can cause swelling of the salivary glands just in front of the jaw. Other symptoms of Sjogren's syndrome include fatigue, arthritis, and a rash (usually on the lower legs, with tiny purple dots that may leave a brown discolouration). Patients may develop damage to the nerves; this shows up as numbness and tingling in the hands, face, and feet.

People with Sjogren's syndrome have a small but increased risk of developing a tumour in the lymph system (lymphoma). If the parotid glands are enlarged, then they need to be monitored.

Investigations

The lab abnormalities include a reduction in the hemoglobin level (anemia), and a low white blood cell and platelet count. The ESR is elevated. Tests for the rheumatoid factor, ANA, and the Ro and La antibodies are usually positive.

Treatment

Treatment is directed at the symptoms. For the dryness of the eyes, artificial teardrops and tear gel are recommended. For the dryness of the mouth, drink lots of water and try chewing sugarless gum. With dryness in the mouth comes an increased problem with dental cavities, so you need to see your dentist regularly. Pain during intercourse due to vaginal dryness can be helped by using a lubricating jelly. Occasionally the eye doctor will put plugs in the ducts that drain the tears from the eye. This helps the dry eyes. Hydroxychloroquine (Plaquenil) may reduce joint pain and fatigue, and a pill called Salagen may increase saliva and tear production.

Polymyositis and Dermatomyositis

Polymyositis is an inflammatory disease of the muscles. It causes weakness of the proximal muscles (neck, back, chest, and shoulder and hip girdles), which will lead to difficulty getting out of bed or a low chair. It can also cause problems with breathing and swallowing.

Dermatomyositis is an inflammatory disease of the muscles and skin. It causes a rash, which is usually in sun-exposed areas. There may be a slightly raised, red, scaly rash over the knuckles and the bony areas of other joints. Rashes can occur on the eyelids, the V-area of the chest, and the shawl area of the nape of the neck and shoulders. There is a childhood form of this disease.

Both of these diseases can be associated with common cancers in adults. Appropriate investigation is recommended as the cancer can be found in an early, curable stage.

Investigations

The most common abnormality is an elevated level of CPK (which is an enzyme released from damaged muscle). Other tests used to make the diagnosis include electrical studies of the muscle (known as EMG, or electromyography) done by the insertion of a needle into the muscle, muscle biopsy, and MRI examination of the muscles.

Several autoantibodies are associated with inflammatory myositis. The anti-Jo1 antibody is associated with interstitial lung disease (inflammation and scarring of the lung) and a scaly rash on the hands.

Treatment

Most people will respond to moderately high doses of corticosteroids. If this fails or if the corticosteroid level cannot be reduced and eventually weaned, then methotrexate and azathioprine may be added. In stubborn cases that do not yield to treatment, intravenous gamma globulin is used. About 85 percent of patients will do reasonably well.

Psoriatic Arthritis

Psoriasis is a skin disease that commonly affects the scalp and the skin of the elbows and knees but it can occur anywhere on the skin. It appears as red patches with silvery to white scales. It is common in some families.

Psoriatic arthritis (PsA) is the arthritis that can occur with psoriasis. The joints can be swollen, reddish or purplish, tender, and warm. It commonly affects the small joints of the hands and feet but any joint can be involved, including those in the back and neck. It also affects the tendons and the attachments between tendons and bones (known as entheses).

Approximately 30 percent of patients with psoriasis have arthritis. Psoriasis occurs in 1–3 percent of the Canadian population, therefore psoriatic arthritis may occur in up to 1 percent of the population. This frequency is similar to that of rheumatoid arthritis. Psoriatic arthritis has been considered to be a mild form of arthritis, and so no specific treatments have been developed for this condition. However, recent studies have shown that the disease can be severe, with deformity and disability affecting about 20 percent of sufferers.

Psoriatic arthritis usually begins sometime after the onset of the psoriasis, but in 20 percent of cases the arthritis begins before the psoriasis, and in 10 percent of cases the psoriasis and arthritis begin at the same time. The common age of onset is between 30 and 50 years, and equal numbers of men and women get this disease. There is a juvenile form of psoriatic arthritis, and this will be discussed in Chapter 3, "Childhood Arthritis."

Causes

Please see Appendix I, "Heredity and Environment."

Symptoms

Most people have psoriasis prior to developing psoriatic arthritis. The affected joints become swollen, tender, stiff, and warm. Pain and swelling can occur in the tendons and ligaments at their point of attachment to the bone (e.g., at the back of the heel where the Achilles tendon inserts; see the illustration on page 39). The neck, back, and buttocks can also be affected. Arising from bed in the morning is difficult due to prolonged stiffness.

Psoriatic arthritis can show up in at least five different patterns, and some people will have a combination of types.

Type 1 primarily involves the DIP joints of the fingers and the toes. (See illustration on page 39.) Psoriasis is usually present in the nails adjacent to the affected joints, and typical changes to the nails would include nail lifting, pitting, and thickening. This type occurs in 10–15 percent of patients.

Type 2, arthritis mutilans, occurs in 5 percent of people with psoriatic arthritis. This is a severe destructive arthritis of the hands and feet in which the bones actually dissolve at the ends. The fingers and toes appear collapsed, which is called telescoping because it looks like you could pull or stretch the digit back to normal length in the same way as you would a telescope.

Type 3, symmetric polyarthritis, looks like rheumatoid arthritis except that the distal joints of the fingers and toes may be involved, the joints sometimes fuse, and the tendons of the hands are more commonly affected. (See illustration on page 19, which shows the joints that are likely to be involved here.) The rheumatoid factor is negative in the blood work.

Type 4, oligoarthritis, involves fewer than five joints (see illustration on page 39). It is associated with a "sausage digit" (when the

Achilles tendon ethesitis

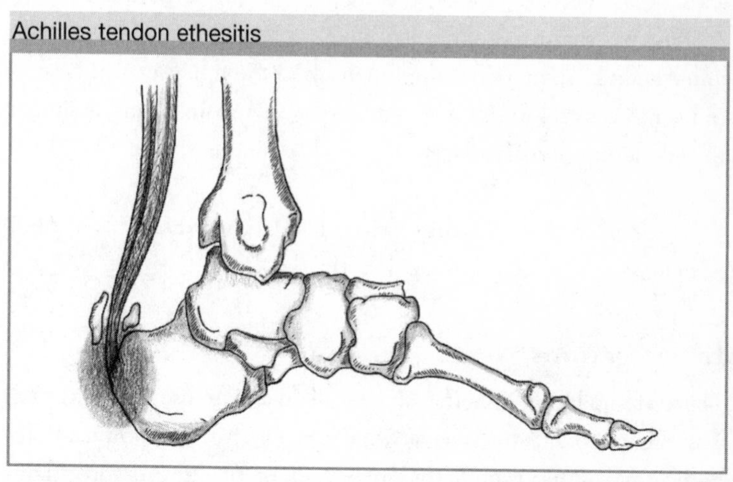

Common joint involvement with psoriatic arthritis

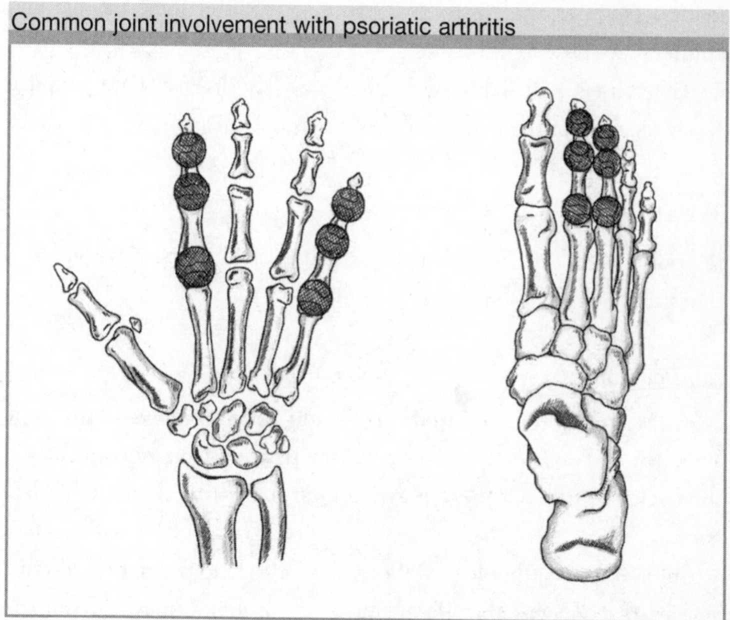

tendon is markedly inflamed, it causes the finger or toe to look like a sausage). This pattern is seen about 40 percent of the time.

Type 5, where there is spinal involvement, affects the sacroiliac joints and the spine (from the low back to the upper neck). It is six times more likely to occur in a man than in a woman, and is similar to ankylosing spondylitis (which is discussed on page 41 of this chapter).

The incidence of other diseases such as Crohn's disease and colitis is higher in people with psoriatic arthritis.

Investigations

There are no blood tests that specifically diagnose psoriatic arthritis. The rheumatoid factor is negative; if it is positive, then you may have both psoriasis and rheumatoid arthritis. The blood tests for inflammation (such as the C-reactive protein, the ESR, and the platelet count) may show high results.

The X-rays will likely be normal in early disease. Later, typical X-ray changes of the hands and feet for psoriatic arthritis may occur.

Treatment

Psoriatic arthritis can be treated with various medications and therapies, which we will discuss below.

Medication

NSAIDs are used to treat the pain and inflammation in psoriatic arthritis, and are particularly useful for treating pain and stiffness in the back and neck. If there is swelling in the joints, then a DMARD is required.

Sulfasalazine and gold have been shown to help psoriatic arthritis. There are concerns that Plaquenil or chloroquine may worsen the skin psoriasis.

Methotrexate is used to treat both the skin and joint disease of psoriatic arthritis. Many dermatologists request a biopsy of the liver to be sure that the methotrexate is not causing damage, but rheumatologists are less likely to require a biopsy. There is some evidence that liver damage from methotrexate may be more common when it is used to treat psoriasis than when it is used for rheumatoid arthritis.

Cyclosporine has been used for the skin and joint disease of psoriatic arthritis. Small clinical trials of the biological agents (etanercept and infliximab) have also shown a very good clinical response.

Sometimes, if the skin disease is well controlled, then the arthritis seems to improve. The use of ultraviolet light therapy combined with retinoids (Vitamin A products) is effective in treating the skin disease.

Ankylosing Spondylitis

Ankylosing spondylitis (AS) is an inflammatory arthritis that primarily affects the spine. The name is derived from the Greek words *spondylos* (spine), *itis* (inflammation), and *ankylosis* (inability to move). It is an ancient disease that has been seen in Egyptian mummies and dinosaurs. It usually begins during the period from the late teenage years to age 35, and affects seven times as many men as women. It is associated with the HLA B27 antigen 90 percent of the time; however, if you have the HLA B27 antigen, your chance of developing AS is still only 10 percent. If a first-degree relative (mother, father, sister, or brother) has AS, then your risk increases to 20 percent. (See Appendix I, "Heredity and Environment.") AS is seen in association with psoriasis, Crohn's disease, and ulcerative colitis.

This disease is characterized by pain and stiffness that are worst upon awakening in the morning and that last more than one hour. Physical activity usually improves the symptoms, which is not the case with the many other causes of low back pain. The first symptom will be pain in the buttock region and posterior thigh arising from the inflammation of the sacroiliac joint (see illustration below).

The pain usually progresses gradually over several weeks. Patients may feel unwell and tired. The inflammation will gradually spread up the spine to the ribs or chest wall and then to the neck. The sacroiliac joints will fuse as bone grows across them. There is no loss of function, however, as these joints barely move even when they are normal. As the joints in the chest wall, spine, and neck fuse, however, there will be loss of movement (see illustration on page 43).

Symptoms

AS progresses differently in different individuals. It tends to be less severe in women, which makes the diagnosis more difficult. How the disease progresses in the first five years usually predicts whether it will

Sacroiliitis

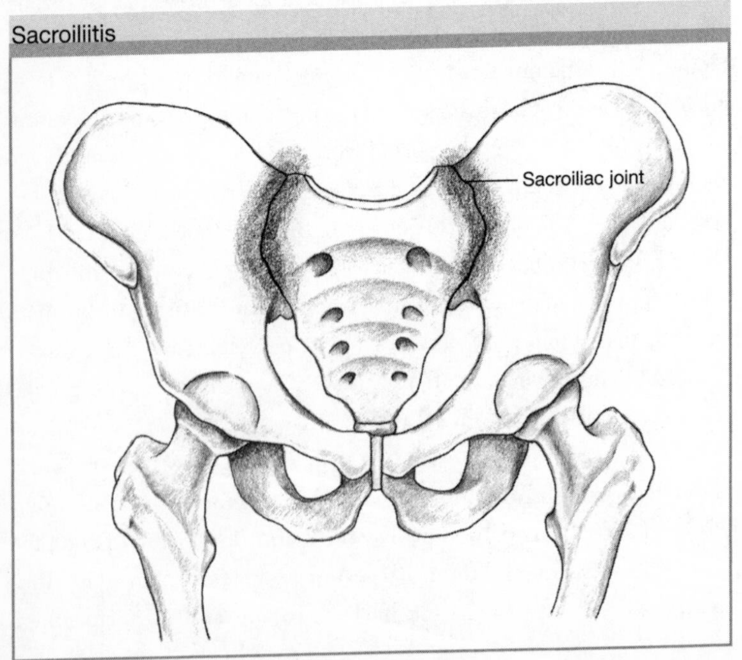

Joint involvement with ankylosing spondylitis

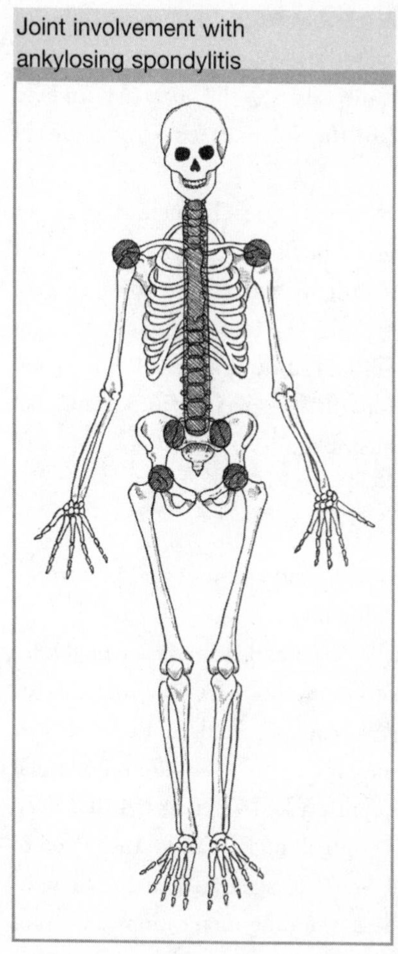

be mild or severe. In severe disease the spine will fuse, beginning with loss of range of motion in the lower back, progressing to decreased chest expansion, and being followed by loss of movement in the neck. The shoulders and hips may be involved as well. Some people will fuse in a bent position so that they are looking at their toes. This can be avoided by paying strict attention to posture and exercise. You will be less disabled if you are fused in an upright position.

Eye involvement is common with AS. The iris becomes inflamed (iritis or anterior uveitis), and the eye will be red, painful, and sensitive to light. This needs to be seen by a physician and treated.

Enthesitis refers to inflammation of the site where a tendon or ligament attaches to bone. This often occurs in AS, most commonly with the Achilles tendon at the back of the heel and the plantar fascia on the base of the heel. (See illustration on page 39.)

The heart valves (especially the aortic valve) are sometimes involved. For some reason, this was more common after the Second World War, when the troops returned from Europe. Some speculate that the difference may be due to the different strains of bacteria that the troops were exposed to. We rarely see this complication today. It is interesting that the valves of the heart are affected where the tendon-like material of the valve attaches to the heart muscle.

Lung involvement is rare. When it does happen, the upper segments of the lung become scarred or fibrous, but patients do not usually have symptoms from this. Patients with AS do, however, have restricted movement of the chest wall. The joints attaching the ribs to the spine can fuse, making it difficult if not impossible to expand the chest wall and clear secretions. It is especially important that people with this condition do not smoke.

Treatment

Treatment is aimed at controlling pain and stiffness, and preventing loss of range of movement and deformity.

The most common treatment for pain and stiffness is a high dose of a fairly potent NSAID. I have commonly used indomethicin or diclofenac at 150–200 mg daily. As many people do not tolerate one NSAID or another, it may be necessary to try a few to find one that works and is tolerated. I am frequently asked whether NSAIDs need to be taken on a regular basis. To control inflammation, they need to be taken for up to three or four weeks to achieve their full benefit. If you have no pain and no stiffness, then the medication can sometimes be stopped. However, if there is pain or stiffness, then it is important to continue taking the NSAID so that you will move better and preserve range of motion.

Several DMARDs have been used to treat ankylosing spondylitis. Salazopyrin helps the peripheral joint disease but not the spine joint disease. Methotrexate has been tried, but there are no good studies demonstrating its efficacy in this disease.

Pamidronate is an intravenous bisphosphonate used to treat

osteoporosis and cancer that has spread to the bone. It has been tried in AS with mixed results, but studies are presently ongoing.

Early studies and experience with the biological agents, etanercept and infliximab, are very promising for the treatment of ankylosing spondylitis. The dosage of infliximab is greater in AS than it is in rheumatoid arthritis, and these drugs are very expensive.

Self-Help

A daily exercise program is essential to maintain range of motion and posture, and will also help to control pain and stiffness. It is important to strengthen the antigravity muscles (front of the thighs, buttocks, and shoulders) and the abdominal muscles in order to maintain an upright posture. Extension exercises are important (such as lying on your stomach and doing press-ups for 20 minutes). A cardiovascular workout will improve your general conditioning and your chest expansion. As you age and the disease changes, you may find that your exercise program needs to be modified. It is important to have the help of a good physiotherapist who is knowledgeable about AS.

Recreational activities are important to all of us. If you have AS, you should avoid activities that keep you in a flexed position (such as bowling, curling, cycling, and hockey). If these activities are very important in your life, however, then balance them with other activities to increase flexibility and promote extension (such as tennis, golf, and tai chi). Please avoid contact sports and play hockey only in a no-checking league (if side-checked, you may be seriously injured due to the loss of flexibility of the spine and supporting tissues).

Keep a straight posture whether you are standing, walking, sitting, or lying down. Patients are encouraged to sleep on their side (but not to curl into a ball), or to sleep on their back with one flat pillow. You should have a firm mattress or a board under the mattress.

A patient with AS should never allow a chiropractor or anyone else to manipulate the spine. In AS, the joints, ligaments, and tendons supporting the spine are fused with bone. Manipulation may cause a fracture through these unmovable bony structures.

Use your medications regularly when the symptoms of inflammation are present. Smoking is absolutely to be avoided: because of the chest wall restriction, smoking will damage the lungs even more than it would in an otherwise healthy person.

As the onset of this disease is in the late teenage and the early adult years, career counselling is an important consideration. In general, you want to consider a career with varied daily activities: someone who must sit all day will be stiff and sore, and heavy physical activity may aggravate the pain. Think carefully before choosing a career. At work, you should stand and stretch every hour. You should avoid driving for prolonged periods of time, but if this is necessary, then stop and stretch frequently.

Reactive Arthritis

This refers to an arthritis that is precipitated by an infection. Most of the time it refers to a triad of symptoms that includes arthritis, urethritis (discharge from the penis and pain when urinating), and conjunctivitis (a red eye). This was previously called Reiter's syndrome but this term is no longer used since it was felt to be inappropriate to honour Klaus Reiter as he was a Nazi and guilty of war crimes in concentration camps.

Reactive arthritis may also refer to any arthritis that develops because of an illness caused by an infectious agent. For example, it may occur after a strep throat. The organism is not found in the joint; it is the body's immune response to the infection that causes the arthritis. The triad of arthritis, conjunctivitis, and urethritis is caused by a urogenital infection, a chlmydial infection, or an infectious diarrhea.

A better understanding of this disease occurred as a result of an unfortunate incident in the 1980s during the Pope's visit to Canada.

A large contingent of the Ontario Provincial Police ate sandwiches that were shipped from Montreal to Toronto in an unrefrigerated truck. As you might anticipate, there was a huge outbreak of salmonella poisoning in the police force, and some individuals went on to develop a reactive arthritis. These individuals were genetically predisposed: they carried the HLA B27 antigen, the same antigen that predisposes you to develop ankylosing spondylitis. Some of the officers developed a chronic deforming arthritis, whereas others had an arthritis only for a few months. See the table below for a list of infections that cause a classic reactive arthritis.

This condition occurs most frequently in young adults aged 20–40. It is more common in males if the infectious source is urogenital or sexually acquired, and equally common in males and females if it is from food poisoning (such as with salmonella or shigella).

Symptoms

Most people develop symptoms about one to four weeks after the infection (which can be very mild or can even pass totally unnoticed).

The arthritis favours the lower limbs. The same joints will not be affected on both sides of the body, and usually fewer than five joints are involved. The inflamed joints are red, swollen, and very tender. The fingers and toes may swell up like sausages (dactylitis), which means that all of the tendons and joints of the digit are inflamed. The

Infections That Cause a Classic Reactive Arthritis

Infection	Bacteria
Urogenital	Chlamydia trachomatis
Diarrhea	Salmonella, yersinia, campylobacter, shigella
Others	Ureaplasma, clostridium difficile, vibrio parahaemolyticus, borrelia burgdorfi (Lyme), neisseria gonorrhoeae (GC)

point where a tendon connects to bone can become inflamed (this is called enthesitis), and therefore Achilles tendonitis and plantar fasciitis are common symptoms. The spine and sacroiliac joints often become inflamed. The typical changes of sacroiliitis and spondylitis will be seen on X-rays in people with longstanding disease.

Other features of reactive arthritis include low-grade fever and weight loss. The front of the eye can become inflamed with either conjunctivitis or the more serious iritis. A rash can occur on the penis (circinate balanitis) and on the soles of the feet (keratoderma blenorrhagicum).

The genital and urinary tracts may be affected by infectious or sterile urethritis, prostatitis, cystitis (inflammation in the bladder), or salpingitis (inflammation in the Fallopian tubes).

Investigations

The diagnosis of reactive arthritis is based on a history and physical examination, and you therefore need to be seen by a physician who is familiar with this condition.

If reactive arthritis is suspected, then the joint fluid should be tested if possible to be sure that there is no an infection in the joint. Swabs should be taken from the man's penis or woman's cervix and tested for chlamydia and gonorrhea. A stool sample should be sent to the lab for bacterial identification.

The blood tests will show an elevation in the CRP and ESR, suggesting an active inflammatory process. Sometimes, blood tests will be ordered to rule out other types of arthritis.

X-rays of the affected joints done early in the disease are not likely to be helpful as it takes some time for them to become abnormal with the typical changes of reactive arthritis.

HLA B27 is not routinely tested as some people will develop reactive arthritis in the absence of B27, and others who are B27-positive can develop other types of arthritis.

Treatment

Reactive arthritis is not a joint infection that would respond to antibiotics. Instead, the immune system is reacting to the infection in the bowel or genito-urinary tract. If an infection is identified then it should be treated with antibiotics, but the antibiotic is unlikely to affect the course of the arthritis.

The arthritis is usually treated with rest and sometimes with splinting. NSAIDs are used at high doses (e.g., indomethacin at 150–200 mg/day). If this does not work, then an injection of corticosteroids into the joint may help. Analgesics can be used for pain control.

This disease will usually go into remission after two to six months. Approximately 20 percent of patients will develop a chronic arthritis and need to be treated with DMARDs. Salazopyrin and methotrexate have been used with some success.

The syndrome can recur with reinfection.

Crystal Induced Arthritis

The two most common forms of arthritis caused by crystals are gout (from urate acid crystals) and pseudogout or CPPD (calcium pyrophosphate dihydrate deposition disease, which is caused by calcium pyrophosphate dihydrate crystals). Calcium hydroxy apatite may cause a marked destructive arthritis of the shoulder and be associated with osteoarthritis and calcific tendonitis (e.g., calcium deposits on the shoulder).

Gout

Gout is caused by there being too much uric acid in the blood, which may then crystallize in the joint. The excess of uric acid is usually caused by the body either producing too much uric acid and/or not passing enough through the kidneys into the urine. An elevated uric acid level can cause arthritis, but it can also cause kidney stones in high excreters of uric acid. In addition, it may lead to some decline in the function of the kidney if the level in the blood is very high over a prolonged period. (Asymptomatic hyperuricemia is a high level of uric acid in the blood that does not need to be treated. The exception to this is if the level is extremely high or if you are receiving chemotherapy for cancer.)

Gout was first described in the fifth century by Hippocrates, although it had been recognized by the Babylonians. The name comes from the Latin *gutta* (drop), because in the thirteenth century it was thought that gout was caused by a drop of evil humour. Gout has been referred to as "the disease of kings," since it was thought that overindulgence led to the development of gout. Certainly, in a predisposed person, alcohol and a diet rich in purines (shellfish, organ meats) will cause an attack.

Van Leeuwenhoek, the inventor of the microscope, first described the urate acid crystals, which looked like small needles. In fact, when they are swallowed up by the white blood cells, their sharp ends rupture the cells, leading to the release of chemicals that stimulate the inflammatory process.

People usually develop gout between the ages of 40 and 50. Gout occurs more commonly in men then women. Some famous people who had gout include Charles Darwin, Sir Isaac Newton, Michelangelo, and Benjamin Franklin. The risk factors for the development of gout include a family history of gout, prolonged use of a diuretic (medication to cause fluid loss), other drugs, alcohol ingestion, high cholesterol, obesity, kidney failure, widespread psoriasis, and low thyroid hormone production.

Symptoms

Usually the first attack of gout comes on suddenly in the middle of the night. Patients will awaken with such severe pain that they cannot even stand the weight of a bedsheet on the joint. The joint most commonly affected is the big toe, because this is the coldest joint and the crystal forms more readily at a low temperature. Other commonly affected joints include the arch of the foot, the ankle, the knee, and the wrist. The joint will be red, swollen, and excruciatingly painful. An attack in the joint lasts several days if treated, and three to four weeks if untreated.

Events that might trigger an attack of gout include alcohol ingestion, increased purine diet (shellfish, organ meats), trauma, surgery, certain drugs, radiation, dehydration, and hemorrhage. Once you have had one attack of gout, it is likely that you will have another, although it may be years later. As time goes by, the attacks become more frequent and last longer, and begin to affect more than one joint at a time. When the attacks begin to become more frequent, it is advisable to begin a drug to lower the uric acid level in the blood and prevent further attacks.

If the disease is not treated, a period of time will pass during which you will not have any attacks. However, some patients then develop chronic tophaeous gout, where the crystals form deposits (tophi) under the skin of the elbows, the ears, the top of the foot, the Achilles tendon, or the joints, causing a destructive arthritis. The tophi can open and drain if untreated. Chronic gout can damage all the peripheral joints and can be mistaken for rheumatoid arthritis. The tophi can be mistaken for rheumatoid nodules. Chronic tophaeous gout can be completely avoided if treated properly. Elderly women who have never had an attack of gout sometimes get tophi over the finger joints where they have changes of osteoarthritis.

Treatment

Gout is a treatable disease, but the treatment has to be done correctly. An acute attack of gout should be treated with ice, rest, and high doses of an NSAID. The usual drug is indomethacin at

150–200 mg per day for three to seven days. There is no reason that other NSAIDs cannot be used. There are times when an NSAID is not a good choice, and other alternatives are available. (For instance, if a patient has had a stomach ulcer or bleed or if the kidney is not functioning well, then an NSAID should be avoided.) Colchicine is an old drug that has been given for acute gout since the mid-1800s. It must be taken every one to two hours as a pill until you are better or until you get diarrhea. Usually, a person would not take more than six doses in a row. Occasionally the best treatment is to inject the joint with corticosteroids or, if many joints are involved, to give a short course of corticosteroids by mouth, intramuscularly or intravenously.

During an acute attack, drugs to lower the uric acid level in the blood should not be started; however if you are already on one of these, then continue it but do not change the dosage. These drugs would include allopurinol, sylfinpyrazone, or probenecid. If you start one of these drugs, increase the dosage, or stop the drug during an acute attack, then you will prolong the attack and make it more severe.

Once you start a drug that lowers the uric acid level, you must take it for the rest of your life. Since a second attack often doesn't come until years after the first attack, I usually do not start medications to lower the uric acid until the attacks become more frequent. The uric acid level must be decreased to at least half the upper limit of the normal range for uric acid in the blood to prevent attacks and dissolve the tophi under the skin. This value will differ in different labs. Once the uric acid is lowered you will have no further attacks, and the deposits under the skin will dissolve. However, as the uric acid levels are being lowered, there may be an increase in the frequency of gout, which can be prevented by small daily doses of an NSAID or colchicines.

There are several medications that lower the uric acid level. Allopurinol causes the body to make less uric acid. The other drugs, probenecid and sylfinpyrazone, lower the uric acid level by increasing the amount that passes out of the body in the urine (these drugs cannot be used if you have a history of kidney stones, reduced kidney function, or if you excrete too much uric acid in the urine to begin with). Please see Chapter 7, "Medications."

Diet alone will not control gout. (Please see Chapter 11, "Diet and Nutrition.") If you have a high uric acid level, then alcohol or a diet high in purines may cause an attack.

Gout can be treated and all further attacks prevented if you take your medications correctly. This means that, for the rest of your life, you will need to take a drug to maintain a low uric acid level. If you stop, the gout will come back: it may take a year or two, but it will return. Often, the attacks of gout may continue even with medication until the tophi under the skin have disappeared, so treatment may take some patience.

CPPD

Calcium pyrophosphate dihydrate deposition disease (CPPD) is a form of arthritis caused by a calcium salt. It is also referred to as pseudogout, because an acute attack causes an acutely painful, swollen joint like gout does. The arthritis is caused by the release of the calcium crystals into the joint. The crystals are engulfed by white blood cells, and this starts an inflammatory response and an arthritis. X-rays usually show calcification of the cartilage (referred to as chondrocalcinosis).

This form of arthritis is often seen in people with osteoarthritis. It is more common with increased age, and by age 90, chondrocalcinosis is seen in 50 percent of X-rays.

Symptoms

CPPD should be suspected if any of the following common symptoms are noticed:

- A joint may be acutely painful, tender, and swollen in an older person. The usual joints to be affected are the knees and the wrists.
- Osteoarthritis symptoms might be experienced, except that the symptoms are also in joints that are not usually affected by primary osteoarthritis (such as the MCP joints of the hands, or the wrists or shoulders).
- Rheumatoid arthritis might appear to be the problem, with chronic swelling of the knuckles (MCP joints), wrists, and knees, but the rheumatoid factor is negative.
- You might have a severely destroyed joint that is out of keeping with typical arthritis.

Diagnosis

The diagnosis is often suggested by the history and physical exam. The X-rays can be helpful to confirm the diagnosis, as they may show typical changes. A swollen joint should be aspirated and the fluid sent for analysis. CPPD crystals can be seen under the microscope. It is very important that the fluid also be sent for culture as an infection and CPPD can sometimes coexist.

If a diagnosis of CPPD is made, then investigations are done to rule out other diseases that can accompany it. These include hemachromatosis, a disorder of iron overload that will damage the liver and other organs unless it is treated with regular phlebotomies (blood-letting) to normalize the iron. CPPD can also be seen in association with hyperparathyroidism (an overproduction of parathyroid hormone, which leads to high calcium levels in the blood) and hypomagnesemia (low magnesium levels in the blood). These are all investigations with blood work.

Treatment

The usual treatment is to take an NSAID. DMARDs are generally not used for this condition. An acute attack in one or two joints may be treated with an injection of corticosteroids, but this should only be done once it is certain that there is no infection in the joint. Colchicine has been used to try to prevent recurrent attacks, but this is only moderately successful. NSAIDs taken on a regular basis may also prevent recurrent attacks.

Most people may have recurrent attacks of joint swelling but usually the attacks are short-lived and spread apart in time. The disease is not progressive like rheumatoid arthritis. If there is joint damage, the outcome is similar to osteoarthritis. Diet does not seem to play a role in the disease, and exercise is important to maintain strength and range of movement.

Polymyalgia Rheumatica and Temporal Arteritis

Polymyalgia rheumatica (PMR) is a disease that is seen after the age of 50 and becomes more common as people get older. This condition can be associated with temporal arteritis (TA), which is an inflammation of the temporal artery (at your temple). Approximately 10–30 percent of patients with PMR will develop TA; however, approximately 60 percent of people with TA will have associated PMR.

The symptoms of polymyalgia rheumatica are severe stiffness and pain upon awakening, and sometimes the pain will wake you from sleep. The shoulder and hip girdles and the neck are all affected, but muscle weakness is not a feature of this condition. There may be arthritis, and patients may have fatigue and feel unwell. However, if there is swelling in the small joints of the fingers in a symmetric pattern, then the diagnosis may be late-onset rheumatoid arthritis.

With temporal arteritis, the symptoms include a headache and scalp tenderness. There may be pain in the jaw muscles when chewing food that is relieved by stopping (this is called jaw claudication). There may be pain down the arms that is made worse by using the arms. There can be swelling, pain, and tenderness of the temporal artery. The major complication of this condition, if not treated, is blindness.

When I first started my practice I had the privilege of seeing a woman in her nineties who came to me with the most severe headache of her life. She had a red, hot, tender artery over the left temple. Her ESR (test for inflammation) result was very high, and the biopsy suggested temporal arteritis. This woman had survived the calamitous December 6, 1917, Halifax explosion, when two ships collided in Halifax harbour; one of them, the *Mont Blanc*, was full of munitions. Many Haligonians went to their windows and watched the fire on board the *Mont Blanc*, unaware that it was about to explode and create the largest man-made explosion before Hiroshima. The explosion shattered windows, and shards of glass pierced the eyes of hundreds. My patient was one of those people, and had had no vision in her right eye since she was a teen; she said that she would rather die than lose her remaining vision. High doses of prednisone took care of the symptoms very well, and fortunately, her vision was preserved.

Diagnosis

The diagnosis of polymyalgia rheumatica is made based on history and examination. The blood will usually show a marked elevation of the ESR. The diagnosis is often confirmed by giving the patient 15–20 mg of prednisone per day: if the diagnosis is correct, then the symptoms will usually disappear in 24–48 hours. The response is dramatic.

The diagnosis of temporal arteritis is made with a history and a physical examination. The ESR is very high. A biopsy is performed of the temporal artery, which should show characteristic inflammatory changes. Sometimes the biopsy is negative, however, because there can be skip lesion (areas of the artery are not involved) and the inflamed area may have been missed in the biopsy.

Treatment

The treatment of polymyalgia rheumatica is low doses of prednisone (usually 15–20 mg once daily). The symptoms should resolve promptly. If the prednisone is weaned too quickly, however, the symptoms will recur. Most individuals require treatment for at least one to two years.

The temporal arteritis will go away after several years. Normally the disease is treated with prednisone at 50–60 mg per day, and when the ESR normalizes, the prednisone is weaned gradually over the course of a year or so.

There are many forms of arthritis, and in this chapter I have attempted to highlight a few of the more common types. It is important to understand what type of arthritis you may have, and how it should be most appropriately treated. If you have an inflammatory arthritis such as rheumatoid arthritis, then prompt diagnosis and treatment will lead to the best long-term results.

2 Not all musculoskeletal pain is arthritis

In the Western world, patients seek out a physician primarily because of pain in their "musculoskeletal" system. Many patients frequently assume that this is the start of arthritis and envision the worst-case scenario: the onset of rheumatoid arthritis, accompanied by severe deformities. As mentioned in Chapter 1, the term *arthritis* merely means that there is inflammation in a joint, and, since there are over 100 types of arthritis, a final diagnosis of "arthritis" should be no more acceptable than a diagnosis of "chest pain." Patients with chest pain want to know if the heart is involved or if it is a lung problem, how serious it is, what is the prognosis, and what can be done. Patients given a diagnosis of arthritis should have similar expectations. It is up to the physician to determine if it is actually arthritis and, if so, what kind.

Patients frequently use the term *rheumatism,* which is not a diagnosis but merely implies that there is pain, aching, or stiffness somewhere in the musculoskeletal system. It is extremely important to understand that not all that aches is arthritis. The diagram of a joint (see page 2) shows other structures around a joint that can cause pain, stiffness, and loss of function. Ligaments, tendons, bursae (sacs that allow structures such as ligaments to glide over each other or over other structures), muscle, and bone can all lead to symptoms that simulate arthritis but have completely different implications for the patient. For instance, an acutely painful, swollen knee may not be arthritis but bursitis, which is an inflammation of a bursa. There are more than 70 bursae on each side of the body, with more than 20 around the knee alone. Bursitis is usually treatable with a restoration of normal function. Moreover, pain around a joint may actually be caused by a problem in some other area of the body, or transferred to the joint by a nerve.

In the next sections, we will discuss some of the more common regional or soft tissue rheumatic disorders, nerve disorders (or neuropathies), and three frequently misdiagnosed conditions (chest pain, reflex sympathetic dystrophy, and referred pain). Next, the most common diffuse pain syndrome—fibromyalgia—will be discussed. Finally, osteoporosis will be mentioned briefly since patients commonly confuse it with osteoarthritis.

Regional Rheumatic Syndromes

There is a huge number of disorders in which tendonitis, bursitis, or soft tissue inflammation causes pain and limits function. The more common examples are described below.

Rotator Cuff Tendonitis and Subacromial Bursitis

Shoulder pain is very common. Patients may notice pain in the outer part of the upper arm, and may be aware of swelling at the top of the shoulder. They often awaken during the night when they lie on the affected shoulder. Trying to lift the arm above shoulder level usually aggravates the pain, and manoeuvres such as reaching back to put on a coat can be excruciating. In spite of all of this, the shoulder joint is actually completely normal. X-rays are usually normal, although they sometimes may show calcium deposits in the tendon. This is a rotator cuff tendonitis, with or without an accompanying subacromial bursitis. Reassurance, pain relief, anti-inflammatory medication, physical therapy, a local injection of corticosteroids, or even time alone usually solves the problem.

Tennis Elbow

Imagine the 67-year-old retired librarian who never picked up a tennis racquet in her life being told that she has tennis elbow. Tennis elbow is caused by inflammation at the site where the tendons that extend the wrist attach to the bone at the outside of the elbow. It usually occurs in people who do not play tennis, but got its name because the backhand stroke in tennis puts repetitive stress on this site. Although a relatively minor problem, it can cause significant disability in someone who needs repetitive use of the arm, such as in operating machinery. It is not arthritis, the joint is fine, and measures such as those described for the shoulder can solve the problem.

De Quervain's Tenosynovitis

A very common wrist problem is swelling, pain, and weakness of grip, especially when using the thumb. An examination shows that the wrist joint is normal, and the problem is actually inflammation in the tendons of the thumb. The impact is huge since the patient feels that the hand is almost useless and even the simplest tasks are difficult or impossible. This is known as de Quervain's tenosynovitis, and simple treatment restores the wrist to normal.

Trochanteric Bursitis

Pain in the hip is usually interpreted as arthritis and, when the pain is severe, patients fear they may have a damaged hip that needs replacement; yet it does not necessarily mean arthritis at all. Typically, patients go to the doctor with severe pain in the outer part of the hip joint. They report difficulty with stairs—especially big steps such as when getting on a bus—that can cause marked aggravation of their pain. Pain interrupts their sleep when they lie on the affected side. Examination reveals exquisite tenderness at the outside of the hip. Hip movements and X-rays are normal, however. This is the typical story for trochanteric bursitis, which responds to simple therapy and can be quickly improved by local injection of corticosteroids.

Bursitis in the Knee

In the knee, pain and swelling may also be due to bursitis with catchy names such as "housemaid's knee" or "preacher's knee." The incapacity is, however, brief and responsive to simple treatment, and the knee joint is normal.

Plantar Fasciitis

Heel pain not only causes misery but makes walking or even standing difficult. The problem is usually inflammation in the soft tissues at the bottom of the foot. Proper orthotics, physical care, and simple measures including local injection usually solve the problem.

Neuropathy

Neuropathy is disease or dysfunction in one or more nerves. An entrapment neuropathy (entrapment of a nerve) can cause feelings of numbness and pain, which often has a burning quality and is accompanied by tingling or "pins and needles." The symptoms are often worse at night or during times of inactivity, rather than with use (as in arthritis or tendonitis). Weakness and loss of muscle mass can also be a late feature. Some of the most common entrapment neuropathies are described below.

Carpal Tunnel Syndrome

Undoubtedly the most common entrapment neuropathy is carpal tunnel syndrome. It is caused by the median nerve being compressed in a tunnel under the palm side of the wrist. The patient commonly complains of burning pain or tingling in the hand. Symptoms are often worse at night and are relieved by holding the hand downward over the side of the bed or by vigorously shaking the hand. Driving, knitting, or holding a book can often produce pain and/or numbness. The pain can spread to the forearm and even the upper arm. It can frequently involve both hands. In mild cases, splinting or local corticosteroids injections can be helpful, but if the symptoms are severe or unresponsive to simpler measures, then surgery is needed to relieve the pressure on the nerve.

Tarsal Tunnel Syndrome

A very similar disorder can occur in the foot, where the posterior tibial nerve is compressed at the ankle. Numbness, burning pain, and pins and needles in the toes and sole of the foot can extend to the ankle. Again, symptoms are often worse at night. Movement can relieve the pain. Shoe corrections, orthotics, and corticosteroid injections can help, but surgery to release the nerve is often required.

Morton's Neuroma

In this disorder, a small nerve that runs between the toes is compressed. It occurs most often between the third and fourth toes. The patient notices a burning, aching pain in the fourth toe, often accompanied by numbness. Walking on hard floors makes symptoms worse, as can wearing tight shoes or high heels. Squeezing the area between the toes can cause exquisite pain. Protection of the metatarsals or a corticosteroids injection into the area of tenderness can solve the problem. If a neuroma (benign tumour) is compressing the nerve, surgical removal of the tumour and a portion of the nerve may be required.

As you can see, not all that aches is arthritis. There is a host of disorders involving soft tissues or nerves that can lead to pain and decreased function. Precise diagnosis and rather simple treatment can reassure the patient and usually solves the problem.

Commonly Misdiagnosed Conditions

Three conditions where misdiagnosis is common are important to mention.

Chest Wall Pain

Few symptoms are more frightening to patients than chest pain: the immediate conclusion is that it means a heart attack. Patients will rush to the emergency room and usually have extensive tests to rule out that possibility. They are initially relieved to hear that the heart and lungs are completely normal, but become dismayed when these frightening symptoms persist.

The pain may actually be in the chest wall, involving musculoskeletal structures and not vital organs. Costochondritis is such a condition. Patients with this disorder feel extreme tenderness where the ribs meet the breastbone. The ribs are, in this location, made up not of bone but entirely of cartilage, and the patient has inflammation of the cartilage. The symptoms can persist for many months. Treatment with anti-inflammatory drugs can help, but time usually solves the problem. The most important parts of treatment are reassurance that it is not the heart, and encouragement to do any activity that the patient finds tolerable.

Reflex Sympathetic Dystrophy

This poorly understood disorder causes severe burning pain in an extremity. It often follows an injury (which can be as trivial as a stubbed toe) or medical condition (such as a heart attack). The hand and foot are most commonly affected, but an entire extremity can become totally useless. The pain is made worse by movement, which the patient tries to guard against at all costs. The affected part is extremely sensitive, even to light touch. Although pain is the predominant feature, other symptoms can occur, such as swelling, purplish discolouration, and mottling. Alternatively, the extremity can be red and warm. Later, muscle weakness and contractures (shortenings and hardenings of the muscle fibres) can develop. The functional impairment is enormous. This disorder can mimic many other disorders such as circulatory or neurological problems or infection, until investigation of the symptoms shows no abnormality in other body systems. Treatment is difficult, and must start early with a team approach in an attempt to reverse the process.

Referred Pain

Without a good history and physical examination, one can be fooled into concluding that the problem is at the site of pain.

For example, a patient seeks treatment for a painful knee but examination and tests reveal nothing at all wrong in the knee, leaving both patient and physician confused. However, moving the hip on that side reveals restriction of movement and reproduction of pain in the knee. The knee pain is actually sent or "referred" from the hip due to irritation of a nerve.

A famous professional golfer's career almost ended because of severe foot pain. Many diagnoses tried to explain the foot pain, including a diagnosis of rheumatoid arthritis. It was eventually discovered that a compressed nerve in the lower spine was causing the problem, although there were no other back symptoms. The nerve was decompressed and the pain disappeared. He is golfing again.

The groin is a typical site for pain from the hip; however, a kidney stone can also cause pain in this region. Acute inflammation of the gall bladder can cause irritation of the diaphragm and pain in the shoulder. In both these situations, the first clue is that examination shows the hip or shoulder to be normal despite the pain at that site.

It is extremely important that a careful history and examination be carried out to diagnose all of the above disorders. In none of them is arthritis the problem, although it is almost always the self-diagnosis.

Fibromyalgia

It is estimated that 2–6 percent of the population suffers from fibromyalgia (FM). In North America, up to 10 million patients may have this disorder, and it accounts for 5 percent of all visits to the family physician. Many of these patients are disabled and cannot work, resulting in profound economic impact on the individuals, their families, and society. The effect on the insurance industry is also enormous, with some insurers indicating that up to 25 percent of patients that make medical claims receive benefits for FM.

Fibromyalgia is not a new disorder. Since its first description in 1904 a great deal has been written about it, and support groups and the Internet provide innumerable other sources of information. The cause of the disorder is unknown and there is no cure, but every new observation or abnormality is seized upon as the long-awaited breakthrough that will lead to a cure.

Yet fibromyalgia remains very controversial. Many physicians feel that the disorder does not even exist, considering it to be simply a set of symptoms that show an individual's inability to deal with the stresses of life. (One might keep in mind the observation of the patient with severe pain, fatigue, and a multitude of other associated symptoms who asks, "Could this be fibromyalgia, doctor?" The physician's response, "I hope so," indicates that the alternatives to explain the symptoms could have far worse implications for the patient's well-being.) Some rheumatologists are champions of the diagnosis of FM; others are detractors who feel that patients are done a disservice when this label is applied to their symptoms. Moreover, many rheumatologists will not see patients who are referred to them for FM, because these patients have no organic musculoskeletal disorder or structural abnormality. Some will see the patient for a single assessment to exclude a disorder such as rheumatoid arthritis or systemic lupus, but will not provide ongoing care.

What about the patients? Daily, patients must deal with overwhelming exhaustion and somehow manage despite widespread deep and aching pain. They are barely able to function and have a variety of other symptoms, such as headaches, bowel problems, unrefreshing sleep, poor concentration, and more. They become extremely worried, seek medical help, and are usually investigated extensively since these symptoms can also point to many serious medical disorders and rheumatic diseases. The results all come back normal, however! The patients are then made to feel that they are imagining the problem, or that they are depressed. Hostility develops between patient and physician, as well as with other physicians whom the patients see of their own accord or by referral. The patients themselves become hostile as they seek—but do not receive—explanations and help with symptoms that they feel are destroying their life. They have an uphill struggle in convincing their employer, family, or insurer that they cannot cope and need help. The vast majority of patients do not respond to therapies with any lasting or sustained results. We are left with frustrated patients and frustrated physicians.

What Is Fibromyalgia?

Fibromyalgia is a chronic pain disorder in which there seems to be a defect in central pain processing. It is not arthritis, nor is it a connective tissue disorder akin to systemic lupus erythematosus (see page 29 of Chapter 1). There are no structural abnormalities in the joints or soft tissues, and laboratory tests and X-rays are normal.

Tender points for diagnostic criteria of fibromyalgia

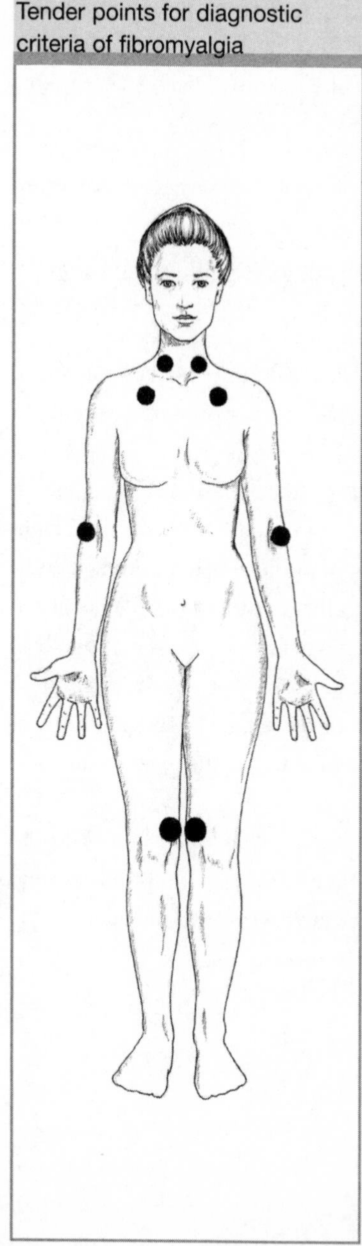

Tender points for diagnostic criteria of fibromyalgia

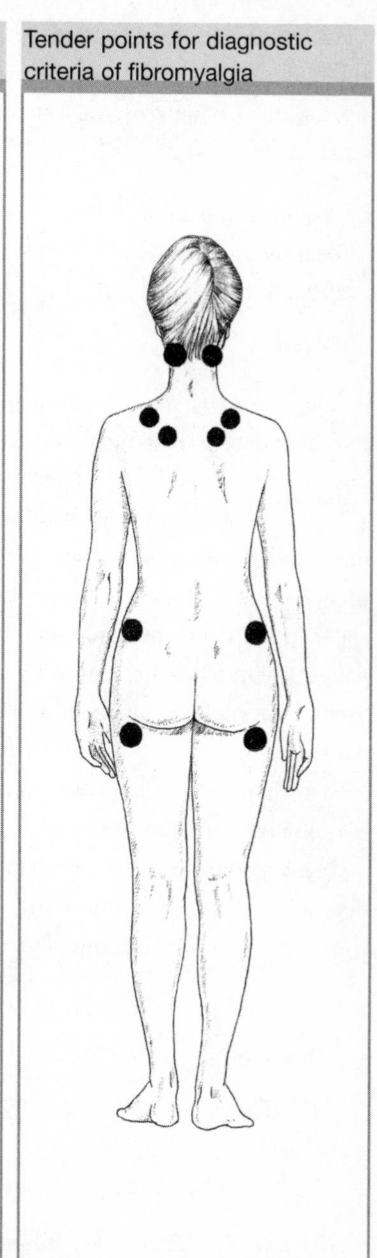

In 1990, the American College of Rheumatology published guidelines for making a diagnosis of fibromyalgia, and these criteria are the most widely used. To meet the diagnostic criteria, patients must have:

- widespread pain in all four quadrants of the body for a minimum of three months
- at least 11 of 18 specified tender points (see illustrations on page 67)

These criteria were established primarily for research purposes, so that groups of patients described in studies would be as similar as possible.

It quickly became evident, however, that physicians came across many other clinical situations: What about patients with only eight tender points? What about patients who did not have enough "official" tender points, but had tender points in other areas? What about patients with tenderness virtually anywhere pressure was applied? In 1996, experts in FM reached the consensus that a patient could be diagnosed and treated for FM with fewer than 11 tender points, as long as there was widespread pain and many of the other symptoms commonly associated with FM.

Many people use a new term, *fibromyalgia syndrome* (FMS), to describe this disorder because patients usually have symptoms beyond pain and tenderness. Commonly associated symptoms include:

- fatigue, often to the point of exhaustion
- disordered sleep
- cognitive or memory impairment
- headaches
- irritable bowel syndrome
- irritable bladder (urinary frequency)

- jaw pain (TMJ or temporal mandibular joint syndrome)
- menstrual cramping in women
- sensations of widespread or fluctuating numbness
- dizziness
- chest wall pain

It is easy to understand how a patient can be overwhelmed by this array of symptoms. He is worried that something horrible is happening and that his life is falling apart. His concerns are justified since many of these symptoms are seen in a variety of serious medical conditions. (The patient with severe chest pain, for example, naturally assumes that this might indicate serious heart disease.) It is very common that such patients see multiple specialists to help with diagnosis and treatment: a neurologist for headaches, a gastroenterologist for symptoms of irritable bowel syndrome, a cardiologist for chest pain, and so on. Many see psychiatrists because they are assumed to be depressed since no other explanation is forthcoming, or they actually do develop a secondary depression because of the impact of their symptoms. (It should be pointed out that patients with FM have been shown to have no higher an incidence of depression than age-matched patients without this disorder. A diagnosis of depression must be made on the diagnostic criteria for depression and not on the simple assumption that, since nothing else has been found to be abnormal, the person must be depressed. Moreover, fibromyalgia is not common in patients with major depression.)

One can also appreciate how the physician is overwhelmed when she encounters such a patient. She must sort through the symptoms—by taking a detailed history, performing a thorough physical examination, and then ordering tests to exclude disease in the various organ systems—to make sure that there is no other underlying disease. Diagnosis is definitely the physician's job, but conditions such as an underactive thyroid gland (hypothyroidism) or even Lyme disease in the right clinical setting can cause similar symptoms and need to be considered and treated.

In the end, we are left with a patient who has diffuse pain, is usually markedly fatigued, and has widespread tenderness in spite of normal lab tests and X-rays. No problem has been identified in any system to explain the symptoms, but he has been diagnosed as having fibromyalgia. By this time, he has already done some research and has gained some understanding of the diagnosis and the nature of the symptoms. Now begins the challenge of doing something about it. At this stage there is a great deal of negativism, since the diagnosis of FM carries the same stigma as mental disorders did (and still do, to some extent).

Fibromyalgia is not an isolated or unique disorder, but is part of the wide spectrum of chronic pain. Many articles dealing with the subject of fibromyalgia begin with the statement that the cause is unknown. Despite this, significant advances have been made in understanding and treating fibromyalgia in particular and chronic pain in general. Active research has shown that there seems to be some problem with the brain's ability to process painful stimuli, and possible contributors to this abnormality are being explored, including the role of growth hormone, and blood flow to the brain and other tissues.

The role of trauma in causing fibromyalgia remains very controversial. A typical scenario involves a patient in a relatively minor motor vehicle accident who experiences neck discomfort immediately afterward. X-rays at the hospital emergency department show everything to be normal, so she is given an analgesic and sent home. The neck pain becomes worse over the ensuing days and weeks. A diagnosis of "whiplash" is made, medication is adjusted, and physiotherapy is usually also arranged. The patient finds that she now has pain not only in the neck but often also in the shoulders and upper back. Headaches develop and she finds that her quality of sleep declines, leaving her feeling unrefreshed in the morning. She then develops pain "all over" and is found to have all of the tender points characteristic of fibromyalgia. She is exhausted, and this intense fatigue and severe pain make her unable to work. She naturally assumes that she was well before the accident, suffered a neck injury, and then developed what has been diagnosed as fibromyalgia. She cannot work and feels that she is entitled to insurance benefits. She then begins the long process of actually trying to prove that this is indeed the case.

The litigation process itself can be damaging to patients, as they must try to prove that they are sick and disabled rather than begin treatment. Often, the issue is not whether the patient has fibromyalgia or not, but rather whether he or she can work. A diagnosis of fibromyalgia does not equate with disability, as the vast majority of patients with fibromyalgia do work despite their symptoms. Since the symptoms are entirely self-reported and subjective, it is difficult to "prove" that the person is indeed disabled. There are no valid tools to measure disability in fibromyalgia, so each case is dealt with on its own merits. It is often found from the past history and medical notes that the patient was not actually perfectly normal prior to the accident, but rather had neck pain, low back pain, diffuse pain, or one of the other symptoms of fibromyalgia. The issue of secondary gain is often raised (i.e., the patient sees an opportunity for payment without work). This process can drag on for years. The opportunity to keep these patients active at work and at home may be lost as the chances for returning a patient to work after two to three years of disability are very poor.

A recent study looked at whether fibromyalgia was more likely to occur after a whiplash injury than after a fracture of the leg. Indeed, 22 percent of patients with a neck injury developed fibromyalgia, compared to 2 percent after a leg fracture. The interesting finding in this study was that all of the fibromyalgia patients were still working

12 months after the onset of their symptoms. One can conclude from this that trauma may cause fibromyalgia, but fibromyalgia does not necessarily cause disability. This study was done in Israel, and results may not be extrapolated to other countries. A survey from Lithuania, for example, not only failed to show any evidence for chronic pain following a motor vehicle accident, but it failed to show any evidence of the "whiplash syndrome." (It should be noted that there is no injury-compensation system in Lithuania.)

On the other side of the coin, we also have no evidence that trauma does *not* cause fibromyalgia. We must admit our ignorance and not try to make a definite statement one way or the other. Where does that leave us? At present, each case must be dealt with on its own merits with input from the family physician, patient, and allied health professionals such as physiotherapists, specialists in pain and fibromyalgia, and others. Once it is concluded that the patient has fibromyalgia and that the accident played a significant role, one still has to make a case for disability. This is rarely awarded unless every effort at treatment has been exhausted. The main objective should be to keep the patient at work at as high a functional level as possible. Only rarely is this not possible.

Prognosis

Currently, the prognosis is not good even if the patient is treated with contemporary treatments. A 1997 survey of 530 patients followed for seven years showed no significant improvement in pain, functional disability, fatigue, sleep disturbance, or psychological status. Half of the patients were dissatisfied with their health. This study confirms the experience of most physicians involved in the treatment of fibromyalgia: the patient must usually cope with pain and fatigue forever, and many do cope, often very well.

Treatment

The list of drugs, physical therapies, behavioural therapies, homeopathic therapies, diets, alternative therapies, sleep therapies, and so on that have been advocated as being helpful in treating fibromyalgia would fill five pages of text. Whenever there is such an extensive list of therapies, it is extremely likely that there is no specific or "best" therapy. (The list for treating pneumonia is, on the other hand, very short.)

Education

The first step in treatment of fibromyalgia is education. The overwhelmed patient must be given some understanding about what is going on. This starts with a patient history and physical examination by a physician. A number of tests need to be ordered since the symptoms are not specific to fibromyalgia, and often, the rheumatologist already has an extensive file of tests done by other physicians to exclude abnormalities in other organ systems. The patient is told that the diagnosis will likely be fibromyalgia, the nature of which is explained. The patient is given some educational material to read at home, and a follow-up appointment is made. At the follow-up appointment, the physician reviews the test results with the patient and confirms that the diagnosis is fibromyalgia. Reassuring the patient that nothing more serious (such as cancer) is going on to account for the misery is very important. The physician asks for the patient's thoughts and questions about the information, and the response is often "That's me, all right," or "Everything fits." The patient must agree with the diagnosis, and this might take a few visits.

Support

No quick fix or magic drug will solve the problem, and it is most likely that the patient will have to cope with symptoms for the rest of his or her life. This is not to say that help is unavailable. Many patients benefit from a therapeutic approach to pain, as outlined in Chapter 5, "Pain and Fatigue." Patients who have a sleep disorder can use a number of medications that will help improve deep or restorative sleep. Some of the associated symptoms (such as irritable bowel syndrome or headaches) can be treated with specific medication, as can associated psychological problems. Pain management clinics can help the patient deal with pain and learn modifying skills (such as pacing themselves as they complete a task) to compensate for their fatigue and pain. Support groups can be helpful, but they are not for everyone. The Internet has a huge amount of information available for those looking for details on fibromyalgia, and, in Canada, the Arthritis Society is an excellent source of information through the Internet, by mail, or at regional offices across the country.

Activity

The basic cornerstone of therapy is self-management and maintaining function, both at work and at play. Patients do not improve when they become sedentary, and can in fact become worse if their level of conditioning decreases. Physical activity remains vital, and aerobic exercise is probably the single most effective intervention to improve symptoms. Patients should not be dismayed if their first brief attempt at aerobics leaves them in incredible pain. Pain is obviously not pleasant, but there is no resultant structural damage and things will improve.

Medications

We live in an age where people believe that there is a pill for everything. Medications have not been terribly effective in fibromyalgia, however, and its patients tend as a group to be extremely sensitive to drugs. (For example, amitryptyline is often prescribed in the low dose of 10 mg in an effort to induce restorative sleep and control pain. People without fibromyalgia given this dose would usually notice no effect and certainly no side effects. Many fibromyalgia patients, however, report that they feel "zonked" the entire next day and unable to function.) It should also be kept in mind that if a sleep disorder is a prominent feature in fibromyalgia, strategies to improve sleep are worthwhile, although it may be necessary to try several medications or combination of medications before success is achieved.

Often, the initial self-diagnosis and physician diagnosis is that the patient has "arthritis" and one of the non-steroidal anti-inflammatory drugs is prescribed. These are rarely effective in fibromyalgia. Regular Tylenol is also largely ineffective, although both groups of drugs are worth a try.

Narcotic medications should generally be avoided except for very short-term use. Patients develop tolerance to these medications so that more and more is required to achieve the same result, and addiction is always a concern. These drugs are also not without side effects. Only in exceptional circumstances with patients suffering from severe chronic pain syndromes should narcotics be used continuously, and this should be done under the supervision of an expert in pain management and the use of these drugs.

Antidepressants are often used in treating fibromyalgia. They are very helpful if the patient is actually depressed (i.e., the criteria for depression are met; physicians cannot merely assume that the patient *must* be depressed over having these symptoms and normal tests). Low doses of various antidepressants may also be helpful in inducing restorative sleep.

It must be kept in mind that if a drug is ineffective, it should be stopped. There is no merit in being on a drug with potential side effects if the drug is not working. Unlike medication for high blood pressure, for example, which must be taken regularly regardless of how the patient "feels," medication for chronic pain should actually be working, not being taken in the hope of preventing problems.

The keys to treatment remain:

- education
- exercise
- pain control
- sleep improvement
- maintenance of function
- anything else that works and is safe

The overall strategy is self-maintenance, whereby the patient takes charge and finds a way to cope with what is definitely a difficult cross to bear.

Osteoporosis

Although osteoporosis is not a type of arthritis, a few brief points should be made about it because patients often confuse osteoporosis with osteoarthritis. Osteoarthritis is definitely a joint problem and is covered well in Chapter 1 and elsewhere in this book.

Osteoporosis, on the other hand, is a bone disorder characterized by a low bone mass and often referred to by patients as "weak" or "thin" bone. Osteoporosis itself causes no symptoms, but this deterioration in bone mass and architecture leads to fractures.

Osteoporosis has been recognized as a major health problem in the elderly. Women are at more risk than are men because women have less bone mass to begin with, and also lose their hormonal protection at menopause. Older white women are at greatest risk, but all elderly women and men may be affected.

Fractures are most common in the spinal vertebrae and the wrist, but fractures of the hip are the most devastating. It is estimated that 1.4 million osteoporosis-related fractures occur each year in the United States and Canada, and about 300 000 of these are hip fractures. The impact is enormous in terms of pain and functional impairment, and medical expenditures in the USA and Canada top $15 billion per year.

Until recently, a steady loss of bone mass was felt to be an inevitable consequence of aging, but things have changed dramatically. We are now aware of the huge impact this disorder has in the elderly population. We now have simple and readily available techniques to determine bone mass precisely and can monitor patients' bone mass over time. This allows us to determine the risk of fracture and thus the necessity for treatment and how aggressive such therapy needs to be. Once a fracture due to osteoporosis has occurred, it is even more imperative to treat aggressively to prevent further fractures.

Aside from a low bone mass, we now recognize a number of other risk factors for the development of osteoporosis, including:

- a previous fracture
- cigarette smoking
- low body weight
- advanced age
- lifetime low calcium intake
- alcoholism
- caffeine intake
- estrogen deficiency
- sedentary lifestyle
- steroid therapy

When possible, these risk factors should be eliminated, and it is imperative that people at risk be screened for osteoporosis.

The most important breakthrough in osteoporosis has been the recognition that therapy can make a difference by *preventing* the deterioration in bone mass and reducing the risk for fractures. Eliminating risk factors, doing weight-bearing exercise, getting enough calcium and Vitamin D, and post-menopausal women's appropriate use of estrogen therapy remain the mainstays of therapy.

A class of drugs known as bisphosphonates has also been shown to have a major impact in decreasing the risk of fractures. Drugs in this class include alendronate, risedronate, etidronate, and pamidronate. Calcitonin and raloxifene are other effective drugs for osteoporosis and fracture prevention.

These drugs are also important in the treatment of arthritis. Corticosteroids (e.g., prednisone) are often used in the treatment of certain types of arthritis. It is now well known that corticosteroids can cause a rapid and significant decrease in bone density and result in osteoporosis. Using a bisphosphonate along with corticosteroids is now common, as it can prevent corticosteroids' negative effect on bone.

This is not the whole story on the nature and cause of osteoporosis, and it raises as many questions as it answers. There are comprehensive sources of information that will provide the details patients with osteoporosis would require. The objective here was to define osteoporosis, differentiate it from osteoarthritis, highlight how common this problem is in the elderly, point out that there are excellent techniques to determine bone mass, and, most importantly, emphasize that there is very effective therapy that will prevent a decline in bone mass and prevent the devastating consequences of fractures. Questions such as how much calcium, how much Vitamin D, which bisphosphonate (if any), and so on are best addressed by consultation with your physician (also see Chapter 7, "Medications," and Chapter 11, "Diet and Nutrition").

3 Childhood arthritis

By Dr. Peter Malleson and Dr. Lori Tucker

Childhood arthritis is a fairly uncommon condition; many families are unaware that arthritis can even occur in children. Parents (and the older child herself) are usually shocked when they are told that their child, for whom they had such hopes and aspirations, has a chronic and potentially crippling disease; their whole lives may seem to undergo an instant, massive change. Being a child with arthritis (or being the child's parent, sibling, or grandparent) can be very difficult; however, most children with arthritis grow up to be active, cheerful, contributing members of society. In this chapter, we will discuss how children and their families can live well with arthritis, so that, despite the problems, life can be great.

What Is, and Isn't, Childhood Arthritis

Although childhood arthritis in its various forms is uncommon, musculoskeletal pain in children is very common indeed. For every child with arthritis whom we see in a specialized pediatric rheumatology clinic, we see many children who have joint and muscle pains due to other causes. These *non-inflammatory conditions* can be very painful, persistent, or severe, so they are discussed further below. True arthritis is caused by inflammation in the joints, and can be due to a number of different diseases, including juvenile idiopathic arthritis, lupus, and dermatomyositis. The role of the doctor is first to make a correct diagnosis—to decide why the child is having joint pain. Once a correct diagnosis has been made, the doctor has to work with the parents and the child to decide on the best possible treatment(s).

How to Make a Correct Diagnosis

When a child has symptoms such as joint or muscle pain, all parents have to decide at what point they should go and see a doctor. That is often not an easy decision, and each family will have a different "threshold" for when to seek medical advice. As a general rule, leg pains that come on with activities such as dancing or soccer (and which go away after an hour or two) are very unlikely to be due to arthritis or any serious disease. On the other hand, a child who wakes up with a fever and an exquisitely painful, swollen, and red joint probably has an arthritis due to an infection, which is a medical emergency.

Initially, parents will take a child with joint pains to the family doctor or pediatrician. In many cases, after the doctor has listened to the story and carefully examined the child, the parents can be told that nothing serious is going on. With this reassurance, they can manage the problem without anything further needing to be done, except perhaps to give the child some painkillers. If the doctor is unsure about what is going on, however, referral to a specialist in bones and joints may be necessary.

There are several kinds of specialists: orthopedic surgeons, adult rheumatologists, and pediatric rheumatologists. Which type of specialist will see the child initially will depend on a number of factors. It should, however, be remembered that children are not simply small adults. Children's diseases are different from adults', and this is true for arthritis too—*arthritis in children is different from arthritis in adults*. Therefore, if a child is given a diagnosis of arthritis, or if she continues to have joint pains that are seriously interfering with her life, it is appropriate for her parents to make sure that she is referred to a pediatric rheumatologist, as this doctor specializes in looking after children with arthritis and conditions that may mimic arthritis. In Canada, each province has at least one pediatric rheumatologist, and therefore it is always possible for a child to be seen, on at least one occasion, by such a specialist.

Non-Inflammatory Conditions

Several non-inflammatory conditions are seen in children that may cause joint and muscle pains.

Activity-Related Pains

Most non-inflammatory limb pains in children are associated with activity and get better after stopping the activity. In some children the pains can be very severe, and can interfere with the child's participation in the activity. The parents (and sometimes the child's teachers) are often concerned that the pain means that something is seriously wrong with the child's bones or joints and that continuing the pain-causing activity will lead to permanent damage to the joints. In reality, the pain does not mean that damage is occurring, and giving up activities means that the child becomes less physically fit and even more likely to get aches and pains when she resumes physical activity.

Therefore, the aim of treatment of this sort of joint pain is to provide pain relief with simple painkillers (such as acetaminophen, which can be given even before the pain-causing activity and a couple of times at four to six hours after the activity). Physiotherapy aimed at strengthening the muscles around the knee is often helpful for activity-related knee pain. Often, children with activity-related pain are hypermobile—that is, they have very flexible joints. They tend to "back-knee" and have flat feet when they stand.

Such children can be helped by the use of good supportive shoes, with a medial arch support and firm heel-cup.

Nighttime Pains

A large number of young children wake up at night with severe leg pains. The pains are usually over the shins or thighs, but can be over the joints. The pains are made better by rubbing (unlike arthritis, in which it is usually painful to rub the affected joints) and by the use of simple painkillers. These pains are often called growing pains, although there is no evidence that they are due to growth. They eventually go away on their own. If the child is having pains almost every night, the pains can often be prevented or minimized by giving the child a painkiller before he goes to bed. Most children are completely well when they get up the next morning. If this is the pattern of pain, then probably no further tests are needed, but if the child has pain when he wakes up, the doctor will probably order some blood tests and X-rays.

Worrying Kinds of Pains

Many types of pains that children complain of are not serious; however, some pains may indicate a more serious condition. When a doctor evaluates a child with pain, he or she will ask questions and do an examination to try to sort out serious from benign problems. The table below shows some of what the doctor might consider in making this decision.

It should be remembered that this is only an outline of the kinds of things the doctor looks for in trying to decide if the pains are due to a serious underlying disease. Just because your child has one or even more symptoms in the serious condition column does not mean that he or she does in fact have something serious. It should also be remembered that the pain itself is serious even though it does not have a serious cause. Pain is unpleasant no matter what causes it!

Considerations in Diagnosis

Less likely to be due to a serious condition	May be due to a serious condition
Pain has been present many months	Pain only started days or weeks ago
Pain worse with activity (sports, etc.) and made better by stopping the activity	Pain present even at rest
Pain is mainly there at the end of the day	Pain and stiffness first thing in the morning that may get better as the day goes on
Pain at night is helped by massage and simple painkillers	Pain at night is not helped, and is even made worse by massage
Bones or joints not painful to touch or to gentle movement	Bones or joints tender to touch
No fevers or weight loss	Fever and/or weight loss present
Normal blood tests and/or X-rays	Abnormal blood tests and/or X-rays

Serious conditions that a doctor tries to rule out when he sees a child with pain are:

- injuries to bones or joints
- infections in bones or joints
- cancer in the bones or joints
- arthritis

Types of Childhood Arthritis

Arthritis means inflammation in one or more joints. Arthritis in children can take several different forms, and these are discussed below. There are no blood tests or X-rays that can be used to diagnose arthritis definitely; a diagnosis can only be made when a doctor finds that a child has a joint that is swollen, unable to be moved fully, and painful to move. Blood tests and X-rays are helpful in ruling out some of the conditions we discussed earlier, and can sometimes help physicians to decide what type of arthritis a child may have. Identifying the kind of arthritis may help the doctor to decide what medicine is best for the child to start taking.

Over the years, a number of different terms have been used to describe chronic arthritis in children: juvenile rheumatoid arthritis, juvenile chronic arthritis, juvenile arthritis, and most recently, juvenile idiopathic arthritis (JIA). This last term is now preferred because it means that the arthritis occurs in a child (juvenile) and that there is no known cause (idiopathic) to explain why the child has arthritis.

It is now very clear that JIA includes many diseases with different clinical and genetic factors, and so under this umbrella term of juvenile idiopathic arthritis are a number of other terms to describe the arthritis more accurately. These terms are:

1. Persistent oligoarticular JIA: the arthritis never affects more than four joints no matter how long the child has arthritis.
2. Extended oligoarticular JIA: although the arthritis initially only affects fewer than four joints, in time five or more joints become inflamed.
3. Polyarticular JIA (rheumatoid factor negative): the child develops arthritis affecting many joints early on in the disease, but blood tests are negative for the presence of an autoantibody called rheumatoid factor.
4. Polyarticular JIA (rheumatoid factor positive): the arthritis affects many joints early on, and the blood contains rheumatoid factor. This is basically the same disease as adult rheumatoid arthritis.

5. Systemic JIA: the child develops high fevers and a rash often before the arthritis appears in the joints.
6. Psoriatic arthritis: the child either has the skin rash psoriasis or the doctors are suspicious that psoriasis is linked to the arthritis in some way.
7. Enthesitis-related arthritis: a form of JIA that often starts off very like oligoarticular JIA, it is often associated with very painful areas where ligaments or tendons join to bone. These children may go on to develop a form of arthritis known as ankylosing spondylitis, which affects the spine and pelvic joints.
8. Unclassified JIA: some children cannot be easily classified into any of these subtypes, so at our present state of knowledge they are called unclassified.

Living Well with Childhood Arthritis

What follows is a short example of one child's experience with arthritis, and how he and his family learned to live well despite the arthritis.

Chris was a 16-year-old boy who loved sports and was working on getting his deep water diving certificate. He suddenly got ill, with high daily fevers, a widespread rash that came and went, very sore and aching joints and muscles, and debilitating fatigue. He lost 10 kg of weight and was having trouble making it through the school day. His parents first brought him to their family doctor, who quickly referred them to the nearest pediatric rheumatology centre.

At the first clinic visit, Chris and his family met the pediatric rheumatologist, clinic nurse, and social worker. It came out that Chris had had an episode of arthritis with fever when he was five years old; it had lasted only six months, and no one knew at the time what had caused it. The pediatric rheumatologist found that Chris had arthritis in many joints, and together with his history of fever, rashes and laboratory test results, she was quickly able to give Chris and his family his diagnosis: systemic juvenile idiopathic arthritis. Chris's parents were upset and worried; but Chris was devastated. He felt that all of his teenaged fun was over.

Chris and his parents spent a lot of time with the pediatric rheumatology team members, learning about childhood arthritis, medications, and the things they could do to help Chris cope and get better. Chris was a determined young man; despite his illness, he went on (with his doctor's OK!) to obtain his diving certificate. He participated in physiotherapy, took his medication, attended school full-time, and somehow maintained a positive attitude and a sense of humour. He dated, bugged his parents about borrowing their car, graduated from high school with honours, and went on to university. He found time to be a volunteer counsellor at the Arthritis Summer Camp. After four years of intensive medical treatment, Chris's arthritis went into remission. His medications were reduced, and eventually discontinued. He no longer had any active arthritis, although he had some limited range of joint motion due to his previous problems.

The diagnosis of juvenile idiopathic arthritis can be devastating for parents, who worry that their child will become permanently disabled and have a life full of pain. Although no one likes to hear that their child has a chronic disease that can be associated with pain and can possibly lead to disability even with the best of treatment, the outcome for most children with arthritis is not quite that bleak. Chris's story is true. His outcome was lucky, but the important lesson is that Chris and his family remained positive, did their best to do what would help Chris's arthritis be manageable (medications and physiotherapy), and didn't forget to let Chris be a normal teenager as well.

A positive outlook is very important, for children as well as for their parents. Don't forget that the child with arthritis is, first of all, a child (or teenager). She needs to do all of the things other children do, with modifications if necessary to accommodate her disease. For children with arthritis, living well with the disease means going to school, playing the piano, joining the Boy Scouts or Girl Guides, having sleepovers with friends, taking horseback-riding lessons, going on special vacations with the family, taking part in the regular chores around the house, and yes, being disciplined as well!

Juvenile idiopathic arthritis may be a part of a child's life, but it should never be her whole life. The pediatric rheumatology team can help parents and children to deal with arthritis and not be overwhelmed by it.

The Team Approach

Many different health professionals provide care for children with arthritis, including the pediatric rheumatologist, family doctor or pediatrician, pediatric rheumatology nurse, physiotherapist, occupational therapist, social worker, and psychologist. Working with a coordinated team of health professionals experienced in the care of children with arthritis is the best way to ensure the best and most comprehensive care.

Parents have an important role as members of their child's health care team. First, they are important contributors during the development of the care plan. No one knows the child and family situation better than the parents do, and the health care professionals need this information to help make the best choices for each specific situation. (For example, if a child has difficulty taking medication at school, an alternative medication may be chosen that only needs to be taken once or twice a day.) Second, parents carry out the health care plan at home with the child, by administering medication, supervising home therapy, and coordinating medical, laboratory, and therapy visits. Parents are able to observe the day-to-day effects of the treatments prescribed, and their impacts on the child's (and family's) quality of life. Other members of the health care team rely on parents' observations to help them do their jobs.

Medications

Most of the medications that are used for children with arthritis are the same as those used for adults. (These are discussed in more detail in Chapter 7, "Medications.") The biggest difference between children's and adults' medication is that the dose of a drug has to be tailored to the child's size. To give a 20-kilogram five-year-old the same dose as a 70-kilogram adult could be dangerous. Children metabolize drugs differently than adults do, however, and are sometimes able to tolerate bigger doses than might be expected. (For example, pediatric rheumatologists tend to use as large or even larger doses of methotrexate in children than do rheumatologists looking after adults with rheumatoid arthritis.) Furthermore, although many of the first-line drugs used in arthritis (the so-called non-steroidal anti-inflammatory drugs such as ibuprofen or naproxen) commonly cause bleeding from stomach ulcers in adults, this is very rare in children (perhaps because they don't also smoke and drink alcohol).

Perhaps the biggest difference between children and adults with arthritis is in the goal of treatment. With most children, pediatric rheumatologists can eventually control the inflammation completely. With adult arthritis, the goal of treatment is usually to lessen the inflammation, but not to suppress it completely. This difference of approach is important because children have to live with their arthritis for very many more years than adults do, and if the arthritis is not really well damped down, over a long period of time even fairly mild arthritis can lead to serious permanent joint damage.

To damp down the arthritis completely often means using several medications together (starting almost immediately after the arthritis has been diagnosed), and also injecting the joints with corticosteroids. Sometimes corticosteroids (e.g., prednisone) given by mouth are necessary.

Corticosteroids have a bad reputation, because people know that they can have serious and very obvious side effects (such as putting on weight, developing a fat, rounded face, getting acne and stretch marks, and, in children, stopping growing). Luckily these side effects tend to occur only if the child is on fairly large oral doses, and if they do occur, they usually get better as the dose of medication is reduced.

Corticosteroids are used because they are the most powerful medicines available for quickly damping down inflammation. Taken by mouth, they can, for example, enable a child who can hardly get out of bed in the morning because of stiffness lasting all day, to feel very much better quickly and be able to get up and go to school. Although doctors don't like children to take corticosteroids by mouth, they recognize that these drugs are often the best means of helping a very unwell child who is in a lot of pain to feel better quickly and be able to start leading a normal life while waiting for some of the other medications to start working. Given by injection into the joint, corticosteroids can very often completely take away the arthritis in that joint for many months—sometimes forever. (The advantage of injecting the corticosteroids directly into the joint is that the side effects described earlier do not occur.)

An important difference in children's and adults' arthritis treatment is in how joint injections are done. Because children dislike injections even more than adults do (or, at least, children are more prepared to kick and scream about having injections than are adults), pediatric rheumatologists tend to give children medications to make them very sleepy, or even give them a general anesthetic before doing the joint injection. This usually means that the injection is not upsetting to the child—in fact, he often has no memory of the procedure, and is therefore not too upset to have it done again later if necessary.

One great disadvantage that children have had compared to adults is that very few studies of antiarthritis drugs have been undertaken in children. Therefore, doctors looking after children have had to use drugs that are not "approved" for use in children, and have not known what is the optimal dose to use, except by trial and error. Recent changes to the rules (particularly in the United States) have made it compulsory for drug companies to study how new drugs work in children as well as adults. This means that new drugs will be able to be used sooner, and with more information about their benefits and side effects, than has been possible up to now.

Finally, it is important to say a little about complementary or alternative treatments in children with arthritis. Some specific substances are discussed in Chapter 7, "Medications," and Chapter 8, "Complementary Therapies." All complementary compounds are chemicals, whether they are from natural substances or not, and as such they are capable of having effects (both good and bad) in children. Almost no proper studies of these compounds have been done in children with arthritis, and therefore it is impossible to know both if these drugs are safe, and if they have any beneficial effect on arthritis. Furthermore, it is impossible to know whether or not these substances may react with any of the prescribed medications.

Although most herbs and homeopathic or naturopathic medications are probably safe, and some may indeed have beneficial effects on arthritis, it is not known for sure; doctors are therefore often anxious about the use of such medications in addition to the drugs that they are prescribing. As families are often aware that doctors "don't like us using these medicines," they often don't tell the doctor that the medications are being given to the child. The physician needs to know what other medicines a child is taking, so that if something unusual occurs, the doctor has a better chance of working out whether this unusual event is due to the conventional treatment, the alternative therapy, or an interaction between these medications. Given the variety of substances contained in many alternative therapies, and the lack of any firm evidence about the effects of these substances, it is usually impossible for the pediatric rheumatologist to say for sure what is going on, but at least the doctor can work with the family to decide together how and when these alternative therapies might be tried, with the best likelihood of helping and not hurting the child.

Physiotherapy and Occupational Therapy

Physiotherapy and occupational therapy are often extremely important for children with chronic arthritis. The role of the physiotherapist and occupational therapist is to work with the child and the family to ensure that the joints are moving as well as possible. Many children are very clever at doing things even though their joints are painful, stiff, and not moving normally. Although this means that the child can often do things that an adult with arthritis cannot, it also means that sometimes not enough effort is made to get the joints back into a normal position and moving normally. Over time, this may lead to joint deformity, muscle weakness, and a greater handicap than if the child had been having regular therapy appointments, doing the exercises, and wearing the splints at home that the therapists would have provided.

In addition to providing exercises to help the joints move properly and strengthen the muscles around them, and providing splints to help keep the joints from getting into a bad position, the therapists work with the family and the school to help the child lead as normal and healthy a life as possible.

Specific Issues

It is worth discussing briefly some other issues that the child with arthritis and her family have to deal with, including eye checks, dental and jaw problems, diet and nutrition, school, transition to adult care, and adolescence and sexuality.

Eye Checks

Children with arthritis, particularly the oligoarticular form of JIA, are at risk of developing inflammation in the eye. Very often this inflammation is very low-grade, so it does not cause a red or painful eye. In fact the child and the parent are usually unaware that there is a problem until relatively serious damage has been done to the eye. Because of this, it is very important that the child with JIA have regular eye examinations by an eye doctor (ophthalmologist) who can look for evidence of eye inflammation with a special kind of microscope called a slit-lamp.

How often examinations need to be done will depend on the child's type of JIA and the child's age. The pediatric rheumatologist will discuss this with the eye doctor, but as a general rule the eye checks (which only take a couple of minutes) should be done every three months to start with, and then if no inflammation develops, their frequency can be slowly decreased. The occasional eye doctor may think that a checkup is necessary only if the eye is red or painful, or if there is a vision problem. This is incorrect advice, and either the parents or the pediatric rheumatologist must explain to the ophthalmologist why it is necessary for the child to have regular checkups.

Dental and Jaw Problems

It is particularly important for children with arthritis to have regular dental checkups, because young people with arthritis have significantly more dental disease than healthy children do. The reasons for this are probably a combination of poor dietary habits, snacking many times a day, being given candies as treats on a very frequent basis, and having jaw disease. It is also possible that some of the drugs used in arthritis may sometimes have an adverse effect on the tooth enamel.

The jaw joints are very often affected in children with arthritis, making it painful to chew solid food. Damage to the jaw joint can lead to difficulty in opening the mouth widely, and therefore also to difficulty in eating and cleaning the teeth normally. An arthritis-affected jaw joint can lead to undergrowth of the jaw, which not only can alter the child's appearance, but can also lead to dental malalignments. For these reasons, regular dental visits are even more important for children with arthritis than they are for other children.

If the jaw growth is seriously affected, surgery can do a marvelous job of improving the appearance (the surgery is performed through the mouth so there are no scars). If the child has limited jaw-opening capability, and particularly if her neck limits her ability to bend her head backwards, it can be difficult to place a breathing tube in her airway if an operation is needed. Before a child with arthritis has any surgery whatsoever, she must be carefully assessed by the anesthetist to make sure that the neck and mouth can move enough to allow surgery to be done safely.

Bone and Joint Surgery

With modern treatments, particularly if they are started early in the disease, it is much less common for children to have surgery on the bones and joints than they did even ten years ago. Very occasionally, an orthopedic surgeon will put a small telescope (arthroscope) into the joint to help diagnose arthritis. Before small enough arthroscopes became available, the orthopedic surgeon had to do a more major operation to look into the joint. The child's knee was left with a large scar, and such stiffness that a lot of physiotherapy was required to straighten it out. No child should need this kind of so-called open surgery as a diagnostic procedure anymore.

Orthopedic surgery may be needed in the following situations:

1. If the joint remains swollen despite the usual conventional treatments, an arthroscopic examination of the joint may help to rule out some other cause for the swelling. Occasionally the surgeon may, through the arthroscope, strip the lining out of the joint (synovectomy) to help decrease the amount of inflamed tissue in the joint.
2. Sometimes, with longstanding arthritis, a bit of the cartilage can come loose in the joint and cause the joint to be painful and lock up. Arthroscopic surgery can remove the cartilage fragment.
3. Rarely, in severe arthritis, one or more joints may become unable to straighten out adequately despite appropriate medications and physiotherapy. In this situation, a surgeon may sometimes cut some of the tissues (muscles and ligaments) around the joint so as to help the physiotherapist work with the child to get the joint straight again.
4. Occasionally—and again, in very severe, long-lasting arthritis—a joint (usually the hip joint, but sometimes the knee) can become so damaged that joint replacement surgery has to be done. This operation can be very successful, but is a major undertaking and is only done if the joint is really totally destroyed.
5. A few years ago it was quite common for children to require surgery because one leg had become very much longer than the other. Nowadays, with the use of medications (and particularly steroid injections into the joint), serious differences in leg length are uncommon, so surgery for this reason is hardly ever needed.

Diet and Nutrition

Children with chronic arthritis often have a relatively poor diet. They should be encouraged to eat as normally as possible, avoiding too many "empty calories" from candies and pop, and eating foods high in protein. Sometimes, if a child is very unwell with the arthritis, high-protein, high-calorie supplements can be prescribed so that he can get adequate calories without having to eat large amounts of food when he is feeling sick. Many children with arthritis are anemic, which sometimes (but not always) can be helped by the doctor prescribing extra iron. There is no good evidence that children with arthritis are usually vitamin deficient, but taking a multivitamin tablet on a daily basis would certainly not be inappropriate. Studies have shown that children with arthritis tend to have osteoporosis (thinning of the bones), particularly if the child has been put on corticosteroids, which themselves can lead to osteoporosis. It is therefore probably helpful to take some extra calcium (the cheapest form of calcium tablet that can be bought over the counter is probably best).

There is *no* evidence that anything in the diet—or anything lacking from the diet—causes arthritis. Many children with arthritis have been put on dairy-free or other restrictive diets (often on the advice of naturopaths or family members), without any benefit. In fact, unusual diets containing inadequate amounts of normal nutrients can cause children to become quite ill.

School

Children spend a great deal of time in school, where they not only learn but also develop confidence, self-esteem, and social skills they will need to succeed as adults. Parents of a child with arthritis may need to pay special attention to their child's school program to ensure that she is able to participate fully and have a positive experience. Arthritis does not interfere with a child's ability to learn, but the pain and disability from arthritis can make it difficult for her to function to the best of her abilities. Fortunately, these are problems that can be overcome; in fact, all children with arthritis, even those with the most severe problems, should be expected to attend school regularly and participate in regular activities with their classmates.

Open communication between parents, the child, and school personnel is critical in ensuring that her needs are met in the school environment. It is important for her teachers and principal to know that she has arthritis, if she is taking medication, and the effects of her arthritis on her ability to participate in school. This communication is often best done in a meeting to develop an Individualized Educational Plan (IEP); even if a child does not need an IEP, the meeting can serve as a mechanism to discuss the issues. Before the school meeting takes place, the parents should discuss the meeting with the pediatric rheumatologist, nurse, and rheumatology team. They may be able to provide resources to educate the school personnel, and sometimes, they are even able to attend school meetings! Some examples of issues that may need to be addressed at a meeting of school personnel are shown in the table on page 97.

For very young children, attending a preschool may be valuable to set normal expectations, help children begin socialization, and identify any problems that come up in a structured learning setting. Attending preschool may also provide a good transition to Kindergarten and Grade 1.

Teenagers face many important issues during their school years, including social pressures, decisions about attending college or university, and vocational choices. These choices may be more complex if a teen has arthritis. Many teenagers whose arthritis is relatively mild are able to attend university full-time, or live away from home with no difficulties. However, for some young adults with arthritis, a full-time university program is too difficult, and plans need to be made carefully to allow for independent campus living. A teenager's vocational choices should take into consideration his current level of disease activity or disability, as well as some realistic estimate of possible future problems.

Transition to Adult Care

All children with arthritis will grow up, and graduate from the pediatric health care setting. Current estimates suggest that at least 50 percent of those with childhood arthritis will continue to have active disease into adulthood; others may have degenerative joint problems from previous arthritis. Therefore, most children with arthritis will, as they enter adulthood, need to find a rheumatologist who cares for adults.

Pediatric rheumatology team care is different from the adult rheumatology care model. In the pediatric setting, parents are

Issues to Address with Educators

Getting to school	Ability to use regular school bus, or need for special transportation
Getting around the school	Optimal locker placement to decrease walking or need for going up and down stairs
	Extra time to change classes
	Use of elevator if necessary
Homework and notes	May need a laptop computer for notes
	Computers may require adapted keyboard, or child may require special typing training
	Extra set of books at home will decrease need to carry heavy books
Participation in physical education	May want to encourage participation in regular phys-ed class, with minor adaptation
Field trips	Need to encourage full participation in all field trips with regular class

initially responsible for decision making and managing the details of their child's arthritis care, and their participation continues even into the child's adolescence. Pediatric care settings may offer parent support, an increased level of understanding concerning the impact of arthritis on child and adolescent developmental issues, anticipatory guidance regarding adolescent health issues, or help with vocation and higher-education planning.

The shift to the adult rheumatology clinic is a big change, both for the young adult and for her family, and one of the important roles of the pediatric rheumatology care team is to begin preparing parents and their adolescent children for the eventual change. The transition to adult care should start early in the child's adolescence, probably long before her parents want to acknowledge that it's time! She needs to begin to learn about her disease, her medications, and how to take good care of herself without her parents' help and guidance.

The pediatric rheumatology team should help with this education process. By the time a child is 14 years old, she should spend part of the clinic visit alone with the rheumatology nurse and doctor. This time away from a parent is important on many levels: the child learns to feel comfortable with the health care professionals on her own; she learns that she needs to know about her medications; she has had private time to ask personal questions; and the team is able to assess her level of independence. Parents can help with this process by encouraging their teenager to spend part of the clinic visit alone with the doctor, by teaching her what they know about arthritis and medications, and by giving her increased responsibility for taking medications. Parents should continue to be included in the clinic visit after the examination, however, to allow them to ask questions and voice concerns.

There is no specific age at which it is universally best for all teenagers to receive adult care; however, many children's hospitals or programs will not care for children over the age of 18 years. Some pediatric rheumatology programs have separate young adult transition clinics, which are ideal for helping to complete this transition process with a continued focus on teen and young adult issues of identity, peer relationships, sexuality, vocation, schooling, and establishing independent living.

Adolescence and Sexuality

The development of a sexual identity is one of the major tasks of adolescence, and this may be a particularly difficult issue for teens with arthritis. Firstly, teens with a chronic disease such as JIA may not receive the same information as their healthy peers about sexual development and functioning from parents, the family doctor, or even peers. People forget that teens with a chronic disease such as arthritis have the same interests, developing desires, and confusion about sex as their healthy friends. Secondly, many teens with arthritis worry about their ability to perform sexually due to their disease, or don't know how to discuss their disease-related sexual needs with a sexual partner. Lastly, their disease or medications used to control it may have a significant impact on contraception choices and future pregnancy planning.

How can we help teens with arthritis with this difficult and important problem? Most important is for parents, doctors, nurses, and other health care providers to discuss sexuality openly as a developmental milestone for teens, and to let the teen know that sexuality is not denied to people with arthritis. Private time for him to ask questions of the doctor or nurse—without a parent being present—is extremely important. The nurse or doctor can assess his level of knowledge and experience, and develop a confidential, trusting relationship that will allow him to ask important questions. A referral to a sexual counselling team or nurse who has experience with chronically ill or disabled people may be helpful for some teens. Accurate and complete information about the impact of the disease and medication on sexual functioning and fertility should be given to the teen and his parents. Some teens will talk about sexual issues with their parents; many will not, but may begin to feel comfortable discussing their questions with the health care team.

A child's arthritis presents many challenges for the child, the family, and, to a lesser extent, the community around the child (friends, schools, etc.). Suddenly, a child who may have been an excellent athlete finds it hard even to get up and walk in the mornings; a child who loves school and has many school friends is unable to get to school in the morning or, when there, finds it difficult to sit and difficult to write. The challenges can be very stressful for all concerned. However, most children and their families, with help from the community and from the pediatric rheumatology team, can cope very well despite these problems. The arthritis can be well controlled, the children can return to school, and very often can go back to doing all the physical activities they were doing before. Most children with arthritis can grow up to be healthy, well-adjusted adults with a job and with a sexual partner. In other words, most children with arthritis can learn to live well with arthritis.

4 Pregnancy, delivery, and arthritis

With most arthritic conditions, conception, pregnancy, and delivery are not a problem. However, there are several considerations that need to be taken into account prior to conceiving a baby, for both the man and the woman, and it is advisable that you meet with your physician to discuss these.

You need to consider whether the disease will worsen or improve during pregnancy and whether your disease will affect the baby. Will you be able to look after the new baby, or will you require assistance? If you are working outside the home, will you be able to continue working through the pregnancy, and will you be able to return to work after the delivery?

A decision needs to be made as to which medications can or must be stopped prior to conception. Some medications need to be stopped (in either the man or the woman) several months prior to conception, while others should be stopped when a woman becomes pregnant. Three months prior to conception, it would be advisable for you to start taking calcium, Vitamin D, and folic acid, to make sure you are immune to German measles (rubella), and to quit smoking.

In addition it is usually advisable for a woman to become pregnant when her disease is under control. Blood tests are usually done a few times during pregnancy whether arthritis is involved or not, and having blood tests done before you conceive will provide a baseline for comparison during the pregnancy.

The next sections of this chapter will discuss the effects of different diseases on the pregnancy, as well as pregnancy's effects on the different diseases. We will also look at common musculoskeletal problems in pregnancy, as well as medications.

Lupus and Pregnancy

Many patients with lupus become pregnant and have healthy, happy babies. However, there are some risks with pregnancy and lupus, and it is important to understand these and to take preventive measures. This means that you will need to see an obstetrician who deals with high-risk pregnancies and a rheumatologist before conception, throughout the pregnancy, and during the postpartum period (the time immediately following the baby's birth).

A preconception consultation is recommended, in which you can discuss the risks of lupus with pregnancy, and weigh the risks against the benefits prior to making a decision to become pregnant. During this consultation, the doctor will review your medications and tell you which ones need to be stopped prior to conception or at the time of conception. Blood tests will be ordered to determine the disease activity, as it is better to become pregnant when the disease is not active. It is important to be as healthy as you can, ensure that you are immune to rubella (German measles), and start taking folic acid before becoming pregnant. (Folic acid contributes greatly to the development of the baby's spinal cord and brain, much of which takes places before you may even know that you are pregnant. Taking folic acid before you begin trying to conceive will ensure that it is available in your system whenever the developing baby needs it.)

There are several circumstances under which pregnancy is not advisable for a woman with lupus. You should not become pregnant if:

- you are taking cyclophosphamide
- you have had a previous stroke as a result of an antiphospholipid antibody; even with treatment, there is a high risk of having another stroke and losing the baby through miscarriage or stillbirth
- your kidneys are affected by active disease; this may lead to kidney failure and premature delivery of the baby
- you have had a major complication from a previous pregnancy and/or severe hypertension
- you have significant lung or heart disease

Birth Control

Oral contraceptives (birth control pills) that contain estrogen should be avoided in all patients with a moderate level of antiphospholipid antibody, although it is not clear that the birth control pills will cause the lupus to flare. Oral contraceptives are also contraindicated if there is active liver disease, Raynaud's phenomenon, complicated migraines, or hypertension (high blood pressure).

The barrier methods of preventing pregnancy (male or female condom, cervical cap, sponge with spermicide) are the safest to use, but they are not totally reliable. An intrauterine device can be used but it may increase your risk of infection, so use it with caution if you are on medications that suppress your immune system. Other contraceptive alternatives include slow-release implants that are placed under the skin, including Depo-Provera and Norplant.

Infertility

Lupus does not increase infertility, but lupus medications can. High regular doses of non-steroidal anti-inflammatory drugs (NSAIDs) may interfere with the implantation of the ovum. Methotrexate can cause miscarriage, and it is recommended that this be stopped three months prior to conception.

Effect of Pregnancy on the Disease

Although the data is not conclusive, most studies suggest there is an increased risk of disease flare anytime during the pregnancy and up to two months after the birth. These flares are mild, however, and usually consist of rash and joint pain. They can be treated safely with low-dose prednisone, hydroxychloroquine, and/or NSAIDs.

If NSAIDs are given past 22 weeks of pregnancy, then the fluid around the baby must be monitored with ultrasound to make sure that the baby's kidneys are working well enough, as the NSAID can temporarily decrease the baby's kidney function. The NSAIDs must be stopped at around 30 weeks into the pregnancy as they can cause problems with bleeding during the delivery and can lead to premature closure of the ductus arteriosum of the baby's heart.

Azathioprine (Imuran) can also be used to treat more severe disease if need be. There is no data to support the routine use of prednisone to prevent disease flares.

Antiphospholipid antibody syndrome (APS)

There is an increased risk for blood clots in veins and arteries during pregnancy. If patients have had a previous clot, then they need to be treated throughout the pregnancy with subcutaneous heparin with or without low-dose aspirin. The possible side effects of the heparin include osteoporosis, fracture, bleeding, and a low platelet count.

At present there are no specific recommendations for treatment of patients who have APS but no history of miscarriage or clotting. Many patients have antibodies to phospholipids and never develop a problem with clotting or recurrent fetal loss (multiple miscarriages or stillbirths).

Effect of the Disease on Pregnancy

Lupus patients with disease flares generally have full-term babies. Your risk of having the baby before the expected end of pregnancy (or preterm) increases if you have:

- active kidney disease
- protein in the urine as a result of pre-existing kidney disease, pre-eclampsia, or renal flare
- a current dosage of prednisone higher than 20 mg per day
- high blood pressure during pregnancy

With lupus and disease flares there is an increased incidence of intrauterine growth retardation (that is, the baby grows more slowly and is smaller than normal). However, despite the fact that the babies may be preterm and small, they usually do very well in the short-term follow-up.

Mothers who carry an antibody to Ro (SS-A) or La (SS-B)—which occurs in systemic lupus ereythematosus or Sjogrens syndrome—can deliver babies with neonatal lupus: that is, the baby is born with some features of lupus. This is uncommon, however, and only occurs in a small percentage of pregnancies of women with these antibodies. Patients with Ro and La should be cared for by an obstetrician, and should have a fetal echocardiogram at 18 weeks and then regularly until 24 weeks. These antibodies cross the placenta and can bind to the electrical conducting system in the baby's developing heart, causing the baby to be born with a heart block (the electrical pulse is not getting through) and possibly to require a permanent pacemaker. A problem with the conducting system of the baby's heart may be found prior to birth and treated by giving the mother dexamethasone (a corticosteroid that crosses the placenta), which may prevent the development of a permanent heart block. Sometimes these antibodies cause the baby to have a rash, enlargement of the liver and spleen, anemia, a low platelet count, and inflammation of the lining of the heart and the lungs. These features—except for the heart block—usually all disappear by the time the baby is nine months old.

Other Problems in Pregnancy

Pregnant lupus patients have a higher than normal likelihood of developing some of the more common problems of pregnancy, including an elevation in blood pressure, diabetes mellitus, pre-eclampsia, placental detachment, and bladder infections. These complications are aggravated or, potentially, caused by corticosteroid therapy.

Antiphospholipid antibodies

If you have antibodies to phospholipids and, in particular, a lupus anticoagulant, then there is an increased risk of fetal loss (most commonly in the second trimester). If there have been previous miscarriages, then patients with antiphospholipid antibody syndrome can be treated with subcutaneous heparin and aspirin to potentially improve the chances of a successful birth.

Delivery

Lupus raises no specific concerns related to delivery other than a very low platelet count, which might result in bleeding in the baby's head as it passes through the birth canal; a caesarian section would have to be performed to try and prevent this. If the mother was taking corticosteroids, then she would need a bolus dosage (large dosage given by slow injection into a vein) during this delivery.

Patients taking corticosteroids are more likely to develop diabetes and hypertension in pregnancy, and both of these conditions can affect fetal growth. Diabetes produces large babies, which can increase the likelihood of a caesarian section. Hypertension can lead to labour being induced before the expected end of pregnancy and an increased likelihood of caesarian section.

Caesarian sections are not routinely done on lupus patients, although they are more common in these women. Patients with lupus are more likely to have their labour induced due to complications of pregnancy, and this can lead to a higher caesarian-section rate.

Scleroderma and Pregnancy

Overall, pregnancy in scleroderma patients is not common due to the fact that scleroderma is an uncommon disease and it usually starts later in life (at around 42 years of age). As women are deciding to have families later in life, however, we are now seeing more patients with scleroderma who wish to become pregnant.

It is advisable that you see a high-risk obstetrician prior to conception to review the risks of pregnancy related to scleroderma. As well, some medications may need to be stopped (such as penicillamine and methotrexate). The pregnancy will need to be managed by a high-risk obstetrical team and rheumatologist.

There are several circumstances under which pregnancy is not advisable for a woman with scleroderma. You should not become pregnant if you have:

- diffuse scleroderma that is active, as there is an increased risk of developing scleroderma renal crisis (kidney failure), serious heart and lung involvement, and death
- a severe restrictive defect of the lungs, serious heart involvement, kidney failure, or malabsorption from the bowel

Infertility

Early studies suggested that, even before the onset of scleroderma, these patients had problems with infertility. However, more recent studies have not shown a decrease in fertility.

Female scleroderma patients do have problems with vaginal dryness and painful intercourse, but K-Y jelly or another vaginal lubricant can help with this. Men with scleroderma have problems with getting or maintaining an erection due to decreased blood flow to the penis. This can be helped by Viagra if the man does not have coronary artery disease or severe hypertension.

Effect of Pregnancy on the Disease

There are several forms of scleroderma, and those with the limited form are usually not affected by the pregnancy, except that heartburn and joint pain may worsen, and the Raynaud's phenomenon will actually improve due to increased blood flow in pregnancy. In one study, 60 percent of patients had stable disease during pregnancy, 20 percent got better, and 20 percent got worse.

Patients with diffuse scleroderma, particularly when the disease had only started recently, had a worse prognosis. They were more likely to have renal crisis, or significant heart and/or lung involvement.

Effects of the Disease on Pregnancy

There is an increased risk for miscarriages and premature infants, especially in the diffuse scleroderma patients. There is also an increased risk of intrauterine growth retardation and fetal death.

Delivery

There is an increased likelihood that labour will be induced as a result of complications from pregnancy. The delivery room should be warm and extra blankets should be available to prevent Raynaud's phenomenon.

Rheumatoid Arthritis and Pregnancy

Rheumatoid arthritis most commonly begins when people are between 30 and 50 years of age, and since some of these years are common childbearing years, there is a fair amount of experience with rheumatoid arthritis and pregnancy. It is important to review your medications with your rheumatologist prior to conception, but no particular problems are related to rheumatoid arthritis and pregnancy.

Infertility

Infertility is not a problem associated with rheumatoid arthritis, but some of the drugs used to treat the arthritis can affect fertility. Non-steroidal anti-inflammatory drugs may interfere with implantation of the ovum, and salazopyrin and cyclosporine can decrease sperm motility.

Effect of Pregnancy on the Disease

Rheumatoid arthritis will improve in 75 percent of women during pregnancy, with the improvement usually beginning in the first trimester. However, the disease may flare six to twelve weeks after delivery.

If your rheumatoid arthritis improves with one pregnancy, then it will usually do so with subsequent pregnancies also.

Effect of the Disease on Pregnancy

Rheumatoid arthritis does not affect the pregnancy. Low doses of corticosteroids, injections of corticosteroids into the joints, sulfasalazine, azothiaprine, gold, hydroxychloroquine, and cyclosporine can all be used during pregnancy.

Delivery

If the hip movements are significantly restricted by arthritis, then a caesarian section may be indicated.

If you are on prednisone or other steroids during the pregnancy, then a bolus (large, slow injection into the vein) of steroid will need to be given during the delivery because of suppression of the adrenal glands.

If you need to be put to sleep for the delivery, a tube will have to be put down your throat to allow you to breathe. In this case, X-rays of the cervical spine in flexion and in extension should be done to assess for vertebral dislocations. Also, the jaw will need to be examined to be sure that the mouth can open far enough for intubations.

Postpartum

As the disease may flare after the baby's birth (postpartum), it is important to follow up with your rheumatologist at about six weeks after the birth.

Fatigue is a problem for any new mother, and with rheumatoid arthritis this may be especially true. Also, with more active disease or damage to the joints, you may experience some difficulty in caring for the baby. You need to plan ahead and arrange for some extra help.

Ankylosing Spondylitis and Pregnancy

Patients with ankylosing spondylitis (AS) do well through pregnancy and delivery. Unlike people with rheumatoid arthritis, however, most people with ankylosing spondylitis do not have an improvement in their arthritis during pregnancy. NSAIDs can be used during the first 30 weeks of pregnancy, but using them after may cause the ductus arteriosum to close prematurely in the baby's heart, and there is also an increased risk of bleeding during delivery. Physiotherapy is often helpful for disease flares but it may be difficult to differentiate the mechanical low back pain of pregnancy from the back pain of AS.

The arthritis has no effect on the pregnancy.

If the disease has significantly affected the mobility of the hips, then delivery may need to be done by Caesarian section. If the neck and/or jaws are involved severely, there may be difficulties if a tube needs to be put down your throat (intubation) to assist breathing while under anesthesia. Placement of epidural catheters for spinal anesthesia can be difficult or contraindicated in some AS patients.

Psoriatic Arthritis and Pregnancy

There is not a lot of information on psoriatic arthritis and pregnancy. It is managed like rheumatoid arthritis, and patients do seem to go into remission during pregnancy.

Common Musculoskeletal Complaints During Pregnancy

Carpal tunnel syndrome is common at any time during the pregnancy. Its symptoms include numbness and tingling of the hand, the thumb, and the index, middle, and ring fingers. There may be pain and loss of strength in the hand. The numbness may wake you from sleep, but shaking your hands usually helps. The treatment is to wear a wrist splint; if the problem is severe, you might consider a cortisone injection. After the delivery of the baby this will resolve.

De Quervain's tenosynovitis is a tendonitis involving the extensor tendon of the thumb. This causes pain in the thumb and wrist when lifting. The treatment includes physiotherapy and ultrasound, NSAIDs, splints, and a cortisone injection.

Low back pain occurs as a result of the weight of the baby in the front and loosening of the pelvic ligaments. After delivery, the pain is usually related to weak abdominal muscles. It is important to do pelvic tilt exercises and to strengthen the abdominal and trunk muscles.

Medications

We will now talk about the various medications commonly used to treat arthritis, and how they might affect fertility, pregnancy, and breastfeeding.

Azathioprine (Imuran)

- Fertility: No effect.
- Safety in pregnancy: This drug can be given. The fetus does not have the enzyme needed to convert this to the active drug. Most of the experience with this medication has been gained in transplant patients.
- Breastfeeding: The drug is not recommended for use while breastfeeding. It does get into the milk and suppresses the baby's immune system.

Cyclophosphamide (Procytox)

- Fertility: This drug causes infertility and ovarian failure, which are dependent on the dosage and length of time taking the drug.
- Safety in pregnancy: This drug is not safe and can cause birth defects, although sometimes in catastrophic systemic lupus erythematosus it has been used in the third trimester.
- Breastfeeding: The drug is not recommended for use while breastfeeding. It will suppress the baby's immune system.

Cyclosporin (Neoral)

- Fertility: This drug has no effect on the woman's fertility, but it decreases sperm motility when the man is taking it.
- Safety in pregnancy: Some experience has been gained using this drug through pregnancy in transplant patients. It requires close monitoring, however, since the drug causes some renal failure and high blood pressure. It has not been associated with birth defects.
- Breastfeeding: The drug is not recommended for use while breastfeeding. The baby may become immunosuppressed.

Corticosteroids (e.g., Prednisone)

- Fertility: No effect.
- Safety in pregnancy: This drug is generally safe. There is an increased risk for high blood pressure, diabetes, cleft palate defects, intrauterine growth retardation, and premature rupture of membranes. This drug should be taken with calcium and Vitamin D to prevent osteoporosis. Very little prednisone gets to the baby. In labour and at surgery, an extra bolus of corticosteroids is required for 24–48 hours.
- Breastfeeding: Less than 10 percent of the prednisone gets into the breast milk, so low to moderate dosages of prednisone can be used.

Gold

- Fertility: No effect
- Safety in pregnancy: It probably does not cross the placenta, and experience with this drug has been favourable. However, in animal studies there were birth defects. Because rheumatoid

arthritis usually goes into remission during pregnancy, gold is generally stopped.

- Breastfeeding: Probably okay.

Hydroxychloroquine (Plaquenil) and Chloroquine (Aralen)

- Fertility: No effect.
- Safety in pregnancy: These drugs have been used by lupus patients throughout pregnancy. There is some concern that the chloroquine can form deposits in the baby's eyes.
- Breastfeeding: The breast milk will taste bitter.

Leflunomide (Arava)

- Fertility: No effect.
- Safety in pregnancy: This drug is *absolutely not safe,* as it is very teratogenic (it causes birth defects). It must be stopped at least 21 months prior to conception, or must be cleared from your system using cholestyramine. This applies to men and women.
- Breastfeeding: The drug is not recommended for use while breastfeeding.

Methotrexate

- Fertility: This drug does not reduce fertility but it does cause abortion or miscarriage.
- Safety in pregnancy: This drug is not safe. It can cause birth defects, and should be stopped three months prior to conception. This applies to men and women.
- Breastfeeding: The drug is not recommended for use while breastfeeding.

Non-Steroidal Anti-Inflammatory Drugs (NSAIDs)

These drugs include aspirin and ibuprofen, which can be purchased over the counter. Pepto-Bismol also contains salicylates and can be a problem if consumed in large quantities.

- Fertility: At high regular dosages, NSAIDs might interfere with implantation of the ovum. Indomethacin may interfere with sperm production.
- Safety in pregnancy: They can be used during the first 30 weeks of pregnancy. They are stopped prior to delivery to eliminate any bleeding complications, to prevent their leading to premature closure of the ductus arteriosum in the baby's heart, and to prevent interference of contractions of the uterus during labour.
- Breastfeeding: If necessary, an NSAID can be used. It is best to use one that is highly protein bound so that very little would enter the breast milk (these would include naproxen, diclofenac, or ketoprofen).

Sulfasalazine

- Fertility: The drug has no effect on female fertility, but decreases the motility of the sperm.
- Safety in pregnancy: There is some experience using this in patients with inflammatory bowel disease and pregnancy. It seems to be relatively safe.
- Breastfeeding: The drug appears to be safe.

Biological Agents

A recent development in arthritis treatment has been the emergence of new biological therapies: these are proteins manufactured in biological systems. Because they are new, there is very little experience or information about their use in pregnancy.

Many of the rheumatic diseases are more common in women than men, and it is therefore common to have to manage these types of arthritis during pregnancy and delivery. It is important that you understand your situation prior to becoming pregnant. A happy, healthy baby and mum is everyone's goal, and this is possible even with arthritis.

5 Pain and fatigue

Pain and fatigue are the two most troublesome and common complaints of people with arthritis, and they are also interrelated: worse pain causes more fatigue, and more fatigue leads to worse pain. This chapter outlines the reasons for pain and fatigue, and then describes remedies such as exercise and mind power strategies that can help in managing both pain and fatigue. Some treatments—like analgesics, heat, and ice—are specifically for pain, and will be discussed in a separate section. The last section of this chapter will deal with treatments specifically for fatigue.

Pain

Pain is an unpleasant sensation that is capable of being recognized by the sensory nerves distributed throughout the body. We are all familiar with the feeling of pain, but may not understand how the body actually responds to it. An explanation of the process is as follows.

Body's Response to Pain

A noxious stimulus (like too much heat, cold, or pressure) triggers the nerve receptors (nociceptors) in the part of the body that is in contact with the stimulus. These activated receptors then send an electrical message along a nerve (by *afferent* nerve fibres, which are nerve fibres that transmit signals *toward* the brain) to an area in the spinal cord called the dorsal horn. A group of these afferent nerve fibres, called C fibres, is particularly sensitive to pain. These afferent nerve fibres connect with another set of nerve fibres that carry messages up the spinal cord to several areas in the brain, which interprets the stimulus as pain and we experience the unpleasantness. Certain chemicals made in the body—like substance P, prostaglandin, and bradykinin—help transmit these impulses. Some other areas of the brain will be alerted by the message of pain and will send an order down the descending nerve fibres of the spinal cord to the ventral horn. Here, a connection is made to another set of nerve fibres that carry the messages from the spinal cord via a peripheral nerve (by *efferent* nerve fibres, which send messages *from* the brain) to the appropriate muscles. This electrical order causes the muscles to move the body part away from the noxious stimulus in order to prevent it from being harmed.

Pain threshold

The pain threshold is the limit below which a stimulus causes no response: it's the level of stimulation that a certain person must get before perceiving the stimulus as painful. Having a low pain threshold means that it doesn't take much before a person perceives that he is in pain, whereas a person with a high pain threshold might not even respond to that same degree of stimulation. No two people experience the same degree of pain even from an identical cause, and men and women perceive pain differently in general.

Pain thresholds are affected by other factors as well, including "gates" in the spinal cord. The gate control theory says that a valve or gate in the spinal cord will open, partially open, or shut to speed, slow, or stop painful nerve signals on their way to the brain. The gate can close if a second irritating stimulus is applied to the same area of the body as the first, thus reducing the sensation of the original pain (counterirritation).

Nerve fibres descending from the brain can also affect the gate. They carry orders from the higher centres of the brain that deal with thoughts and emotions, and as a result, positive attitudes, distractions, depression, anxiety, expectations, memories, cultural attitudes, fatigue, etc., can alter the gate to change our pain thresholds. For instance, if one is fearful that pain in a limb is due to cancer rather than arthritis, the anxiety perceived in the brain will send impulses down the spinal cord to open the gate wider. More pain impulses will now get to the brain, increasing the perception of this pain.

Also, if pain receptors are continually exposed to painful stimuli as in chronic arthritis, new sensory fibres will sprout and the chemical mediators of pain will change so that more pain impulses reach the brain. The pain threshold becomes lower.

On the other hand, the body produces a family of chemicals called endorphins. They are natural narcotics that reduce the perception of pain and raise the pain threshold. Exercise, massage, and acupuncture are examples of therapies that can increase the production of endorphins.

Sources of pain

The synovium (joint lining), bones, joint capsules, ligaments, tendons, entheses (locations where tendons attach to bone), and muscles are all potential sources of pain in arthritis. However, cartilage and discs are not painful because they do not contain nerve fibres.

The stimuli for pain can be physical and chemical. Chemicals play a larger role in inflammatory arthritis, in which inflammation leads to the production of chemicals (such as bradykinin, prostaglandins, cytokines, substance P, and serotonin) that trigger the afferent nerves to light up the pain pathway. Physical factors play a larger role in non-inflammatory arthritis. Physical stimuli include bone-on-bone contact when the cartilage is gone from the ends of the bones, bony cysts containing joint fluid under pressure, microscopic fractures of the bone just under the eroded cartilage, loose bodies (e.g., fragments of cartilage) getting caught in the moving joint, stretched and torn joint capsules and ligaments, muscle spasm and strains, and repetitively irritated tendons and entheses.

Pain due to inflammation is accompanied by local tenderness, heat, swelling, and redness. Tenderness is pain that occurs when an affected area is pressed, and usually means that the problem is actually in the structure that is painful when pressed, such as the synovium of an inflamed joint or the bursa of a shoulder with bursitis. Pain at one location in the body isn't necessarily caused in that location, however. Referred pain is pain that is felt somewhere other than where the source of the problem is. Pain felt in a knee might be referred (or sent) from an osteoarthritic hip, pain in the shoulder blade might be referred from arthritis in the neck, or pain in the buttock might be referred from a slipped disc in the lower back.

Describing pain

It is important to describe your pain clearly and objectively so that your health care professionals can picture it. Some of the things that they will want to know about the pain are as follows:

- Degree or amount—The degree or amount of pain can be measured from 0 to 10, with 0 being no pain, and 10 being the worst pain.
- Location—The location of the pain should be as accurate as possible. Sometimes, it is best to point to the area of pain or circle it with a pen.
- Onset—The onset of the pain (when it came on and how) should be noted.
- Course—The course of the pain from the onset should be summarized (e.g., constant, intermittent, daytime, nighttime, sporadic, worsening, improving).

- Quality—You should be able to describe the quality of the pain in a word or two (e.g., burning, crampy, tingling, sharp, or dull).
- What makes it worse, and what makes it better—You should be aware of the factors that worsen and lessen the pain (e.g., medications, positions, and activities).
- Associated symptoms, localized and generalized—You may have other symptoms along with the pain, and they should be noted. Sometimes they are localized—such as swelling, redness, and heat. Sometimes they are generalized—such as fever, rashes, and diarrhea.

Fatigue

More than 20 percent of visits to family physicians are for fatigue. It is a more common complaint of women than men, and needless to say, it is a very common problem in arthritis. Fatigue is tiredness and, if it is severe, exhaustion. Fatigue is both mental and physical, and interferes with memory, concentration, thinking, mood, being active, coping, motivation, and immunity. Fatigue is not the same as weakness, which refers to muscles not being strong. Muscle weakness also occurs with arthritis, however, and contributes to fatigue. Another allied symptom is reduced stamina, which refers to the inability to use muscles for a sustained period of time and to the inability to carry on an activity for very long. It is due to poor generalized fitness, and it too is associated with arthritis and fatigue.

Many factors contribute to fatigue, and some of them are listed in the table on page 122. Those directly related to arthritis include pain, inflammation, muscle weakness, poor physical fitness, joint inefficiency requiring more energy to do activities, and anemia. Those that might be indirectly related to the arthritis include nonrefreshing sleep, depression, anxiety, stress, boredom, and lack of motivation. Inadequate nutrition, too much sugar, and obesity also contribute to fatigue. Overexertion can result in fatigue. A person can have other illnesses (co-morbid diseases) besides the arthritis that add to the fatigue (e.g., heart failure). Medications such as antihistamines can also cause fatigue.

When describing fatigue to others, you should differentiate amongst tiredness, muscle weakness, lack of stamina, shortness of breath, and dizziness or light-headedness. Quantifying fatigue—or describing exactly how much fatigue you are feeling—is difficult. It can be measured by noting the approximate times of the day that you feel the most tired. If you are tired when you awaken, then you have a sleep disturbance.

Treatments Directed at Both Pain and Fatigue

The amount of pain and fatigue that you experience will go up and down, and identifying the factors that influence your pain and fatigue will help you manage them. Treatments for managing pain and

Contributors to Fatigue

Pain	Anxiety
Inflammation	Stress and daily hassles
Muscle weakness	Boredom
Poor physical fitness	Lack of motivation
Lack of exercise	Poor diet
Overexertion	Obesity
Inefficient joint mechanics	Co-morbid illnesses
Anemia	Medications
Sleep disorders	Substance abuse
Depression	Drug or substance withdrawal

fatigue can be divided into four categories: medical, surgical, physical, and psychosocial. Because the following are common to the management of both pain and fatigue, they will be discussed in this section: controlling the arthritis, exercise, rest and relaxation therapy, being positive and motivated, overcoming obesity, dealing with stressors, managing anxiety, depression, and anger, breaking bad habits, joint protection, and the self-management program.

Controlling the Arthritis

It is important to learn about your type of arthritis, including its symptoms and treatment, as such knowledge will make it easier to manage the pain and fatigue. This process of self-education should never stop. Information is available from your doctors, other health care workers, support groups, lectures, public forums, and the Arthritis Society. You can tap into the public library system and the Internet. There are many informative books, pamphlets, videotapes, and websites. Unfortunately, there is a lot of unreliable information, too: information from the Internet, news reports, personal anecdotes, and testimonials may or may not be true. You must learn to distinguish the facts from the myths.

Some treatments are directed specifically at one type of arthritis. For instance, gout can be controlled by drugs like allopurinol that lower uric acid levels. Rheumatoid arthritis can be controlled by DMARDs like methotrexate, gold, hydroxychloroquine, and sulfasalazine. Polymyalgia rheumatica can be treated by Prednisone and infected joints by antibiotics. By controlling the arthritis with these specific therapies, the pain and fatigue can be alleviated.

Exercise

Exercise plays a big role in the management of pain and fatigue, and it is discussed in greater detail in Chapter 12, "Exercises and

Activities." Stronger muscles will protect arthritic joints from pain and make activities less strenuous so that energy is conserved. (For example, strengthening the thigh muscles in a person with osteoarthritis of the knees will lessen the pain and the energy needed to walk or climb stairs.) The endorphins released during exercise will also reduce pain. Exercise helps shed the excess weight that places more pressure on the lower extremity joints. Aerobic exercise improves your fitness level and stamina, raises your pain threshold, and helps you to sleep better, which will diminish your pain and fatigue. The sense of well-being and the reduction of depression, anxiety, anger, and stress that are derived from exercise will help the pain and fatigue. The intensity and frequency of exercise may be more important than the type of exercise.

Rest and Relaxation Therapy

Appropriate periods of rest will prevent overtiredness and will allow pain in the involved joints to subside. Try not to nap too much or too close to bedtime, however, or getting to sleep at night will become more difficult. You can rest sitting up or lying down, while watching television, listening to music or the radio, reading a book, or doing nothing.

Relaxation and meditation will calm the body and mind as you enter a deep physical state: stress, tension, and anxiety will lessen, muscle tightness will ease, endorphin production will increase, and heart rate and blood pressure will drop. Several relaxation and meditation techniques are available, and you should choose the ones that suit you the best. They can be done individually or in groups, and some that you might like to try are as follows:

- tensing then relaxing muscle groups in a particular order such as from head to toes (at first, the tensing might cause muscle cramps or pain)

- slow, regular, deep breathing at a rate of four to eight breaths in and out per minute using your full chest expansion and abdominal muscles (this might cause some lightheadedness at first)
- listening to an audiotape with sounds from nature, soothing voices, or gentle music
- concentrating on bodily sensations (like warmth, heaviness, and tingling), on a key word or phrase (mantra), or on a pleasant mental picture or memory
- sitting or lying comfortably in a quiet, dark room that has no distractions; set aside a time when you will not be disturbed and try to do this at least once a day
- Eastern or Western styles of meditation taught by an instructor

It takes practice to learn these skills, but after a few weeks your pain, fatigue, and need for medications should improve. Stress, depression, negative thoughts, blood pressure, and panic attacks can lessen. The benefits are even more far-reaching than that, however: rheumatoid arthritis, fibromyalgia, psoriasis, and irritable bowel syndrome all improved in controlled studies where the results of relaxation were tested. The effects can linger, and improvement from these strategies can continue even after you've stopped the actual activity itself. These are not the only ways that a person can relax, of course. Relaxation can result from doing such enjoyable physical activities as walking the dog, swimming, stretching, tai chi, and yoga. Whatever type of relaxation therapy you choose, the important thing is that you do it.

Biofeedback can help you learn relaxation therapy. Sensors are painlessly attached to the appropriate areas on your body and connected to electronic equipment that measures heart rate, blood pressure, skin temperature, and muscle tension. You will be taught mental techniques that can change a physical outcome (such as relaxing tensed muscles), and the machine will let you know when the outcome has been achieved. With practice, the machine will not be needed. Biofeedback can improve pain, blood circulation, stress, anxiety, and muscle tightness. It has been shown to help rheumatoid arthritis, juvenile rheumatoid arthritis, and Raynaud's phenomenon. It has reduced the need for drugs and physician and hospital visits.

Being Positive and Motivated

You must learn to accept the reality of having arthritis, its symptoms, and its limitations. Create a new self-image, and do not dwell on what was. Turn this setback into a springboard for developing new interests and learning new skills. Being positive, self-motivated, and busy will help you distract yourself from the pain and inspire you to get beyond your inertia and fatigue. Being creative about your limitations and solving problems will enhance your self-image. Emphasize the positives and minimize the negatives. Look for the good in life—the arts, scientific discoveries, charities, good deeds, favourite sports events, etc. Change your reactions to the negative: where there is black, see colours. Instead of thinking, "This pain is terrible. I can't stand it," think, "I've dealt with this before. I can control the pain. It will get better." It's not what happens to you that is important, but how you react to what happens to you.

Make a realistic daily schedule. Include a task or two that you need to do but can easily accomplish. Make room for an enjoyable activity such as a hobby, sport, social event, entertainment, opportunity to volunteer, lecture, or community centre program. Pamper yourself from time to time with a new hairstyle, new clothes, a spa treatment, beauty care, or the purchase of a non-necessity. Do bigger projects in smaller steps over several days. Make some time for socializing with family and friends and celebrating holidays. But do not overdo it or you will get tired, stressed, and achier. If you can't do it today, do it tomorrow or next week.

Overcoming Obesity

If the arthritic joints in the legs, feet, and lower back have to carry more weight, they will become more painful. Obesity will make fatigue worse because it causes problems with sleep (obstructive sleep apnea), mobility, and breathing. It also takes more energy to carry around the extra weight. The only ways to lose weight are to eat fewer calories and to exercise more.

Dealing with Stressors

Stress makes pain and fatigue worse. Unfortunately we often fail to identify stressors or we bury them somewhere in our mind, and stressors cause the most havoc when they are not obvious to us. It is important to be honest about what is bothering us. Some stressors can be altered when we face up to them; other stressors cannot be altered, but our response to them can be. Chronic stress leads to depression, anxiety, tension, anger, fear, and frustration.

Stressors come from the ordinary things in life. There are the family problems: marriage, sexual difficulties, children, elderly parents, and relatives. There are the problems at work and at school. There are financial problems. There is someone close to you who is involved in troubling behaviour: criminal activity, substance abuse, or alcoholism. There is child abuse: sexual, physical, and emotional. There is the self-imposed stress: perfection, too many obligations, workaholism, keeping up with the Joneses, and great expectations. You might be surprised to discover how many other people are in the same boat.

There are ways to change your reactions to stressors. Be more flexible and humorous. Avoid exaggerating the worst outcomes and amplifying your worst fears. Be realistic and put things into perspective. Try to turn a problem into an opportunity or challenge. Don't be ashamed and isolate yourself. Communicate and seek help from family, friends, health care workers, and counsellors. If you find it difficult to talk, write your heart out. Writing therapy has been shown to improve arthritis. Learn to be pleasantly assertive. Say no without guilt. Don't turn yourself into a complaining, helpless victim. Don't try to do everything yourself. Delegate and seek help. Make a chore fun and include others.

Social workers are usually part of the arthritis treatment team. They can connect you with the resources available for people with arthritis. They can help you fill out forms and deal with the red tape. They can help with housing and placement, home care, funds for medical needs (such as drugs and assistive devices), parking stickers, transportation issues, and workplace problems. They can give you advice about medical coverage, insurance, and tax benefits and rebates. They are knowledgeable about domestic, vocational, and psychological problems, and can direct you to other professionals who specialize in these issues.

Managing Anxiety, Depression, and Anger

Anxiety, depression, and anger affect all of us to different degrees, and they often occur together. It is important to recognize these feelings and deal with them, as they have a negative effect on pain and fatigue. The diagnosis of arthritis may elicit the cycle of grief: denial, anger, bargaining, depression, and acceptance. Denial of the diagnosis will only delay the proper care of your condition. Anger should be channelled constructively into getting and following proper care. Bargaining will help you deflate the anger but it may prevent you from facing reality. Regaining control and hope will defeat depression. Acceptance will allow you to cope, set new goals, and get on with life.

Depression causes sadness, discouragement, weeping, guilt, feelings of worthlessness, poor sleep, listlessness, apathy, increased or decreased appetite, trouble concentrating, forgetfulness, indecision, loss of sexual interest or performance, irritability, drooped head and hunched shoulders, hopelessness, and suicidal thoughts. Depressed people experience low self-esteem, frequent failures and losses, unobtainable goals, feelings of inadequacy, preoccupation with physical complaints, and a tendency to social withdrawal and isolation.

Depression can be caused by difficult-to-explain internal problems of the emotional system (endogenous depression), by reactions to things that happen to us (reactive depression), or a combination of both. The development of a disease like arthritis with its limitations, symptoms (such as pain and fatigue), and change in appearance can cause depression. Chronic stress is another cause. Alcohol, cocaine, and other illicit drugs—as well as prescribed drugs like sedatives, sleeping pills, corticosteroids, and heart and blood pressure pills—are also associated with depression. Winter depression (also called SAD, for seasonal affective disorder) is related to a lack of light. Hormone problems like diabetes mellitus, low thyroid function, increased corticosteroids secretion, and elevated calcium levels can cause depression. Depression can also accompany surgery or childbirth, neurological diseases, infections, and certain vitamin deficiencies.

Anxiety (nervousness) is stepped up by adrenaline. It can cause a fast heart rate, palpitations (heart pounding), chest discomfort, elevated blood pressure, rapid breathing, hyperventilation, faintness, muscle tension, tightness around the neck, shoulders, and upper arms, clenching or grinding of teeth, cold, clammy soles and palms, sweating, dry mouth, headaches, knots or butterflies in the stomach, diarrhea and/or constipation, tremor, and restlessness. Anxious people can exaggerate and dramatize their symptoms, be overly concerned and vigilant about their body, worry and fret a lot, panic, be hysterical, depend on the medical system too much, rely on too many medications, and be hypochondriacs (people who imagine themselves to be afflicted with illnesses they don't actually have).

Anxiety can result from the arthritis and fears about its effects and treatments. Drugs and chemicals like corticosteroids, digoxin, some psychiatric drugs, caffeine, MSG (monosodium glutamate food additive), amphetamines, cocaine, and ephedra (in health foods and supplements) can worsen anxiety. So can drug and alcohol withdrawal. Anxiety can result from medical conditions like unrecognized heart rhythm abnormalities, hormonal problems like overactive thyroid or adrenal glands (adrenaline or corticosteroids), menopause, trauma, and various brain diseases.

Another emotion that needs care is anger. Anger can increase pain and fatigue whether the anger is expressed or bottled up. The frustration and uncertainty of the arthritis can feed anger, and the anger can alienate family members, friends, and health care workers. Instead, this energy should be channelled into doing something constructive or changing the system. Release the anger by exercising, punching a bag or pillow, or yelling. Find someone to whom you can express your anger. Don't dwell on "Why me?" or self-pity.

Treatment of depression, anxiety, and anger includes medications, psychotherapy, behaviour therapy, education, support, techniques for coping with stress, methods for controlling the arthritis, and elimination of alcohol and depressing illicit and prescription drugs. Better sleeping habits, exercise, socializing, being active, gaining insight, and using relaxation techniques also help. Brighten up your appearance, attitude, and environment.

Breaking Bad Habits

Alcohol, smoking, illicit drugs, and poor eating habits can intensify pain and fatigue. These habits interfere with sleep and with prescribed medications. If you can't break these habits, seek help: don't make lame excuses for continuing them.

Joint Protection

Physiotherapists and occupational therapists will teach you how to avoid joint pain and damage. Physical stress and overuse of arthritic joints will worsen the pain. Improving body mechanics (ergonomics) will lessen the stress on joints. Ergonomics involves adopting proper techniques for bending, lifting, reaching, sitting, and standing by using the largest and most stable joints and the largest muscles (e.g., lifting with your legs; holding items close to your body when lifting or carrying them; using your forearms to get out of a chair after sliding forward in the seat and putting your feet flat on the floor; using your palms to press water out of a wet rag rather than wringing it out with your wrists and fingers). When going up the stairs, lead with your stronger leg, and when going down the stairs, lead with your weaker leg. Good posture and positioning will protect joints as well (e.g., not sleeping on your stomach because it will twist your neck; supporting your neck with a neck pillow while sleeping; sitting in a raised chair with a back and arm supports; using a headset phone instead of a hand-held phone with your neck tilted and elbow and shoulder bent up). You should sit with your knees, hips and ankles at right angles (90 degrees).

Your activities should be moderated, simplified, and done gradually. Take frequent breaks so as not to strain the joints. Use devices that make tasks easier and get help rather than irritate your joints. Canes, crutches, and walkers protect the joints in your legs, but if weight bearing is greatly impaired, an electric scooter or wheelchair may be needed. Do not get any of these ambulatory tools without the input of the physiotherapists and occupational therapists who know how to tailor these aids for each individual. Enlarging handles and grips on utensils, tools, golf clubs, keys, and pens will lessen the stress on your hands. Snaps and Velcro instead of buttons, zippers, and laces make dressing easier on your joints. A variety of long-handled aids such as shoehorns, dressing hooks, combs, and tap turners will reduce the stress on your upper extremity joints. Powered devices are better for your joints than manual ones. Lifting lighter devices is easier than lifting heavy ones, so use lightweight vacuum cleaners, etc. An automatic-transmission car and electric garage opener are better for your joints, too.

Make your environment user-easy (e.g., live in a house with minimal stairs if you have arthritis in your hips or knees, and keep things within easy reach if you have arthritis in your elbows or shoulders). Raised chairs, toilet seats, and beds are easier to get into and out of. Grab bars in the tub and shower and beside the toilet provide a measure of safety. Also, remove clutter and scatter rugs to prevent falls. Use the rails on your stairs for support and balance.

The Self-Management Program

The Arthritis Society has helped thousands of people with arthritis improve their lives through the Arthritis Self-Management Program (ASMP). ASMP is a health promotion program designed to help you better understand your arthritis, learn ways to cope with chronic pain, and take a more active role in managing your arthritis. It will teach you new skills and information about exercising, managing pain, preventing fatigue, protecting joints, taking medications, dealing with stress and depression, evaluating alternative treatments, and solving problems. Participants of ASMP have less pain, better ability to move around, and an increased understanding of arthritis. They have learned new ways to cope with arthritis and get more involved in managing it. You can register in the program by contacting your provincial office of the Arthritis Society.

Treatments Applicable to Pain

The medications and surgery mentioned in this section are dealt with in more detail in Chapter 7, "Medications," and Chapter 10,

"Surgery." Finding an effective treatment program is often a process of trial and error. The benefits and adverse effects of therapies will vary from one person to the next.

Non-Narcotic Analgesics

Acetaminophen is a non-narcotic analgesic (pain reliever). If your pain is fairly constant, then analgesics should be taken on a regular basis to prevent the pain from getting out of control by waiting too long before taking the next pill.

Non-Steroidal Anti-Inflammatory Drugs (NSAIDs)

In low doses, NSAIDs have analgesic properties only: that is, they only reduce or relieve pain. In higher doses, they also reduce inflammation and fever. If your symptoms are constant, then the NSAIDs should be taken on a regular basis. If side effects occur or if the pain and inflammation are not much better after two to three weeks, stop the NSAID and consider trying a different one.

Narcotic Analgesics

Narcotics are not a good idea for most people with arthritis. Whether you use narcotics or not should be a decision between you and your physician, and, if necessary, a specialist in pain should be consulted. Individuals taking narcotics get greatly varying degrees of pain relief and occurrence of side effects. Furthermore, a person can respond differently to each of the available narcotics.

Codeine is the narcotic most commonly used for chronic arthritis. It cannot be metabolized to an active drug in 10–20 percent of the white population, however, and although these people will derive no benefit from the codeine, they can experience any of its side effects. The next most popular narcotics are oxycodone and morphine. In chronic arthritis, hydromorphone, fentanyl patches, and methadone are rarely used. Narcotics can be administered by mouth, rectum, skin injection, skin patch, muscle injection, intravenous injection, pump, spine injection or cannula (small tube), and joint injection.

For chronic pain, the goal is to use a slow-release form of the drug only once or twice daily. Sometimes, a delay between two doses might trigger a "mini withdrawal." Pain in the muscles and joints can be a symptom of withdrawal, but such pain could be mistaken for a flare-up of the arthritis. Also, some people may develop an allergic reaction that shows itself by painful or inflamed joints.

Co-analgesics

Sometimes other medications can be added to analgesics to increase their effect. These co-analgesics include antidepressants, anti-epilepsy drugs, membrane stabilizers, clonidine, and muscle relaxants. Antidepressants and muscle relaxants are the co-analgesics most commonly used to treat arthritis. Examples of antidepressants include amitriptyline, imipramine, and nortryptiline. Examples of muscle relaxants include cyclobenzaprine, methocarbamol, and orphenadrine.

Liniments

Various liniments, creams, and patches can be rubbed on sore areas with temporary relief of pain but little to no harm (see table on page 135). It is not practical to use them when there is widespread arthritis unless they are applied to just a few key areas. Counterirritants probably work by closing the gate to pain. Anti-inflammatory creams are absorbed through the skin and reduce the pain and inflammation locally. NSAID creams are not generally available in Canada, but some pharmacists can compound them for you using such agents as diclofenac. Capsaicin cream is derived from cayenne peppers, and it reduces pain by depleting the nerves of

Topical Agents for Pain

Type	Active ingredients	Some trade names
Counterirritants	Wintergreen, camphor, menthol, eucalyptus oil, turpentine oil	Tiger Balm, Absorbine Jr.
Anti-inflammatory creams	Aspirin, NSAIDs	Ben Gay, Aspercreme
Substance P depleter	Capsaicin	Zostrix, Capzasin-P, Capsin
Local anesthetics	Lidocaine	Lidocaine 4% patch or 10% in Glaxal base cream

substance P. Osteoarthritis in the hands is an ideal place to try it. When first applied, it may cause local tingling and burning, and to be effective it must be applied regularly, three to four times per day. Local anesthetic patches or creams can also be applied to sore areas. Avoid getting any of these substances into open skin areas or eyes, however, and stop them if they cause skin irritation.

Injections

Injections relieve pain rapidly, and are helpful when there is pain in only one to a few areas. The benefits can last for a few hours to a few months. Local anesthetics or long-acting corticosteroids or a combination of both can be used. Corticosteroid injections reduce pain and inflammation, whether the arthritis is inflammatory or degenerative. A joint should not be injected with corticosteroids more than four times per year, although exceptions for more frequent injections can be made (e.g., an elderly person who cannot have surgery). It is common for areas around the outside of an osteoarthritic joint to be a source of pain too. These areas are quite tender to pressure and can be bursae (fluid-filled sacs that allow soft tissues like tendons to glide smoothly over bony surfaces) or tendon and ligament insertions into bone (entheses). Injections of these tender areas are very effective at relieving pain. Tendonitis and bursitis respond well to injections but this should not be done more than three times as the soft tissue structures will be weakened by the corticosteroids. Injections into the epidural space or facet joints of the spine can relieve pain from osteoarthritis, degenerative disc disease, and lumbar spinal stenosis. Back pain can also be due to enthesitis and other soft tissue problems that can be injected. Sclerotherapy or prolotherapy involves multiple injections of certain chemicals (glucose, glycerin, phenol, and others) into painful and tender ligaments or tendons in the neck, back, pelvis, or areas adjacent to certain joints. The injections are supposed to stimulate the production of collagen to strengthen and tighten the lax ligaments and tendons. If the therapy works, the pain relief can last for some time. To some physicians, prolotherapy is a controversial form of treatment. Pain from muscle knots and trigger points can be relieved by injections of local anesthetic alone or just needling the area without injecting anything.

Sometimes when the source of someone's pain is not clear, local anesthetic can be injected into the suspected areas in sequence to pinpoint the origin of the pain. For example, in a person with unexplained right knee pain and osteoarthritis in the right hip, anesthetic could be injected into the right hip joint. If this injection causes the knee pain to disappear, it is likely that the knee pain is referred from the osteoarthritic hip joint. In some cases, X-ray or ultrasound may be needed to guide the needle into the joint.

Sometimes, nerve blocks with local anesthetic are done to control pain. Epidural and spinal blocks are also effective. The anesthetic can be administered by repeated injections or by intermittent or continuous infusion through a cannula (a small tube inserted into the body).

Experimental Painkillers

Cannabinoids (marijuana and its derivatives) appear to be able to reduce pain and inflammation. Oral forms (used to treat nausea and vomiting) are not effective for pain, but alternative methods of delivery such as nasal spray, skin patches, and inhaled aerosol are being tested.

Botulinum toxin (Botox®) injections are presently being used to treat muscle spasm. They may prove helpful for treating painful muscle disorders like tempero-mandibular joint (TMJ) problems, myofascial trigger points, and chronic neck pain.

Other chemicals like adenosine, epibatidine (from secretions of South American tree frogs), and spinal cord calcium channel blockers (including one found in the venom of sea snails) may also prove to be of value in treating pain.

Surgery

Joint surgery is very effective at relieving the pain of arthritis. It is discussed in detail in Chapter 10, "Surgery."

Rarely, neurosurgical techniques are used to stop chronic, unremitting pain in people suffering from arthritis. These techniques are designed more for treating the pain of cancer or neurological conditions. Intraspinal drug delivery systems can be implanted to deliver drugs to the spinal cord to ease pain. Spinal column stimulators can be inserted to give mild doses of electricity to block the transmission of pain impulses to the brain. Other techniques are permanent. A sensory nerve carrying the pain impulses can be cut, or a sensory area in the spinal cord transmitting the pain impulses can be removed surgically.

Heat

Heat applied to an arthritic area can reduce pain, stiffness, and muscle spasm. The benefit is short-lived; however an active exercise program following the application of the heat will prolong its effect. The heat can be superficial (depth less than 1 cm) or it can penetrate deeper (up to 5 cm). Limit heat to 20 minutes, and put a towel between your skin and the heat source to prevent burns. Hot packs, heating pads, hot towels (heat in microwave for one minute), hot water bottles, wax (paraffin) baths, heat lamps, hot baths and tubs, hot showers, hot springs, saunas, whirlpools, and Jacuzzis provide superficial heat. The pools also provide buoyancy for easier movements, reduced weight bearing, and space for exercising. Wax baths and washing dishes in warm water are suited for arthritic hands. Heating clothes in the clothes dryer before putting them on is also nice. Using an electric blanket for a few minutes in the morning before getting out of bed can relieve morning stiffness.

Deep heat is provided by ultrasound or diathermy but must be given by a therapist. It probably does not help the pain of arthritis but can help soft tissue pain caused by bursitis or tendonitis.

Remember that heat can worsen swelling and inflammation.

Cold

Cold applied to arthritic joints reduces pain, swelling, inflammation, and muscle spasm. The cold can be provided by ice packs, frozen vegetables, popcorn kernels, or ice cubes in a plastic bag, frozen gel packs, and vapocoolant sprays (e.g., ethyl chloride, fluoromethane). A towel or padding should be put between the skin and ice pack to protect the skin. The cold should be applied for 20 minutes. Because it can constrict blood vessels, do not use cold therapy if you also have Raynaud's phenomenon (in which the fingers and toes turn white and purple in the cold or with anxiety), vasculitis (inflammation of the blood vessels), or poor circulation. Do not use cold therapy if you have cryoglobulinemia. If you get hives (cold urticaria) from the ice, discontinue it.

Electrotherapy

Electrical currents can diminish pain, relax muscle spasm, and stimulate and strengthen muscle. Electrotherapy should be avoided in someone with phlebitis, a pacemaker, hemorrhage, or recent fractures. It can be given as TENS (transcutaneous electrical nerve stimulation) by a physiotherapist, and if this treatment is successful, you could learn to use a portable TENS unit. It probably works by stimulating the afferent sensory nerve fibres to close the pain gate in the spinal cord and by releasing endorphins. Although electrotherapy can reduce pain coming from muscles and nerves, its benefit for arthritis is not as clear-cut. Its pain-relieving effect may last 2 to 18 hours. If electrotherapy worsens your pain, discontinue it.

Laser Therapy

The evidence for the effectiveness of low-energy or cold-laser therapy to reduce pain in arthritis is contradictory.

Acupuncture

Acupuncture probably reduces pain by stimulating the afferent nerve fibres to close the gate and by producing endorphins. There is contradictory evidence as to whether it works in chronic arthritis but it seems to help myofascial pain, facial pain, and headaches. Very fine needles are inserted through the skin at specific points on the body. These points are then stimulated by twirling the needles or by the application of herbal medications, low electrical currents, or laser. It is a relatively safe procedure and worth trying. However, make sure that the practitioner is licensed and well trained and that the sterilization techniques are scrupulous. Disposable needles should be used to prevent the transmission of infections.

Mobilizations

Mobilization refers to the gradual movement of a joint through its range of movement and then stretching the capsule at the end of each range in order to increase the joint mobility. It can also reduce the pain that a joint encounters when it reaches a barrier to normal movement. Physiotherapists can do mobilizations.

Manipulation

Manipulations or adjustments are high-velocity thrusts to joints to move them as far as they can go. There is evidence supporting their use in chronic low back pain, especially if they are combined with an active exercise program. Evidence for manipulation in chronic neck pain and chronic soft tissue shoulder disorders is contradictory. There is little evidence for its use in arthritis.

Chiropractors, osteopaths, and sometimes physicians and physiotherapists perform manipulation. If the spine is fused (as in ankylosing spondylitis), manipulation should *not* be used because the spine might fracture. If the spine is unstable (as is the cervical spine of people with rheumatoid arthritis), manipulation should not be done because it might dislocate the vertebrae further, causing permanent damage to the spinal cord. A serious but rare complication of neck manipulation is injury to the vertebral arteries, which could result in a fatal stroke.

Massage Therapy

Massage therapy is the application of touch or force to the soft tissues (muscles, tendons, ligaments) without causing movement or change in position of a joint. The purpose is to reduce pain, stiffness, soft tissue tightness, muscle spasm, and tension. Massage can also help depression and anxiety, increase endorphin production, and improve sleep. It should not be used for inflamed joints, however.

There are many different types of massage: acupressure, connective tissue, rolling, deep frictions, Swedish, Asian, Reiki, and therapeutic touch. Various oils and creams can be used. A trained registered massage therapist should do it. Some chiropractors and physiotherapists also have experience with massage.

Traction

Manual or mechanical traction with weights and pulleys can be applied to the neck or back. It is done in the lying position, but the neck can also be done in the sitting position. There is contradictory evidence as to how well it works. It should not be painful. If it works, pain will be eased promptly, and the pain relief may last for hours to a few days. It should not be done if there is a fracture, a tumour, infection, or instability in the spine. A physiotherapist can institute traction. You can learn to do it at home using an over-the-door traction device in the sitting position for two to five minutes once or twice daily.

External Devices

The occupational therapists and physiotherapists will help you with external devices that protect your joints from pain and damage. These external devices should not be worn all the time. They must be removed at appropriate times during the day so that the joints are put through range of movement and strengthening exercises for at least one session daily. If not, the joints will lose their ability to move and the muscles will waste and weaken.

There are resting and working splints. The resting splints will reduce pain and possibly prevent the worsening of deformities. They are worn when the joint is not being used, and are stiffer and harder than the working splints that are worn when the joint is being used. They reduce pain and improve function but they may impair dexterity. Resting splints are made from plaster of Paris or hard plastic. Working splints are made from polyethylene, leather, or neoprene. Splints are used most commonly for the hands and wrists, and are used less often for the elbows, knees, and ankles.

Braces reduce pain by stabilizing and realigning joints and by shifting the forces away from the problem joints. They are made from combinations of materials such as metal, leather, plastic, neoprene, and tensor bandage material. The knee is the most frequently braced joint.

Compression gloves (such as Isotoner) improve the pain, stiffness, and swelling of the arthritic joints in the hands. Farabloc may also reduce pain; it is a fabric made from a woven mesh of stainless steel and nylon thread that blocks electromagnetic fields. It can be wrapped around muscles and joints.

Neck collars, made out of soft or hard and rigid materials, often reduce neck pain. They will restrict the range of movement of the neck to varying degrees. Lumbar corsets, back braces, and sacroiliac belts may help control back pain. Again, these measures should be coupled with an active exercise program.

Problems with the jaw joints and muscles can be treated with bite guards and occlusal splints. Dentists make and fit them.

Well-fitting footwear, inserts, and exterior shoe modifications are used to reduce the pain caused by arthritis in the feet. Good shoes should be lightweight and have extra depth and width, an extended counter to increase the stability of the hind foot, and good shock-absorbing soles. They will prevent pressure on the deformed areas so that painful corns, calluses, and blisters will not form. The heels should be less than one inch high. Insoles or orthotics and heel pads will lessen pain. Lifts, metatarsal bars, and rocker bottoms can be applied to the soles of the shoes to reduce pain as well. Podiatrists and occupational therapists can be very helpful with suggesting appropriate footwear and modifications, if necessary.

Support Groups

There are many support groups. Your health care workers and the local branch of the Arthritis Society can recommend the most appropriate one for you. Support groups are made up of individuals with a similar condition who meet on a regular basis to discuss common concerns. They should provide up-to-date education about the condition, as well as emotional support, encouragement, and social interaction. You may also pick up valuable practical tips from the old-timers. However, if the support group is making you feel depressed or worried, then quit: support groups are not for everybody.

Cognitive Behaviour Therapy

Cognitive behaviour therapy is not designed to eliminate your pain. It teaches you to manage your pain, reduce your suffering, regain a sense of control, and lead a more meaningful life. Your thoughts, feelings, and beliefs about pain and your learned responses to pain are modified. Passivity, helplessness, and loss of control over life are replaced by resourcefulness, competence to manage suffering, and better control of your life. Coping skills—such as distraction, relaxation, and pacing—are taught. Self-confidence is strengthened. You learn to anticipate problems and to plan solutions.

Self-Efficacy

Self-efficacy is the belief that you are capable of making the choices and of putting in the effort to organize, initiate, and persist in carrying out the actions needed to manage your arthritis. You know that you are capable of starting and carrying on with an exercise program, a medication regimen, and a plan of continuous self-education. You will achieve goals that are meaningful for you. As a result, a self-image of competence will develop that will be therapeutic in itself. It will help you combat the feelings of helplessness, and you will experience less pain and disability, better mood, and more confidence.

Hypnosis

Dr. Mesmer started modern hypnosis in the 1770s in Austria. It can be done with a hypnotist or without (self-hypnosis); it is related to visualization and meditation, and allows you to enter a state of mind or trance for relaxing and focusing attention away from your pain. You can will the pain to leave your body or to be blocked from reaching your brain. Hypnosis can lessen the need for analgesics and it may help fibromyalgia. Hypnosis is safe.

Distraction Therapy

You can distract your mind from perceiving pain by being active, by thinking, or by getting involved in activities with which you get carried away (e.g., doing arts or crafts, music, cooking, other hobbies, reading, surfing the Internet, volunteering, helping others with their problems, watching sports, or arguing about politics).

In distraction by thinking, one usually begins with relaxation, meditation, or breathing exercises. Guided imagery and visualization are methods of imagining that should be used in a quiet, relaxing place. With guided imagery, you transport yourself to a pleasant place with pleasing sights, sounds, smells, and feelings, or you imagine yourself as a superhero. Your attention will shift from the pain, and endorphin production will actually increase. With visualization, you picture your disease and its symptoms, "see" the pain in your joints, and then "push" the pain out of your joints into your arms and legs and then out of the ends of your fingers and toes until all of the pain has left your body. These methods can be done alone or in a group, with an instructor, audiotape, or book.

Humour

Watching funny movies or TV shows or listening to jokes can make you laugh. Laughter can lessen pain, anxiety, and depression; it can make you feel happy and sleep better. It also causes endorphins to be released.

Spirituality

Prayer and spirituality can provide comfort, calming, and inspiration. They can help you cope and reduce pain and stress. Regular attendance at religious services can lessen anxiety and depression.

Pain Management Clinics

Only rarely do people with arthritis need to attend a pain clinic. A pain clinic is staffed by a team of various health care workers (e.g., physicians, psychologists, physiotherapists, occupational therapists, social workers, nurses). The goals of these inpatient or outpatient clinics are to withdraw some of the drugs, make the patient take charge of controlling the pain, and return the patient back to an active life. This will involve adjusting medications, education, active exercise, rehabilitation for work and activities of daily living, psychosocial assessments, teaching of coping skills, treating depression and anxiety, and many other techniques.

Treatments Applicable to Fatigue

There are several treatments that act on the fatigue in particular. They will be discussed below.

Treating Co-Morbid Diseases

The co-existence of other illnesses can add to the fatigue of the arthritis. Such diseases include heart failure, chronic lung disease, anemia, hypothyroidism, diabetes mellitus, adrenal gland insufficiency, chronic diarrhea, kidney failure, hepatitis, liver cirrhosis, infections, and neurological conditions like multiple sclerosis or myasthenia gravis. It is important to have these conditions treated expertly in order to lessen fatigue.

Medications

Medications can contribute to the fatigue. Sleeping pills, tranquilizers, certain antidepressants, and narcotics can cause tiredness. Heart and blood pressure pills like reserpine, clonidine, methyldopa, digoxin, and beta-blockers like propranolol could add to the fatigue. Antihistamines and anti-epilepsy drugs can cause sleepiness. In fact, any medication that was started just before your fatigue increased could be the culprit. Suddenly stopping or withdrawing from certain drugs like steroids, narcotics, caffeine, alcohol, and illicit drugs can lead to tiredness.

Stimulants

Stimulants should be avoided, other than caffeine in moderation (such as in tea, coffee, and soft drinks, which should all be avoided before bedtime because they will interfere with your sleep). Avoid herbal stimulants that contain ephedra because it has numerous side effects. Siberian ginseng (eleuthero root) is worth a try.

Dietary Intake

Eating large meals will make you tired, as will skipping meals. It may be best to eat smaller meals six times daily for more energy. Also, increase your energy by losing excess weight.

Minimize your intake of alcohol and do not smoke. Foods high in sugar or simple carbohydrates may contribute to your fatigue. It is best to avoid excess sugar and fats and eat complex carbohydrates like rice and pasta. Some people are less fatigued when they take supplements containing vitamins (especially the B complex) and minerals.

Adequate Fluids

Fluids are lost constantly in sweating, urinating, and breathing. Diuretics (water pills) cause more fluid loss. Mild dehydration can contribute to fatigue, apathy, and reduced mental skills (such as in memory). It is worth drinking two litres or more of fluid over the day to keep well hydrated.

Energy Conservation

By following the tips for energy conservation, you will prevent yourself from becoming overtired. These tips fall into two categories: simplifying activities, and pacing yourself.

Make tasks easy by using assistive devices as described previously. Have family, friends, and hired help assist you. Maintain good posture and positioning so that jobs like lifting take less energy. Organize by time and place and prioritize by importance your activities for the day and for the week. Lump all the activities that need to be done on one floor of your house together so that you do not have to use the stairs as often. Organize all your errands so that you only have to make one trip outside the house. Plan an efficient route. Pay bills and do your banking on the computer. Use lightweight rather than heavy things. Use power machines rather than manual ones. Make dressing easy with Velcro instead of buttons, zippers, and laces. Put things where they are easy to reach. Do not turn taps or jar tops too tightly. Get a handicap parking sticker.

Take rest breaks during the day just before you tend to experience your lowest ebbs of energy. Rest or take a nap for about 20 minutes. Do your most taxing activities when your energy is at its highest.

Alternate periods of physical work with sedentary work, and the most difficult and unpleasant jobs with the easiest and most enjoyable jobs. Say no to requests that will overburden you and stress you out. Divide big projects into smaller parts that can be done over several days.

Environment

Warm, stuffy, dull surroundings will make you tired. Make the room or house cooler. Let fresh air in and let it circulate, or go outside for a walk in the fresh air. Make sure you take frequent deep breaths to fill your lungs fully—expel the carbon dioxide and inhale the oxygen. Surround yourself with bright paint and good lighting from outside and inside. Move around. Play lively music.

Sleep

Sleep disturbances may be the most common cause of fatigue. Sleep problems include less sleep, not enough restful sleep, and interrupted sleep. Fatigue on awakening is due to sleeping poorly. It is important to identify the causes of your poor sleep pattern (see table on page 149). The causes can be divided into the following categories: primary (cause unknown), situational, emotional problems, substance-related, medical conditions, and sleep-associated.

Caffeine may be one of the ingredients in your pain pills (as it is in Tylenol #3). If you have trouble sleeping, use analgesics without caffeine. Beta-blocker drugs (like propranolol) can sometimes cause nightmares. Some people experience painful cramps (usually in the feet and calves) while sleeping. Restless leg syndrome causes the legs to move or jump uncontrollably during sleep. Obstructive sleep apnea is manifested by snoring, periods of no breathing, and obstruction to breathing (such as a thick neck and obesity). Fibromyalgia is characterized by a non-refreshing sleep pattern.

Some Causes of Sleep Disturbances

Situational	Emotional	Substances	Illness	Sleep-associated
Stress	Depression	Cocaine	Overactive thyroid gland	Nocturnal cramps
Pressured lifestyle	Anxiety	Caffeine	Nocturnal arthritis pain	Restless leg syndrome
Late-night TV watching	Nocturnal panic attacks	Alcohol	Chronic lung disease	Obstructive sleep apnea
Small baby	Nightmares	Amphetamines	Asthma	Central sleep apnea
Shift work		Sleeping pills	Post-nasal drip	Fibromyalgia
Grief		Tranquilizers	Esophageal reflux	
Jet-lag		Cigarettes	Plugged nose	
Noise			Corticosteroids-like drugs	
Menopause				

Improving your sleeping pattern will lessen your fatigue. It is important to stop taking any substances that keep you awake at night. Eliminate noise and bright lights. Painkillers, splints, neck pillows, and proper positioning should reduce your night pain. Antidepressants can improve your sleep by helping depression, fibromyalgia, and pain. Try to avoid sleeping pills, as they disrupt healthy sleep hygiene, suppress normal dreaming, cause dependency, and result in rebound insomnia when they are stopped. Nocturnal cramps can be treated with quinine, Vitamin E, and some other drugs. Restless legs can be treated with clonazepam, levodopa, or some other drugs. Obstructive sleep apnea can be treated by weight loss, a continuous positive airway pressure apparatus (C-PAP) worn overnight, surgery to remove obstructions of the airway (e.g., enlarged tonsils and adenoids), and relieving nasal obstruction with appropriate nasal sprays. Medical illnesses causing insomnia can be treated. If your problem with sleep is serious, then investigate it further at a sleep laboratory.

During the day, you should engage in a regular exercise program, be active, and spend less time napping. Before bedtime, relax or meditate, or try a warm bath or shower. Do not do vigorous exercise or eat a large meal for two to three hours before going to sleep, but you can have some warm milk, Ovaltine, or herbal tea (without caffeine).

Sleep in a quiet, dark room with the temperature around 18 to 20 degrees (Celsius). Use earplugs and nightshades if necessary. Turn the clock away from you. Do not use a ticking clock. Use a comfortable pillow and mattress. Satin sheets or pajamas may help you sleep better. Read, listen to restful music, or watch a pleasant movie or television show if you have trouble falling asleep. Do not get stressed out if you cannot fall asleep right away, as the stress will make it even more difficult to sleep. In fact, some people concentrate on staying awake in order to fall asleep!

6 Your health care team

As most arthritis is of a long-term nature, it is important that you surround yourself with a group of health care experts. This chapter is intended to introduce you to these people and describe how they may be able to assist you.

Always remember that, as the person with arthritis, you are at the centre of the health care team, and it is your responsibility to choose people with the expertise to assist you. You must be able to work with these individuals for the long term. It is also your responsibility to be informed about your disease and therapies, to make decisions, and to participate fully in mutually agreed-upon therapies (there's no point in a doctor prescribing a medication if you have no intention of taking it). These are some of your responsibilities as set out by the Canadian Arthritis Bill of Rights.

Family Physician

People seeking help with arthritis generally see a family physician first, and this doctor is pivotal in the ongoing management of the disease. Most family physicians are comfortable diagnosing and treating osteoarthritis, gout, and fibromyalgia. In more difficult cases, they may ask for an opinion from an arthritis expert (a rheumatologist), or if the problem requires surgery, they may consult with an orthopedic surgeon. In rheumatoid arthritis and the connective tissue diseases, a rheumatologist is usually involved with the family physician in the ongoing management. They communicate by mail, or by telephone if there is an urgent situation. The family physician will usually follow the blood work, arrange for gold or methotrexate injections, and deal with any acute problems.

Rheumatologist

A rheumatologist is a physician who has completed training in internal medicine and then rheumatology, all after medical school. A rheumatologist cares for patients with arthritis, connective tissue diseases, and osteoporosis. A patient would initially see a rheumatologist at the request of another physician (who would make a referral). Sometimes patients may need to be seen only once, but with a chronic inflammatory disease like rheumatoid arthritis, they would be seen repeatedly. If there are complications or if the disease is very active, the visits would be more frequent.

Usually a rheumatologist would prescribe the medications and make the decisions about continuing or changing them. On a patient's initial visit, a rheumatologist would take a history of the disease and the patient's other health problems, and do an examination not only of the joints but also of the lungs, heart, abdomen, head, and neck, as many forms of arthritis and connective tissue disease affect other organs. In addition, the rheumatologist must determine if there are any reasons why the patient could not take certain medications or if he is unfit for surgery. Blood work and X-rays are frequently required to determine the diagnosis, to help in making management decisions, and to monitor for drug toxicity.

A rheumatologist's whole career revolves around arthritis: looking after patients, teaching students, and doing research into causes and cures. Rheumatologists are experts in the diagnosis and management of arthritis, and are very familiar with the medications they prescribe because they see the medications in use every day. They constantly update their knowledge and keep abreast of new therapies by attending conferences, lectures, and hospital rounds, reading journals and websites, and talking with colleagues and researchers.

If you have questions or concerns about a medication that your rheumatologist has prescribed, you should talk to her before making a decision to stop or start it. For example, methotrexate is the drug most commonly used to treat rheumatoid arthritis: every day, rheumatologists write prescriptions for it, see patients who have been taking it, and monitor their blood work. Most arthritis patients take this drug with a non-steroidal anti-inflammatory drug. Some pharmacists will advise patients not to take an anti-inflammatory with methotrexate, however; on the pharmacist's computer, this combination of drugs is listed as an interaction because when methotrexate is used at high doses for treating cancer, the anti-inflammatory may increase the blood's methotrexate concentration to a toxic level. At the low doses used in arthritis, however, it is safe to combine the two. It is not that the pharmacist is wrong, but because the pharmacist may not have the familiarity with this prescription that the rheumatologist has gained through seeing many arthritis patients, more information might be needed in order to advise a patient taking this drug for rheumatoid arthritis.

The rheumatologist can help you to coordinate your health care team. She knows the surgeons and allied health professionals in the community who have expertise in the care of patients with arthritis. However, you must help to choose the people with whom you can work to get the best possible results. This includes your rheumatologist.

Nurse

The nurse is a very important member of the team. He is often involved in the clinic setting of a hospital unit or in a physician's office, has extra experience in arthritis care, and is a valuable resource for educating patients about arthritis. He may also administer and facilitate therapies and may coordinate clinical trials. Nurse practitioners are becoming increasingly popular as physician extenders. These individuals will have done extra training at university and will be actively involved in the decision-making process. They may do the history and physical exam, and they work alongside the rheumatologist.

Physiotherapist

Physiotherapists can do a full examination of the joints and an assessment of functioning. They are trained at a university and receive a Bachelor of Science in Physiotherapy.

Physiotherapists can treat pain and swelling with a mild electric current (a therapy called TENS, for transcutaneous electrical nerve stimulation), interferential therapy, ultrasound, pool therapy, and the use of ice and heat. Some perform acupuncture, or will do joint mobilizations and back and neck manipulations. Many are also involved in teaching patients about their arthritis.

Physiotherapists will guide you through a rehabilitation program after surgery, and will teach you how to protect your joints and use walking aids like canes and crutches properly. They will work with you to design a self-managed home program that includes physical treatments for pain, and an exercise program to improve your range of movement and flexibility, muscle strength and stamina, and general conditioning. This can only be done with your cooperation, however: a mutually agreed-upon course of action is necessary, and you must do the stretching and exercises as prescribed. A passive approach to physiotherapy is not helpful. (For example, if you go to physiotherapy, have a hot pack put on your shoulder, but never do the stretching or exercises, then the benefit will only last until the hot pack is removed.) Finding a good physiotherapist with whom you work well is invaluable, and you will benefit most if everyone has a positive attitude.

Occupational Therapist

Occupational therapists have much to offer a person with arthritis. They will assess your daily activities and ability to cope, and then provide treatment to improve your ability to function. They are trained at a university and graduate with a Bachelor of Science in Occupational Therapy.

Occupational therapists will arrange for splints to help reduce pain, improve function, and prevent deformity in the hands, wrists and some of the other joints. They can recommend and fit appropriate bracing of the neck and back, and insoles, orthotics, or special shoes to accommodate foot and ankle problems. They will help with walking aids such as canes, crutches, walkers, and wheelchairs.

They can also visit the home or workplace and recommend changes to help you function better. In the home, such changes might be a raised toilet seat, railings in the tub, or a seat in the shower stall; extra-grip utensils and an electric can opener might be suggested for the kitchen. In the workplace, they might find you a more appropriate chair, adjust your computer height, and order a new keyboard that is designed for comfort and efficiency. They usually do not do job counselling. Their role is to come up with practical solutions to make your life easier.

Orthopedic Surgeon

An orthopedic surgeon is a physician trained in the assessment and surgery of the bones and joints. The orthopedic surgeon will see patients with osteoarthritis, rheumatoid arthritis, and other forms of arthritis when conservative treatment has failed and surgery is recommended. For more information on various forms of surgery available to patients with arthritis, please see Chapter 10, "Surgery."

A visit to an orthopedic surgeon does not mean that you have agreed to surgery. A consultation with an orthopedic surgeon will make you aware of the options available for surgery, the risks of having or not having a procedure, and the likelihood of a successful outcome. No one can make a decision without this information. Even if you are dead set against surgery, it is worthwhile finding out what is involved and what are the consequences of doing nothing.

Plastic Surgeon

Surgery on the hands and wrists is often done by a plastic surgeon. In some centres, the orthopedic surgeon has special training in hand surgery. You should see whichever surgeon is most experienced with hand surgery, whether this is a plastic surgeon or orthopedic surgeon.

Neurosurgeon

A neurosurgeon will usually do any spine surgery, especially if there is involvement of the nerves or the spinal cord. However, in some centres orthopedic surgeons will do neck and back surgery.

Physiatrist

A physiatrist is a physician with special training in rehabilitation medicine who will help improve function and independence. Patients are sometimes referred to a physiatrist for intensive therapy and rehabilitation. This may be after surgery, or if there are many damaged joints or if there is a complicated mechanical problem.

Social Worker

Depending on where you live, finding out what resources are available to you can be a difficult task. Social workers can help with this. They can help with disability insurance, pensions, tax exemptions, funding of medications and other medical supplies, and other financial problems, and can arrange for assistance in the home or placement in a nursing home or other personal care facility.

Social workers are also helpful in dealing with employers and difficulties at the workplace. They have experience in counselling for family-related and personal problems.

Pharmacist

A pharmacist is a trained professional who has completed four years of university and obtained a Bachelor of Science in Pharmacy. Pharmacists study disease processes and the effects of medications on them. They keep track of your medications and the potential interactions, and can tell you if an adverse effect is likely related to one of the medications you are taking. Often when a new medication is introduced, the potential adverse effects, how to use it, and why it is being used are not completely understood: there is often simply too much information to absorb in the physician's office. The pharmacist can review those details with you. If you are still confused or if you are uncomfortable with the medication, then you will need to contact the physician who wrote the prescription.

Podiatrist

A podiatrist is trained in diseases and conditions of the feet. Podiatrists are required to get a Bachelor of Science degree and then a four-year degree in podiatric medicine, which is available only in the United States. They will help reduce pain and discomfort of the feet by providing insoles, shoe modifications, or prescription shoes. They are qualified to do minor procedures on the feet, including bone surgery on the forefoot. They will treat corns, calluses, toenail problems, and infections.

Chiropodists receive a diploma after completing a three-year course of study after high school. They can do minor procedures, but are not as extensively qualified as podiatrists.

There are, of course, many other heath care professionals whom you may need to see, but this chapter has outlined the potential roles of those involved in the care of arthritis patients.

7 Medications

Today more than at any time in the past, we have effective medications to treat many forms of arthritis. The recent development of the biological response modifiers to treat rheumatoid arthritis, psoriatic arthritis, and ankylosing spondylitis has given many patients their lives back. Not only have we seen control of the inflammatory process, but there is also a reduction in the degree of joint damage, as the process of damage to the cartilage and bone of the joints has been slowed. With the development of these drugs, we have learned much about the immune system and its role in the development of all forms of arthritis (including osteoarthritis). I believe that this has opened the door for the development of new treatments that are better and safer than anything we have seen in the past.

Most of us do not like taking medications. For most people with arthritis, daily medication is a fact of life: for the pain, to control the disease, to sleep, and to prevent osteoporosis caused by the disease or the other medications. It is important to take the medications as directed and to have blood work done regularly if required.

In diseases with a significant inflammatory component, like rheumatoid arthritis, the medication prevents further damage and disability. *Not* taking these medications *leads to* progressive deformity and disability. Damage to the joint can take place within three months of the onset of the disease, and 50 percent of patients with untreated rheumatoid arthritis will be disabled from work within 10 years of the onset of disease. We know that this can be prevented by early, effective management of the disease process. In diseases such as systemic lupus erythematosus, medication will prevent kidney failure, arthritis, lung disease, stroke, and even death, to name a few of the possible disease effects that most people would like to avoid. There is no good evidence that diet or alternative and complementary products will significantly alter the course of many forms of arthritis, and if they did, then we would use them.

Choosing to take a medication for arthritis can be a big decision, especially when it will be required for an indefinite period. If you have concerns about the medication, talk to your physician, pharmacist, or clinic nurse. It is important to understand why you will be taking the medication, what response to expect, and potential side effects to watch for. Medications do have potential side effects, and many people wonder, "Is this worth it?" If you have an adverse effect, it is important to let your physician know. Most people do tolerate the medications, but if they are not tolerated, they are stopped and something else is tried.

This chapter outlines the common medications for treating arthritis, osteoporosis, and pain. The effects of the medications while pregnant or breastfeeding are covered in Chapter 4, "Pregnancy, Delivery, and Arthritis."

Treatments for Inflammatory Arthritis and Immune Mediated Diseases

Therapies commonly used to treat inflammation include non-steroidal anti-inflammatory drugs (NSAIDs), disease modifying anti-rheumatic drugs (DMARDs) and immunosuppressant drugs, the biological response modifiers, and corticosteroids.

Non-Steroidal Anti-Inflammatory Drugs (NSAIDs)

Non-steroidal anti-inflammatory drugs (NSAIDs) are medications commonly used for treating inflammation, fever, and pain. They are often the first medications used to treat arthritis. They work quickly for pain, but the full anti-inflammatory effect may take up to two weeks.

NSAIDs do treat the symptoms of inflammation, including stiffness, swelling, and pain. They do make you feel better, but they do not treat the underlying disease, nor do they halt or slow down joint damage. In some forms of arthritis such as ankylosing spondylitis or osteoarthritis, other medication may not be necessary or available. In a disease like rheumatoid arthritis, almost all patients require a disease modifying drug.

The first NSAID, aspirin (a derivative from willow tree bark), was developed over 100 years ago by the Bayer Company. Traditional NSAIDs may cause ulcers and bleeding in the stomach lining. NSAIDs work by inhibiting an enzyme called cyclo-oxygenase (COX), of which scientists have found two forms: COX-1 and COX-2. The COX-1 protects the lining of the stomach and allows the platelets to clot, whereas the COX-2 promotes inflammation. The traditional NSAIDs block both COX-1 and COX-2. Therefore newer NSAIDs—called COX-2 selective or COXIBs—were developed that mainly inhibit COX-2. These drugs, including celecoxib (Celebrex) and rofecoxib (Vioxx)—were developed specifically to reduce the risk of ulcers and bleeding in the stomach, and to allow the platelets to do their job of stopping bleeding normally. However, they are no more effective than the traditional NSAIDs and have the same adverse effects on kidney function, high blood pressure, and fluid retention.

Approximately 30 million people use NSAIDs today. They can be purchased over the counter (as aspirin or ibuprofen) or by prescription. (See tables on pages 163 and 164 for the list of NSAIDs available in Canada.) One may ask why there are so many of these drugs. The reason is that it has been found that different individuals may find one medication more effective or more tolerable than another.

The NSAIDs are usually given in a pill form, but some are also available as suppositories. Pennsaid, a lotion containing diclofenac, is applied to the skin that overlies an affected joint. Skin patches and creams are available in some countries but not in Canada, unless a pharmacist has specially prepared them for you. The NSAIDs are absorbed in whatever form the drug is given, so there is still potential for adverse events, including peptic ulcers.

Potential side effects

Approximately 4 percent of patients on NSAIDs will have a symptomatic stomach or duodenal ulcer or a bleed. The risk factors for this include increased age, previous stomach ulcer or bleed, other serious health problems, or use of a corticosteroid with the NSAID. Patients at high risk for an ulcer or bleed should avoid NSAIDs if possible. If it is necessary to use them, then the patient should be given a medication to protect the stomach (such as misoprostol or a proton pump inhibitor [for example omeprazole]) or be switched to a COX-2 selective NSAID.

NSAIDs can cause such nuisance symptoms as nausea, bloating, and stomach upset. Up to 5 percent of people will have to stop the drug because of the nuisance side effects. Another NSAID may be tolerated, however, and should be tried. These symptoms do not predict a stomach ulcer. Many patients with an ulcer or bleed will have no prior symptoms. NSAIDs can sometimes cause mild reversible derangements in liver enzyme tests.

Traditional NSAIDs may prolong bleeding by their effect on platelets, and they should be avoided if the patient is on blood thinners such as warfarin (Coumadin). The use of a COX-2 selective drug is preferable, but these too might interact with warfarin, so the blood clotting time needs careful monitoring after starting the medication.

All NSAIDs can potentially increase the risk of cardiovascular disease (heart attack and stroke). This risk is small and is dose related

Traditional Non-Steroidal Anti-Inflammatory Drugs

Medication	Dosage	Supplied
Aspirin	1300–5200 mg/day	Oral, or cream
Diclofenac (Voltaren)	100–200 mg/day	Oral, slow release, or suppository
Fenoprofen (Nalfon)	1200–2400 mg/day	Oral
Flurbiprofen (Ansaid, Froben)	100–300 mg/day	Oral
Ibuprofen (Motrin, Advil)	1200–3200 mg/day	Oral
Indomethacin (Indocid)	50–200 mg/day	Oral, or suppository
Ketoprofen (Orudis)	150–300 mg/day	Oral, slow release, or suppository
Meclofenamte (Meclomen)	200–400 mg/day	Oral
Nabumetone (Relafen)	1000–2000 mg/day	Oral
Naproxen (Naprosyn, Anaprox)	500–2000 mg/day	Oral, slow release, or suppository
Piroxicam (Feldene)	10–20 mg/day	Oral, or suppository
Sulindac (Clinoril)	150–300 mg/day	Oral
Tolmetin (Tolectin)	1200–1800 mg/day	Oral
Etodalac (Ultradol)	400–600 mg/day	Oral
Ketorolac (Toradol)	40 mg/day	Oral
	30–120 mg/day	Intramuscular injection (for maximum of 2 days)
Tenoxicam (Apo-Tenoxicam, Novo-Tenoxicam)	10–20 mg/day	Oral
Oxaprozin (Daypro)	600–1800 mg/day	Oral
Tiaprofenic acid (Surgam)	300–600 mg/day	Oral, slow release
Diflunisal (Apo-Diflunisal Novo-Diflinisal, Nu-Diflunisal	500–1000 mg/day	Oral
Choline magnesium trisalicylate (Trilisate)	1000–3000 mg/day	Oral
Meloxicam	7.5–15 mg/day	Oral

COX-2 Selective Non-Steroidal Anti-Inflammatory Drugs

Medication	Dosage	Supplied
COXIBs:		
Celecoxib (Celebrex)	200–400 mg/day	Oral

(the higher the dose, the greater the risk). In patients with multiple risk factors for cardiovascular disease, the potential benefits of the NSAIDs need to be weighed carefully against the risks for cardiovascular disease. All NSAIDs can raise blood pressure, cause fluid retention, and reduce kidney function. They should be used with caution in the elderly.

Some NSAIDs may cause ringing in the ears, reversible hearing loss, altered moods, confusion, headaches, or drowsiness; switching the NSAID or lowering its dose is usually effective in relieving these adverse effects. They can cause mouth sores, rashes, or skin sensitivity to the sun, and they sometimes make asthma worse.

COX-2 selective anti-inflammatory drugs

The advantage of COXIBs, or COX-2 selective NSAIDs, over the traditional NSAIDs is the reduced frequency of stomach ulcers and bleeds. In the large clinical trials of rofecoxib (Vioxx) and celecoxib (Celebrex), there was a 50 percent reduction of the risk of ulcers and ulcer complications. The use of misoprostil (Cytotec) with a traditional NSAID also reduces the risk of developing ulcers and ulcer complications. The addition of a proton pump inhibitor will also reduce the chances of developing stomach ulcers and bleeds. For people taking blood thinners, the use of celecoxib is safer than the use of the traditional NSAIDs.

As a result of the VIGOR clinical trial, comparing Vioxx to naproxen, and a subsequent trial testing the role of COXIBs in the prevention of polyps from growing in the colon, Vioxx was voluntarily removed from the market because of increased incidence of heart attacks and strokes in those using Vioxx compared to those taking naproxen or a placebo. The FDA and Health Canada have reviewed all available data and have determined that all NSAIDs, traditional or COXIBs, are associated with an increased risk of cardiovascular events. Accordingly, warnings have been placed on their labels. Celebrex is now the only COXIB available in Canada. Any patient at risk for a heart attack or stroke should be treated with 81 mg of aspirin (a baby aspirin) per day even if another NSAID is required for arthritis.

Disease Modifying Anti-Rheumatic Drugs (DMARDs) and Immunosuppressant Drugs

Disease modifying anti-rheumatic drugs (DMARDs) and immunosuppressant drugs are used to treat inflammation and to control the immune process. It is hoped that they will control the arthritis, slow joint damage, and alter the natural course of the disease. Some of these include methotrexate, gold, sulfasalazine, penicillamine, hydroxychloroquine and chloroquine, leflunomide, cyclosporine A, cyclophosphamide, and azathioprine.

Methotrexate (Rheumatrex)

Methotrexate is the DMARD most commonly used to treat rheumatoid arthritis in North America. It may be used alone or in combination with other agents. It was originally developed to treat cancer, but it has been used to treat rheumatoid arthritis, psoriasis and psoriatic arthritis, reactive arthritis, polymyositis, dermatomyositis, Wegener's granulomatosis, systemic lupus erythematosus, and scleroderma. Methotrexate controls joint inflammation, allows the reduction of corticosteroids and NSAIDs, and prevents joint damage as seen on X-ray.

Potential adverse effects There is a lot of experience with methotrexate, and generally speaking, methotrexate is well tolerated, few people will develop serious adverse effects because of it, and it works well. This is why it is the most widely used DMARD in Canada. It does, however, have the following adverse effects:

- A rash can occur with any medication; with methotrexate, a serious rash is uncommon.
- Mouth sores occur with methotrexate and can sometimes be treated by taking up to 5 mg of folic acid by mouth each day.
- Methotrexate can cause nausea, stomach upset, and diarrhea. Folic acid can sometimes help with this, as can changing from an oral to an injectable form of the medication. Some people find that it helps to take an antinauseant (such as Gravol) before the dose of methotrexate.
- A low white blood cell count (WBC), platelet count, or red blood cell count (RBC) can accompany methotrexate usage and is usually the result of suppression of the bone marrow. The addition of trimethoprim-containing antibiotics like Septra or Bactrim may increase the risk for this to happen.
- Methotrexate can be toxic to the liver, and you must avoid drinking alcohol while taking the drug. Other factors that might put you at risk for liver disease while on methotrexate include obesity, diabetes, and underlying liver disease. Underlying liver diseases like hepatitis should be screened for before starting methotrexate. The liver enzymes must be monitored. A liver biopsy is not routinely required but may be requested if there is a concern about liver function or if the total dose of methotrexate over time is high.
- Rarely, methotrexate will affect the lungs, causing cough, shortness of breath, and fever. A chest X-ray will show pneumonitis. It is important to be aware of this adverse effect so that if you have these symptoms, you will contact your physician. Do not assume that it is a cold or flu.

A daily dose of folic acid (1–5 mg/day) may prevent some of the adverse effects of methotrexate without interfering with the therapeutic action of the drug.

Dosage and monitoring Methotrexate is prescribed at a dosage of 7.5–25 mg one time per week for rheumatoid arthritis. The dosage may be higher for myositis, vasculitis, and psoriasis. The dose may need to be reduced if the kidneys are not functioning normally. Methotrexate is quick-acting for a DMARD, and will generally be beneficial within four to six weeks of starting it. The drug can be given by mouth or by injection under the skin, into muscle or through a vein. Methotrexate is sometimes not tolerated or is only partially effective, in which case injecting it may be more helpful than taking it orally as many people do not absorb this drug well by mouth. Patients can be taught to give themselves the injections. Methotrexate may be combined with other drugs to treat arthritis.

The American College of Rheumatology recommends that patients should have their blood monitored for adverse effects every four to six weeks. This includes a complete blood count (CBC) and measurement of the liver enzymes.

Gold

Gold was used for the treatment of rheumatoid arthritis for much of the twentieth century, and is now used to treat rheumatoid arthritis and psoriatic arthritis. Gold can be as effective as methotrexate, sulfasalazine, and penicillamine in the management of rheumatoid arthritis, and is one of the only agents that can put the disease into remission. Exactly how gold controls rheumatoid arthritis is unknown, but it does have several effects on the immune system that dampen the inflammatory process. The benefits should be reduced joint pain and swelling, reduced morning stiffness, and an improved energy level.

It may take up to six months to know if gold is working. A nurse or doctor administers an injection into the muscle weekly for the first six months, and then the frequency is reduced, in some patients to only every four to six weeks. A blood test and urine sample must be taken before every injection.

Potential adverse effects Some people find the risks involved with gold therapy to be unacceptable; potential adverse effects include:

- decreased white blood cell count (WBC), red blood cell count (RBC), and/or platelet count
- protein in the urine (if this is severe, it can cause diffuse swelling in the body; this side effect will disappear after the gold is stopped, but it may take up to a year to clear completely)
- an itchy rash, which may be severe enough to require hospitalization
- sores in the mouth
- irritation of the liver and an increase in the liver enzymes
- lung inflammation (which is very rare)

Dosage and monitoring Gold comes in two equally effective injectable forms: gold sodium thiomalate (Myochrysine) and gold thioglucose (Solganal). The Myochrysine has a water base and the Solganal is oil based. One side effect of gold therapy is that you may become flushed, dizzy, sweaty, and nauseated just after the injection, but this is less frequent with Solganal than with Myochrysine. Gold also comes in an oral form called auranofin (Ridaura), but it does not work as well.

The dosage is usually 50 mg per week for six months, and then an attempt is made to reduce the frequency. Some patients' disease is well controlled on dosages as low as 10–25 mg every six weeks. A few patients will have a complete clinical remission on this drug.

Note, however, that if you are doing well on the medication, it should not be stopped even if your dosage is very low. Often, stopping the drug allows the disease to become active again, and the gold does not always work as well when it is reintroduced.

A complete blood count and urinalysis should be done before each injection. You and your physician should have a chart where the results of the blood tests and the cumulative dosage of gold are recorded. There is no limit to the amount of gold you can receive.

Sulfasalazine (Salazopyrin)

This medication is used to treat rheumatoid arthritis, psoriatic arthritis, reactive arthritis, and the peripheral joint disease of ankylosing spondylitis. It has been demonstrated to be effective and, when given in combination with methotrexate and hydroxychloroquine, it works better than methotrexate does alone.

A female Swedish physician developed sulfasalazine in the 1940s, by combining aspirin (the only available anti-inflammatory) with sulfa (the only available antibiotic). The bond between the drugs breaks in the large bowel; most of the aspirin leaves the body in the bowel movement, and the sulfa is absorbed. This drug fell out of favour when corticosteroids were discovered, but came back into use when the toxicity of corticosteroids was recognized. Sulfasalazine is also effective in treating inflammatory bowel disease (such as Crohn's disease and ulcerative colitis).

Sulfasalazine usually begins to work after about six weeks of therapy. It can be expected to decrease pain, swelling, morning stiffness, and fatigue.

Potential adverse effects Anyone with an allergy to sulfa should not use this medication. The common side effects include:

- allergy, effects of which may be a rash, wheezing, or anaphylaxis (an allergic reaction that results in shortness of breath, wheezing, rash, and drop in blood pressure)
- irritation to the liver, which is reversible and should be monitored with regular blood tests
- a low white blood cell count, platelet count, or red blood cell count; this should be monitored by blood work
- decreased appetite, nausea, and abdominal bloating

Dosage and monitoring The medication is given at a dose of 1500–3000 mg per day. Some physicians will start at a low dosage (500 mg per day for a week) and gradually increase the medication to 2000–3000 mg per day. This may help you to tolerate the drug better.

The blood work is usually monitored every six to eight weeks. The complete blood count and the liver enzymes are tested.

Penicillamine

This is an older medication that has been used to treat rheumatoid arthritis. It may help soften the skin and prevent progression of the disease in scleroderma, but more studies are required.

This medication is given by mouth. It is often tried when other medications have failed to treat rheumatoid arthritis, because it takes up to six months to work and it has a number of adverse side effects. How it works is not completely understood.

Potential adverse effects Adverse effects that may be seen with penicillamine include the following:

- a rash of any sort, often itchy
- protein in the urine, which can lead to swelling of the body (fluid retention); this will gradually disappear when the drug is stopped

- loss of taste
- drug-induced lupus
- low white blood cell count, red blood cell count, and platelets
- myasthenia gravis (a neurological condition with muscle weakness)
- mouth sores
- nausea and abdominal pain

Dosage and monitoring Penicillamine is usually given by mouth at a dosage of 125–1000 mg daily. It is started slowly and gradually increased.

A complete blood count and urinalysis should be done every two to four weeks when starting the medication or when changing the dosage.

Hydroxychloroquine (Plaquenil) and chloroquine (Aralen)

These two medications are closely related, having similar effects and side effects and having been originally used to treat malaria. The hydroxychloroquine has less toxicity to the eyes. Chloroquine is an older drug and sometimes is better tolerated or is effective when hydroxychloroquine fails.

These medications are used to treat milder forms of rheumatoid arthritis and systemic lupus erythematosus. In rheumatoid arthritis, they can be used in combination with methotrexate and sulfasalazine and should reduce the joint swelling, pain, and stiffness. They help with the rash, joint pain and swelling, and fatigue associated with lupus. They are sometimes helpful in Sjogren's syndrome. They can be used to treat psoriatic arthritis, but they may cause the psoriasis to worsen.

It is usually three to six months before these medications are fully effective.

Potential adverse effects These medications are very well tolerated and the risk of an adverse effect is low. The following are potential problems with the medication.

- Deposits of chloroquine on the cornea (outer layer of the eye) may develop and cause blurred vision, halos around lights, and light sensitivity. This is not dangerous, will disappear after lowering the dosage of the medication, and is not a reason to stop the medication.
- Permanent damage to the retina at the back of the eye may occur in extremely rare instances. This can lead to loss of colour vision and central vision. Regular eye examinations can pick up changes in the retina before visual loss occurs.
- Photosensitivity can occur. This means that you will burn more easily and/or develop a rash in the sun, and should always use sunblock and protective clothing. In addition, the skin and hair can sometimes discolour.
- If muscle weakness occurs, the medication should be stopped and the weakness will disappear.
- Some people will experience loss of appetite, nausea, abdominal pain, or diarrhea.

Dosage and monitoring The usual dosage for hydroxychloroquine is 6.5 mg/kg/day, not to exceed 400 mg daily. The dosage for chloroquine is 4 mg/kg/day, not to exceed 250 mg/day.

While you are on these medications, your eyes should be examined and your peripheral fields tested every six to twelve months by an ophthalmologist. The ophthalmologist should give you a copy of an Amsler Grid, which you can use very easily at home to detect visual field disturbances between visits.

Leflunomide

Leflunomide is a relatively new medication for the treatment of rheumatoid arthritis. Clinical studies have shown it to be as effective as methotrexate, and in practice it is effective for some patients when methotrexate fails, is contraindicated, or is not tolerated. It can be combined with methotrexate; the combination may work better than either medication alone, however, there is more potential toxicity when the two are combined.

The medication is given orally and eight to twelve weeks are needed to know if it is effective. It works by inhibiting some of the actions of the immune system cells.

Usually this medication would not be given to patients who are of childbearing years; however, if a patient is taking the medication and wishes to have a child, then cholestyramine can be given by mouth to clear the leflunomide from the body faster, as it may otherwise take two years to clear. This applies both to women and to men who wish to become parents.

Potential adverse effects Potential adverse effects of leflunomide include:

- stomach upset, nausea, abdominal cramps, and diarrhea, which can sometimes be controlled by reducing the dosage of medication
- irritation of the liver, which is identified by an elevation of liver enzymes above normal levels in the blood work (there have been recent reports of serious liver toxicity on this medication, and therefore careful monitoring of the blood work and identification of other risk factors for liver disease are required)
- a low white blood cell count, red blood cell count, or platelet count, although this is rare
- a rash, usually between the second and fifth months of treatment
- mild hair loss

- an increased risk of infection
- the possibility of birth defects if either the mother or the father is on this medication at the time of conception

Dosage and monitoring The usual dosage is 100 mg daily for three days and then 20 mg daily thereafter.

Monitoring includes a complete blood count, and testing for liver enzymes and creatinine every two to four weeks initially and then every eight weeks.

Cyclosporine A (Neoral)

This medication is used primarily to prevent rejection in organ transplant patients. It has been found to be effective in the treatment of rheumatoid arthritis when combined with methotrexate, and is also used to treat psoriasis and psoriatic arthritis. This drug may be used in patients with serious eye and lung problems, secondary to rheumatoid arthritis, scleroderma, or other connective tissue diseases.

It takes about eight to twelve weeks to know if this medication is effective. It has a number of adverse effects, requires close and frequent monitoring, and is expensive. These factors have limited its use in rheumatoid arthritis to those with more severe disease for whom a number of other medications have failed.

Potential adverse effects Grapefruit juice should be avoided as it can increase the cyclosporine levels in the blood, unless your doctor instructs you to drink it regularly in order to lower the dose of cyclosporine needed. There are interactions with other drugs, so check this with your physician and/or pharmacist. Other potential adverse effects include:

- high blood pressure
- decreased function of the kidney (this occurs in almost everyone on the medication, and needs to be monitored with regular blood work)

- thickening of the gums
- increased hair growth
- decreased numbers of blood cells (this is rare)
- liver toxicity (this is rare)
- increased risk of cancer of the lymph glands (lymphoma)
- increased risk of infections
- increase in uric acid levels and gout
- tremor, headache

Dosage and monitoring The usual dosage is 3–5 mg/kg/day in one or two divided doses. The dosage is adjusted depending on the response to therapy and the development of adverse effects.

The blood levels of the drug can be monitored as they are in transplant patients, although this is not usually necessary when using it in arthritis therapy. It is, however, necessary to monitor the blood pressure and do blood tests for the kidney function and blood cell counts.

Cyclophosphamide (Procytox)

This immunosuppressant drug is frequently used in chemotherapy to treat cancers, and is also used in serious and life-threatening diseases of the immune system.

Cyclophosphamide is given in a daily oral dose to treat serious lung disease associated with rheumatoid arthritis, scleroderma, and polymyositis, and in vasculitis (polyarteritis nodosa and Wegener's granulomatosis). In lupus associated with serious disease of the kidney or brain, it is given as a monthly infusion for three to six months and then less frequently depending on the response to therapy.

Potential adverse effects Cyclophosphamide is used for a limited amount of time because of its toxicity. The following are potential adverse effects.

- It can cause hemorrhagic cystitis, which is an inflammation of the bladder lining that causes bleeding and discomfort. Sometimes it can cause fibrosis or scarring of the bladder so that the capacity of the bladder is reduced, causing the need to urinate frequently. In order to prevent these complications, it is important to take the medication in the morning and to drink large amounts of water during the day to dilute the drug when it gets to the bladder. If cystitis develops, then the drug may need to be switched from an oral to an intravenous form. Mesna is a drug that can be given intravenously with intravenous cyclophosphamide to prevent cystitis.
- There is an increased risk of cancer of the bladder, which may occur up to 15 years after receiving the drug. The risk is dependent on the degree of exposure of the bladder to the drug.
- There is a small but increased risk of cancer of the lymph glands (lymphoma) and leukemia.
- Cyclophosphamide can cause nausea, vomiting, and stomach upset. This is more of a problem when it is given intravenously, but can be treated with a drug for nausea (for example, Zofran) and dexamethasone (a corticosteroid).
- Cyclophosphamide can cause a low white blood cell count, but if the white blood cell count drops too low, the chance of infections occurring is increased. The medication can also lower the platelet count (so that bleeding is prolonged) and the red blood cell count (resulting in anemia).
- Fatigue can be due to the medication itself or to the anemia that might develop because of this medication.
- Hair loss is common. It can range from thinning of the hair to complete baldness. A short haircut often helps hide the thinning, but a wig may be desired. After the drug is stopped, the hair will grow back, often thicker than it was previously.

- Infections are more likely to occur, especially when cyclophosphamide is combined with corticosteroids. Often, Septra, three times a week, is added to these medications to prevent the development of *pneumocytis carnii pneumonia*.
- Menstrual periods may stop transiently or permanently. Both men and women can become infertile. If you still plan on having children, sperm or eggs can be put in storage before the cyclophosphamide is started. The ovaries may become fibrotic to the point that there is a deficiency of estrogen. Hormone replacement may be recommended to prevent menopausal symptoms and premature osteoporosis.

Dosage and monitoring The oral medication is given at a dosage of 2 mg/kg once per day. The intravenous dose is 500–750 mg/m2 given every four weeks for three to six months and then less frequently. The dosage may need to be reduced if the kidneys are not functioning normally.

A complete blood count and a urinalysis need to be done every week at the start of therapy, then monthly. If the drug is given intravenously, testing should be done weekly for two weeks, and then monthly. The creatinine (a test for kidney function) and liver enzyme tests need to be monitored regularly as well.

Azathioprine (Imuran)

This immunosuppressant drug is used to treat patients with organ transplants, inflammatory bowel disease, rheumatoid arthritis, systemic lupus erythematosus, other connective tissue diseases, and vasculitis.

Azathioprine is sometimes referred to as a corticosteroid sparing agent because, if it is effective, it may allow for a reduction in the dose of corticosteroids. Because of the adverse effects of corticosteroids, rheumatologists prefer to use them at the lowest possible dose for the shortest time. However, the disease will recur if the corticosteroids are simply stopped. Corticosteroids work right away, while azathioprine takes three to six months to be effective. Therefore the corticosteroid is used to get the situation under control quickly, and the azathioprine is introduced to allow the patient to be weaned from the corticosteroid and to keep the disease under control for the long term. Methotrexate is often used in a similar way.

Potential adverse effects The potential adverse effects of azathioprine are:

- fever, diffuse joint pain, irritation of the liver, and rash that develop when the drug is started and are resolved when the drug is stopped
- a low count of white blood cells, red blood cells, and platelets
- mouth sores
- rash
- stomach upset, nausea, and vomiting
- an increased risk for infection
- a potential risk for cancer of the lymph glands (lymphoma), although this may not be a risk when azathioprine is used to treat rheumatic diseases
- inflammation of the pancreas (pancreatitis)
- the toxicity of azathioprine (especially a drop in the blood cell counts) is greater if it is used in combination with allopurinol; therefore the azathioprine is given in a reduced dose

Dosage and monitoring The usual dosage is 2 mg/kg/day. The drug takes approximately three months to begin to be effective, and six months to be fully effective.

When starting the drug, blood work should be done to check the complete blood count and liver and kidney function. A complete blood count should be done every one to two weeks until the dosage is stabilized, and then every one to two months thereafter.

Tetracycline, doxycycline, and minocycline

Tetracycline, doxycycline, and minocycline are antibiotics of the tetracycline family. For some, minocycline is effective for the treatment of mild to moderate rheumatoid arthritis, particularly if started early in the course of the arthritis, and ongoing studies are looking at its potential benefit in osteoarthritis. It is of questionable benefit in psoriatic arthritis and reactive arthritis.

Potential adverse effects These medications are generally well tolerated, but among their few side effects are:

- loss of appetite, nausea, vomiting, abdominal pain, diarrhea, and inflammation and ulcers of the esophagus
- rash, and bluish-black discolourations of the skin (mainly with minocycline)
- photosensitivity
- allergic reactions including hives, fever, joint pains, and a lupus-like syndrome
- hepatitis, jaundice (in very rare instances)
- oral yeast infections (thrush), and in women, vaginal yeast infections

Dosage and monitoring The usual oral dosages are: minocycline 100 mg twice daily, doxycycline 100 mg once daily, and tetracycline 250 mg four time daily. They should be taken on an empty stomach. No specific monitoring is necessary.

The Biological Response Modifiers

The biological response modifiers are a new group of medications that are produced in cell cultures. They are very effective in controlling rheumatoid arthritis, even in patients for whom all other medications have failed. The cost to the consumer is very high.

Previous medications have suppressed the immune system but have not specifically targeted the cytokines (hormones or chemicals secreted by cells in the immune system that regulate immune responses by stimulating or inhibiting other cells to behave in a specified manner) that are responsible for the disease. Three currently available biological response modifiers—adalumimab (Humira), etanercept (Enbrel), and infliximab (Remicade)—take aim at a specific cytokine: tumour necrosis factor (TNF). This cytokine has been found to be very important in rheumatoid arthritis, ankylosing spondylitis, and psoriasis. Another biologic agent, anakinra (Kineret), targets the cytokine interleukin-1 (IL-1). Suppressing these cytokines improves the pain and swelling of rheumatoid arthritis and has been shown to prevent joint damage.

TNF, in rheumatoid arthritis, is responsible for recruiting more immune cells to the site of inflammation, and increasing the production of other cytokines responsible for the disease and more enzymes and cells that damage the cartilage and bone. In order for TNF to act on a cell, it must bind to the cell, which it does through a receptor on the cell's surface. To illustrate this, imagine that each TNF molecule is a key, and that each cell has a lock (the receptor) that lets in anything that has the right key. Sometimes the TNF levels can get out of control, so the body naturally produces extra receptors (locks) that float freely, catching TNF molecules (keys) so that they cannot be used in the receptors (locks) of the cells. This reduces the action of TNF on the cells.

Etanercept (Enbrel)

Etanercept is a soluble receptor for TNF that mops up the free TNF so that it can't work on the cells. This medication can be used in patients with moderate to severe rheumatoid arthritis, psoriatic arthritis, ankylosing spondylitis, and juvenile rheumatoid arthritis. It has been shown to work in patients for whom methotrexate has failed and it has benefited 60–70 percent of patients. It is more effective in combination with methotrexate.

Potential adverse effects Potential adverse effects of etanercept include the following:

- A hive or redness with or without pain or itchiness may develop at the site of injection, and it may get worse with each injection. Hives may also break out where the previous injections were given. This reaction will subside over the course of four to six weeks.
- There is an increased risk of infection. Etanercept can cause the reactivation of tuberculosis and histoplasmosis.
- A rash may develop.
- There may be an increased risk of lymphoma; this is not yet known.
- Patients with multiple sclerosis should not use etanercept, as it may worsen multiple sclerosis.
- A reduction in the white blood cell count has been reported, usually when the medication is given with methotrexate or leflunomide.
- Autoantibodies like those in lupus may develop (antinuclear and anti-DNA antibodies).

Dosage and monitoring The usual dosage is 25 mg injected under the skin twice a week. The patient or a family member or friend can give the injections.

Before starting therapy, you will require a chest X-ray and a skin test for tuberculosis. If you have previously had a positive skin test for tuberculosis, you don't need the skin test again. If there is evidence of old, untreated tuberculosis, then you will need to be treated with antibiotics when starting the etanercept. A complete blood count is done initially, then every few weeks, and then every few months.

Infliximab (Remicade)

Infliximab is used to treat rheumatoid arthritis, Crohn's disease, juvenile onset rheumatoid arthritis, psoriatic arthritis, and ankylosing spondylitis. Like etanercept, this drug also decreases the effect of TNFα on the cells. However, infliximab is actually an antibody to TNFα that is grown in the laboratory in cell cultures combining human and mouse antibodies. The infliximab binds to the free TNFα so that it cannot bind to cells. It can also bind to the TNFα already attached to cells. When the antibody has bound to the TNFα, the TNFα cannot work on the immune cells and the inflammation is improved. Infliximab works better when combined with methotrexate. Approximately 40–60 percent of patients who take methotrexate and infliximab together will receive additional benefit over those who are taking only methotrexate.

Potential adverse effects The following are potential adverse effects of infliximab:

- An allergic reaction to the infusion may occur, including hives, shortness of breath and anaphylaxis (which is rare). Some doctors will give an antihistamine (e.g., Benadryl) before the infusion to prevent such a reaction.

- The infusion can cause a headache, which is usually treated with acetaminophen.
- There is an increased risk of infections, including tuberculosis and histoplasmosis.
- This drug should not be given to patients with multiple sclerosis as it may worsen this condition.
- There may be an increased risk of lymphoma.
- The drug can cause a low white blood cell count.
- The drug can cause a worsening of congestive heart failure.
- The drug may cause a lupus-like syndrome, with antinuclear and anti-DNA antibodies.

Dosage and monitoring Infliximab is given as an infusion (a slow injection into a vein) over what is called a "loading phase"—the drug is given initially, then again at two weeks, and again at six weeks at a dose of 3 mg/kg. After this loading phase, it is given every eight weeks. The dosage may need to be increased to 5 mg/kg every six weeks. The cost is $1000 per 100 mg.

Before starting the medication, a chest X-ray and skin test for tuberculosis is done. If there is evidence of old tuberculosis that was not treated in the past, then an antibiotic will need to be taken to prevent a reactivation of the tuberculosis. Complete blood counts should be performed regularly.

Adalumimab (Humira)

This is a fully human antibody to TNF. It works similar to infliximab. It is effective for the treatment of rheumatoid arthritis, ankylosing spondylitis, and psoriatic arthritis. As this drug is a fully human antibody, there should be fewer allergic reactions.

Potential adverse effects These are similar to infliximab.

Dosage and monitoring Adalumimab is given 40 mgs subcutaneously once every two weeks and in resistant cases once every week. It is given in combination with methotrexate for best results. All patients must be screened for tuberculosis.

Anakinra (Kineret)

This drug blocks the action of a different cytokine, IL-1. It is used for the treatment of rheumatoid arthritis but in clinical trials is not as effective as the TNF inhibitors.

Potential adverse effects Patients may experience injection site reactions (hives). There is no increased risk of tuberculosis.

Dosage and monitoring It is given subcutaneously daily. No routine monitoring is necessary.

Corticosteroids

These medications are very effective in controlling inflammation, but have a number of serious adverse effects that are usually dose-related (meaning that, the higher the dose and the longer you take the drug, the greater the chance of adverse effects). Whenever a medication is prescribed, the potential benefits are weighed against the risks. Corticosteroids can be life-saving, and are very effective at settling many of the diseases involving inflammation.

There are various forms of corticosteroids and these may be given by mouth (orally), into a vein (intravenously), into a muscle (intramuscularly), into a joint (intra-articularly), as a lotion, cream, or ointment, or into the lungs by inhalation from a puffer (for asthma). The table on page 185 lists some of these.

Indications

In severe cases of connective tissue diseases with major organ involvement, corticosteroids may be necessary at high doses, possibly as a single dose of medicine given intravenously (this is known as a bolus). Pulse therapy (1 gm of methylprednisilone daily for three days) is sometimes used in very aggressive disease that needs rapid control. In rheumatoid arthritis, moderate to low doses of corticosteroids are sometimes used to bridge treatment, that is, to keep the patient functional and in less pain while he is waiting for another drug to kick in. Some patients require low-dose corticosteroids on a regular basis for their arthritis. In diseases like polymyalgia rheumatica and temporal arteritis, regular corticosteroids may be required for up to several years.

Intra-articular corticosteroids are very useful for treating an acutely swollen joint or a persistently inflamed joint. An infection in the joint needs to be ruled out prior to injecting a corticosteroid into it, however. A joint should not be injected with corticosteroids more than four times a year, although exceptions for more frequent injection can be made. If the joint is inflamed, then there is potential

Corticosteroids

Preparation	Anti-inflammatory potency	Common name
Hydrocortisone	1.0	Cortef
Cortisone	0.8	Cortone
Prednisone	4.0	Prednisone
Methylprednisolone	5.0	Medrol
Triamcinolone	5.0	Aristocort
Betamethasone	25.0	Celestone
Dexamethasone	25.0	Decadron

for damage. Injecting the joint will help control the inflammation and will therefore benefit the joint, not damage it further.

Our adrenal glands are directed by the pituitary gland to produce our own cortisone. The pituitary gland only orders this production if it sees the need for it, though; if you have been on a regular dose of corticosteroids for even a month, then the pituitary gland will have gone on vacation and will not tell the adrenal glands to produce cortisone. Corticosteroids should therefore not be stopped abruptly, but must rather be gradually reduced in order to give the pituitary gland time to adjust and the adrenal glands the opportunity to produce their own cortisone again.

During times of stress on the body (such as surgery or illness), an extra amount of cortisone may be required. The adrenal glands would normally produce extra corticosteroids at these times, but if they are not responding normally because you have been on a corticosteroid, you will require a boost in your usual corticosteroid dose.

Contraindications

Some relative contraindications to the use of corticosteroids include diabetes mellitus ("sugar diabetes"), infection, old, untreated tuberculosis, osteoporosis, high blood pressure, and active stomach ulcers. If the corticosteroids are really needed in these situations, they can be used with precautions.

Adverse effects

Some adverse effects that might be seen in various body parts are as follows.

Hair

- Corticosteroids may cause thinning of the scalp hair, and the growth of fine facial hair called lanugo. This will disappear when you get off the medication.

Eyes

- Prolonged use of corticosteroids can cause cataracts.
- These drugs might increase the pressure inside the eyes, causing or worsening glaucoma.

Body

- The corticosteroids can cause increased appetite, weight gain, and a redistribution of body fat to the torso and face. When the face becomes full it is called a moon face. Fat pads can develop at the base of the neck (called a buffalo hump) and above the collarbones. These will disappear once you are off the medication.
- Bluish lines or stretch marks (called striae) sometimes develop on the abdomen, legs, and arms.

Suppression of growth

- Corticosteroids can stunt the growth of children.

Menstrual periods

- Menstrual irregularities can develop due to corticosteroid usage.

Musculoskeletal system

- Corticosteroids cause osteoporosis and susceptibility to fractures. The dosage and length of time on the drug will determine the degree of osteoporosis, but we do know that bone loss from corticosteroids occurs early in the course of taking the medication. It is recommended that if you are taking more than 7.5 mg of prednisone per day or its equivalent for more than three months, you should take a bisphosphonate drug to prevent bone loss. (Bisphosphonates are discussed later in this chapter; see page 197.) All patients should also be taking 1500 mg of calcium and 400–800 IU of Vitamin D daily.

- Another complication of corticosteroid use is osteonecrosis, where the blood supply to a section of bone gets cut off and the bone dies. This happens most commonly to the ball of the hip joint, but can also occur in other joints. Osteonecrosis in a joint may lead to the necessity of joint replacement.
- The prolonged use of corticosteroids can cause muscle weakness, usually in the hip girdle region, making it difficult to rise from a chair. This improves after the medication is stopped or the dosage is lowered.

Skin

- Prolonged use of corticosteroids can cause poor healing and thinning of the skin.
- The medication can cause acne and easy bruising.

Infection

- Corticosteroids suppress the immune system. As a result, you will become more susceptible to acquiring new infections or worsening underlying infections. Rheumatologists sometimes have to use these drugs in spite of an infection, and it is then important to use appropriate antibiotics as well.
- If you have had previously untreated tuberculosis (as diagnosed by a chest X-ray or a positive skin test), then you may need to take a course of antibiotics to treat tuberculosis when you start the corticosteroids.

Diabetes mellitus

- In patients with diabetes, corticosteroids will increase the blood sugar levels. Diabetes is sometimes unmasked by the addition of corticosteroids.

Cardiovascular system

- Corticosteroids have been associated with accelerated atherosclerosis (hardening of the arteries), elevated levels of cholesterol, aggravation of high blood pressure, fluid retention, and potassium deficiency.

Psychologic

- Corticosteroids can cause depression, euphoria, anxiety, agitation, and psychotic behaviour. These changes are dose dependent, and people might be affected differently by the same dose. I once gave prednisone to a child in hospital, and returned to find the child jumping from bed to bed. Some of my patients report similar feelings; some of them are up all night rearranging closets that have been ignored for a quarter-century. Many people experience difficulties with sleep and increased sweating. These symptoms will improve when the dosage is decreased and will disappear once you are off the medication.

Stomach

- Some people develop symptoms of heartburn, stomach upset, abdominal distension, and nausea. This can usually be controlled with medication.
- Rarely people will develop inflammation of the pancreas (called pancreatitis).

What you really need to know

1. Do not stop the corticosteroids on your own: you could make yourself very sick. Consult with your physician on how the drug should be decreased gradually.
2. If you are ill, have had an accident, or require surgery, you may need an extra amount of corticosteroids. You must tell

the physician that you are taking prednisone or another corticosteroid. A medic-alert bracelet is a good idea if you are taking these medications for a prolonged period.

3. If you use corticosteroids, discuss with your physician the need for a bisphosphonate, calcium, and Vitamin D to prevent osteoporosis.

Radioactive Synovectomy

An alternative to a surgical synovectomy (see Chapter 10), is a radioactive synovectomy. Radioactive material, usually yttrium-90 or dysprosium-165, is injected into the knee (because of the very short half life of the products, very little material escapes from the joint). This usually decreases the synovial lining and leads to decreased swelling, improved pain, and movement. These result last one to two years. A surgical synovectomy can be performed if this fails.

Treatments for Gout

Gout is a disease in which there is an excess of uric acid in the body and blood. As a result, crystals of urate will form in the lining of the joints. If enough crystals are suddenly released into the joint space, an acute attack of gout will occur, causing a very painful, red, hot, swollen joint. The joints of the great toe are the most frequently affected, followed by the ankle, arch of the foot, and knee. An acute attack of gout is usually managed with NSAIDs. Colchicine can be used to treat acute gout or to prevent recurrent attacks. Allopurinol (Zyloprim), sulfinpyrazone (Anturan), and probenecid (Benuryl or Benemid) are used to lower the uric acid levels in the blood and body, prevent recurrent acute attacks of gout, and treat chronic gout.

Colchicine

Colchicine has been used for over two centuries to treat gout. It is given as an oral medication, at a dosage of 1.0–1.2 mg for the first dose and then 0.5–0.6 mg every two hours, to control the pain and swelling of an acute attack to a maximum of six doses or until toxicity (nausea, diarrhea, and vomiting).

Colchicine is also used to prevent recurrent attacks of gout while your physician is trying to lower the uric acid levels with other medications (allopurinol or probenecid). It is also used to prevent attacks in people who do not tolerate the drugs that lower uric acid levels. The dosage used to prevent attacks is 0.5–0.6 mg taken orally once or twice daily. In elderly patients or patients with kidney failure, the dose may be 0.3 mg per day or 0.6 mg every other day. This dose rarely causes diarrhea or nausea.

Potential adverse effects There is no antidote for colchicine, so care must be taken to avoid an overdose. It should always be kept away from children. The adverse effects of colchicine are dose related, and include:

- nausea, vomiting, diarrhea, and abdominal pain
- muscle weakness and nerve damage (these are usually seen with chronic dosing in patients with kidney disease)
- suppression of the bone marrow, causing anemia, and low white blood cell and platelet counts
- hair loss

Drugs to Lower Uric Acid Levels

Two types of drugs are commonly used to lower the level of uric acid in the blood and stop recurrent attacks of gout; these are the uricosuric agents and the xanthine oxidase inhibitor. They should not be started, stopped, or dosage-adjusted during an acute attack, as any of these actions will prolong the attack and make it worse. They are usually started one month after an attack has settled.

Uricosuric agents: sulfinpyrazone (Anturan) and probenecid (Benuryl or Benemid)

The uricosuric agents—sulfinpyrazone and probenecid—lower the blood levels of uric acid by causing the kidneys to excrete more uric acid from the blood. The uricosuric agents cannot be used in patients with kidney stones or kidney failure.

Potential adverse effects Potential adverse effects of the uricosuric agents are:

- acute gout
- kidney stones
- rashes
- fever
- headaches
- stomach upset
- allergic reactions
- bone marrow toxicity (rare)
- liver failure (rare)

Dosage Sulfinpyrazone is started at a dose of 50 mg twice per day, and can be increased to 300 mg/day. Probenecid is started at 500 mg twice per day, and can be increased to 3 g/day.

Xanthine oxidase inhibitor: allopurinol

Allopurinol (Zyloprim) causes the body to make less uric acid. This normalizes the blood levels of uric acid and prevents further attacks of gout. This drug must be taken indefinitely.

Potential adverse effects Approximately 20 percent of patients will have an adverse reaction to this medication. Only 5 percent will have to stop the medication, however.

- The common side effects are nausea, diarrhea, rash, elevated liver enzymes, headache, and acute gout.
- Many different types of rashes occur with this medication, including exfoliative dermatitis, a severe all-over rash that frequently requires hospitalization.
- There may be bone marrow suppression.
- There may be fever.
- A hypersensitivity reaction may occur, which includes severe rash, fever, liver changes, elevated white blood cell count, and worsening of kidney function. Those with kidney failure are at increased risk for this complication.

Dosage and monitoring Allopurinol is usually started at a dose of 100–300 mg/day, and can be increased to as much as 600 mg/day.

While on this medication, a complete blood count and liver and kidney tests should be done at least yearly.

Treatments for Osteoarthritis

There are no commercially available medications for osteoarthritis that prevent cartilage loss or restore lost cartilage. Treatment is available to help with the symptoms of osteoarthritis, including acetaminophen for pain control and NSAIDs for control of pain and secondary inflammation. Additional treatment might include viscosupplementation, as discussed below.

Viscosupplementation

Our joints are filled with a naturally occurring joint fluid that lubricates and protects them. The fluid is usually thick, having the consistency of egg white. Hyaluronic acid (hyaluronan) makes up part of the joint fluid, and causes the fluid to have its normal sticky thickness. In osteoarthritis and joint inflammation, the fluid has thinned and does not work as well as it should.

Viscosupplementation—injecting synthetic hyaluronans into the joint—once a week for three weeks can benefit the symptoms of an osteoarthritic joint for up to six months. The treatment is usually used for osteoarthritis of the knee, and offers some help with walking and pain control. Viscosupplementation is an alternative for patients with mild to moderate osteoarthritis of the knee, but may be tried in patients with advanced osteoarthritis when surgery is contraindicated. Some clinical trials have shown long-lasting benefit from these injections, while others have not; this may be related to the patients selected for the trials, or to which specific hyaluronan preparation was injected.

The products available for viscosupplementation in Canada are Hylan GF-20 (Synvisc), Orthovisc, and Supplasyn.

Potential adverse effects Occasionally a joint may react to an injection by becoming more painful, swollen, and tender for up to a week. As with any intra-articular injection, there is a small risk of infection.

Treatments for Osteoporosis

The treatment of osteoporosis includes modifying your risk factors: stop smoking, decrease alcohol consumption, increase exercise, and consume 1000–1500 mg of calcium and 400–800 IU of Vitamin D daily.

Normally, our bodies build up and break down bone on an ongoing basis. Osteoporosis occurs when we break down more bone than we form. We measure osteoporosis by assessing bone density, which is an indirect indicator of how strong the bone is.

It is important that osteoporosis be treated to prevent fractures of the spinal vertebrae, hips, and other bones. Present medications work by decreasing bone breakdown or absorption.

Estrogen Replacement

Once a woman has gone through menopause (or more specifically, upon the withdrawal of estrogen from her system), her bones will lose strength rapidly for a period of approximately eight years. The purpose of hormone replacement therapy is to delay the bone loss seen at the time of menopause. Estrogen therapy may not be for everyone, however, and you should discuss with your family physician or gynecologist if it is appropriate for you.

The benefits of hormone replacement therapy are that it lowers the risk of fracture of the vertebrae, and it stops hot flashes and other menopausal symptoms. Hormone replacement may also decrease the risk for ovarian cancer.

The potential risks of hormone replacement therapy include:

- a small but increased risk of breast cancer
- an increased risk of cancer of the endometrium (lining of the uterus); if you have not had a hysterectomy, then you need to take progesterone with the estrogen
- an increased risk of blood clotting; if there has been a previous recent stroke, heart attack, or a blood clot to the lung or leg, then this therapy is generally not recommended
- bloating, increased incidence of gall bladder disease, weight changes, vaginal bleeding, breast tenderness, headaches, and mood changes

If you choose to take hormone replacement therapy, then your doctor needs to give you a yearly mammogram and breast exam, pelvic exam, and Pap smear.

Selective Estrogen Receptor Modulators (SERMs)

Selective estrogen receptor modulators (SERMs) are now available to treat and prevent osteoporosis in postmenopausal women. Selective estrogen receptor modulators should not be used if you are still having menstrual cycles. The original SERM was tamoxifen, a medication used to treat breast cancer. Raloxifene (Evista) is an example of a SERM currently in use to treat osteoporosis. SERMs have both positive and negative effects on the estrogen receptors of cells. They have the following benefits:

- SERMs decrease the incidence of vertebral fractures.
- They may provide protection against breast cancer.
- There is no increase in the incidence of cancer of the uterus.
- They do not adversely affect cholesterol.

The downside is as follows:

- SERMs do not prevent hot flashes or other menopausal symptoms; in fact, they may worsen those symptoms.
- SERMs should not be used if there has been a previous blood clot.

Calcitonin (Miacalcin)

Calcitonin is a hormone that helps to regulate bone density by decreasing the amount of bone that is reabsorbed. It is usually given as a liquid sprayed into the nostrils in a dose of 200 IU daily, although it sometimes needs to be given by injection.

The benefits of this therapy are that it causes a decrease in vertebral fractures, and that it is helpful for bone pain associated with a fracture (although the dosage may need to be doubled for it to have this effect).

The potential adverse effects include increased bone pain, a sore nose, and nausea.

Bisphosphonates

Bisphosphonates reduce the amount of bone that is reabsorbed by decreasing the action of the cells whose job it is to break the bone down (the osteoclasts). These drugs are used to treat osteoporosis, high calcium levels in the blood from cancer, Paget's disease of bone, and reflex sympathetic dystrophy.

Oral bisphosphonates are poorly absorbed, so they need to be taken on an empty stomach. Because they can cause ulcers in the esophagus, you should take them with a full glass of water and remain in an upright position for half an hour. These drugs are generally well tolerated and are taken regularly, with the exception of Didronel. (Didronel cannot be taken regularly because it will cause osteomalacia [abnormal bone]; it is taken daily for two weeks every three months.) The bisphosphonates can cause stomach upset, ulcers in the esophagus, abdominal pain, and diarrhea; in rare instances, they may cause a rash. See the table below for a summary of their dosages and effects.

Forteo

Forteo is a new treatment for osteoporosis. It is used in patients who have failed bisphophonates and is given as a subcutaneous injection daily for 18 months. Forteo is well tolerated.

Bisphosphonates

Drug	Dosage	Effect
Etidronate (Didronel)	400 mg daily for two weeks of every three months	Decreases vertebral fractures
Alendronate (Fosamax)	10 mg daily or 70 mg once a week	Decreases vertebral and non-vertebral fractures
Risedronate (Actonel)	5 mg daily or 35 mg once a week	Decreases vertebral and non-vertebral fractures

Pain Medications

The common medications for pain include the non-opioids (which are acetaminophen and the NSAIDs), the co-analgesics (which include antidepressants, anticonvulsants, muscle relaxants, and some topical agents), and the opioids. The medications used depend upon the severity of the pain. The World Health Organization has developed an "Analgesic Ladder" that is used worldwide as an aid in determining the pain medications that would be appropriate to prescribe (see the table below).

Non-Opioids

The non-opioid drugs include the non-steroidal anti-inflammatory drugs (NSAIDs), which were discussed earlier in this chapter (see pages 160–165), and acetaminophen, which is discussed below.

Acetaminophen (Tylenol, Atasol)

Acetaminophen is effective for the management of mild pain and fever, but does not have an effect on inflammation. It does not damage the lining of the stomach and is therefore not associated with stomach ulcers, and does not interfere with platelet or kidney function.

Pain Medications

Pain level	Analgesic given
Mild	Acetaminophen
	NSAIDs
Mild–moderate	NSAID + low-efficacy opioid
	ASA + codeine
	Acetaminophen + codeine
Moderate–severe	Opioids + co-analgesic

Acetaminophen can be given regularly or intermittently, with the usual adult dosage being 325–650 mg every four hours or 500–1000 mg every six hours to a maximum of 4 g per day. If the pain is chronic, then a regular dosage is preferable, with a maximum of 3.2 g being taken each day. There is a separate dosage schedule for children.

If an overdose of acetaminophen is taken, or if it is regularly taken in excess of 4 g per day, there is a risk of fatal liver damage. In elderly patients or patients with heart or kidney failure, the maximum dose should be 2.6 g per day.

Co-Analgesics

A co-analgesic is a medication that works together with acetaminophen, an opioid, or an NSAID to improve pain. Among the commonly used co-analgesics are tricyclic antidepressants, anticonvulsants, muscle relaxants, and topical agents.

Tricyclic antidepressants

The effect of these drugs on pain is independent of their effect on depression. These medications are useful for constant, burning pain, and they also help with sleep. Their potential adverse effects include dry mouth, drowsiness, low blood pressure, weight gain, and an irregular heartbeat. The occasional patient will become depressed on these medications.

Amitriptyline (Elavil) This is the most commonly used tricyclic antidepressant, with a usual dosage of 10–200 mg per day. It is sometimes not tolerated because of drowsiness and dryness of the mouth, but if this happens, another drug of this class may be tried.

Other tricyclic antidepressants Desipramine, doxepin, imipramine, and nortriptyline are other tricyclic antidepressants. Their dosage range is 10–200 mg per day.

Anticonvulsants

These medications are used to treat sharp, stabbing pain. Some of the more common drugs of this class are valproic acid (Epival), carbamazepine (Tegretol), phenytoin (Dilantin), and gabapentin (Neurontin). They are used to treat neurological pain rather than arthritis.

Muscle relaxants

These medications are used mainly to treat muscle spasms. Some of the more common drugs of this class are described below.

Baclofen Baclofen is used for muscle spasms. The usual dosage is 5 mg three times per day, but this can be increased to a maximum of 80 mg per day. It is associated with dry mouth, dizziness, and dependence (see the discussion that follows on page 202 for a description of dependence, addiction, and tolerance).

Cyclobenzaprine (Flexeril) This drug is derived from the tricyclic antidepressants, and is used for muscle spasms and for fibromyalgia. It can cause dry mouth, drowsiness, and dizziness, and when used with some antidepressants, it can cause convulsions. Other commonly used muscle relaxants are methocarbamol (Robaxin) and orphenadrine (Norflex).

Topical agents

Topical agents are medications that are rubbed into the skin. Capsaicin cream is a topical pain medication—derived from cayenne pepper—that is used to treat osteoarthritis. It must be applied four times per day, but not to the face as it will burn. It may cause a rash.

Pennsaid is a mixture of DMSO (a solvent) and diclofenac (a NSAID) and is applied externally to the joint for the treatment of osteoarthritis.

Commonly Available Narcotic Drugs

Generic	Trade name	Available forms
Morphine sulphate	Morphine sulphate, Statex MS Contin	Regular acting and sustained release
Oxycodone	Supeudol	Regular acting and sustained release
Hydromorphone	Dilaudid	Regular acting and sustained release
Codeine phosphate	Codeine phosphate, Codeine Contin	Regular acting and sustained release
Meperidine	Demerol	Regular acting
Propoxyphene	Darvon	Regular acting
Fentanyl		Patch
Methadone		Regular acting

Narcotics (Opioids)

Narcotics can be considered for the treatment of moderate to severe chronic pain even if it is not caused by cancer. They can be used by people who are reliable and have no history of drug dependence or abuse, and for whom reasonable alternative treatments have not worked.

Narcotics were originally derived from the poppy seed and have been used since ancient times. They were used at first to treat dysentery, but were also found to help pain and cause euphoria. Today, many different forms of narcotic drugs are available. Which one should be used depends on the degree of pain, whether the pain is intermittent or continuous, and whether it is acute or chronic. The table above lists some of the commonly available narcotics. It should be noted that 10–20 percent of the Caucasian population will have no painkilling effect from codeine despite experiencing all of its side effects.

The adverse effects of the opioid analgesics include the following:

- decreased breathing
- mood changes (high or low) like depression
- sedation, confusion, and impaired thinking
- nausea and vomiting
- increased pressure in the brain, headache
- constipation
- retention of urine
- dry mouth
- hives or itching, and increased sweating
- tolerance, dependence

Before deciding to use opioid therapy to control pain over the long term, it is necessary to understand drug tolerance, addiction, and dependence.

Tolerance is the body's adaptation to the drug over time, so that the drug's effectiveness decreases. Most people will adapt or develop tolerance to some of the adverse effects such as sedation, nausea, and decreased breathing; this is desired. However, some people develop a tolerance to the analgesic effect of the drug and require larger amounts of drug for the same effect on pain; this is not addiction.

Addiction is a disease that is influenced by such things as the person's genetic makeup, environment, and interactions with others. Signs of addiction include poor control of drug use, craving, compulsive use, and continued use despite harm.

Dependence is also a state of adaptation to a drug. With drug dependence, not only may the body have developed a tolerance to the drug, but it has actually come to need it, to the point that if the drug is suddenly stopped, a withdrawal syndrome will occur. The features of an opioid withdrawal syndrome are:

- craving for the opioid
- restlessness and irritability
- increased sensitivity to pain
- nausea, cramps
- low mood
- inability to sleep
- anxiety
- sweating, dilated pupils
- racing heart and high blood pressure
- fever
- diarrhea and vomiting

These medications should be administered by a physician who deals with pain and is familiar with the use of narcotics. For chronic pain, a long-acting agent should be used and a short-acting drug may be prescribed for breakthrough pain. There is no evidence of any long-term organ toxicity from the long-term use of opioids; in fact, there is growing evidence that long-term opioid use significantly reduces pain in some people, with no significant adverse effects and a low potential for addiction. The College of Physicians and Surgeons of Ontario reviewed the literature on the long-term use of opioids in non-cancer pain, and concluded that sustained-released opioid therapy helps selected patients with chronic musculoskeletal pain and neuropathic pain (pain caused by diseases of the nerves).

New Therapies

Several new therapies have recently been developed for the treatment of rheumatoid arthritis, psoriatic arthritis, and ankylosing spondylitis. Some of them will be discussed below.

Immunosuppressive Therapy

Some immunosuppressant drugs were discussed previously in the chapter, but there is a new one, mycophenolate mofetil, that is used to treat severe kidney disease in patients with systemic lupus erythematosus.

Mycophenolate Mofetil (CellCept)

Recent studies have shown that this medication (when combined with corticosteroids) is effective in the management of severe kidney disease in systemic lupus erythematosus patients. It is more selective than cyclophosphamide in its suppression of the immune system, as its effects are concentrated on specific cells' multiplication, not on the immune system as a whole.

This drug's effectiveness was compared over a one-year period to that of cyclophosphamide and prednisone, and the results achieved with all three drugs were the same. The advantage of using mycophenolate mofetil over the others is that it is less toxic: compared to cyclophosphamide it is less likely to cause cancer, hair loss, and menstrual problems. Mycophenolate mofetil has not yet replaced cyclophosphamide in the management of patients with severe kidney disease (i.e., diffuse proliferative glomerulonephritis) associated with systemic lupus erythematosus, however, as further studies are necessary.

Potential adverse effects It increases the risk of infection, including lung infections and shingles. Some patients experience diarrhea, vomiting, and reduced white blood cell counts.

Prosorba Column

This treatment proved to be ineffective for the treatment of rheumatoid arthritis until a prosorba column was added into the system recently. Basically, the patient's blood is run through a plasmapheresis machine to separate the plasma (the clear fluid part of the blood) from the blood cells. The plasma then passes through a prosorba column (a tube containing silicon beads to which are attached highly purified protein molecules), where the protein binds to the rheumatoid factor and removes it from the plasma. The plasma is then recombined with the blood cells and put back into the patient.

Clinical trials have shown this treatment to be beneficial to patients with moderate to severe rheumatoid arthritis for whom at least two other DMARD therapies have failed. In the trials, the procedure was done every week for 12 weeks and the patients were evaluated after the therapy had been stopped for eight weeks. The procedure can be repeated, but it is not yet known for how long it will benefit patients.

The most common side effect is increased joint pain and swelling, which improves after the first few treatments.

Endothelial Receptor Antagonists

Endothelin is a naturally occurring chemical that causes constriction (narrowing) of the blood vessels. The chemical itself acts like a key, finding the receptor (lock) on the cells that make up the blood vessels, and acting upon the cells with receptors that it fits. If the blood vessels are too constricted, however, the blood pressure increases; this condition is known as hypertension.

Bosentan (Tracleer)

High blood pressure in the blood vessels of the lungs is referred to as pulmonary hypertension. It can be a complication of scleroderma, systemic lupus erythematosus, and mixed connective tissue disease. The symptoms are progressive shortness of breath, fatigue, chest pain, and Raynaud's phenomenon. There had been no effective treatment for pulmonary hypertension until the advent of bosentan. It is a new drug that binds to the cells' receptors for the vessel-squeezing endothelin; since the receptor is already occupied by the bosentan, the endothelin can't bind, and therefore it can't cause constriction of the blood vessels. This lowers the blood pressure in the pulmonary artery (the large blood vessel leading from the heart to the lungs).

Potential adverse effects Potential adverse effects of the drug are:

- elevation of the liver enzymes; bosentan should not be used in patients with serious liver disease
- interaction with several drugs, including warfarin, glyburide, and cyclosporin
- a fall in hemoglobin (anemia)

What Is in the Pipeline?

Although the cause of rheumatoid arthritis and other forms of arthritis is not known, scientists have worked out many of the mechanisms of the diseases, which has lead to promising new therapies that will be on the market in the next few years, including:

- Anti CD20 (rituximab) is an antibody against B cells that produce antibodies, including rheumatoid factor. Other important antibody mediated diseases include SLE, Sjogren's syndrome, Wegener's granulomatosus, and polymyositis. This drug was originally developed for B-cell lymphoma and has been available since 1997. Studies have shown it to be effective for 48 weeks after two intravenous infusions for the treatment of rheumatoid arthritis. Studies are now being done for its use in SLE, MS, Sjogren's, and Wegener's granulomatosus.
- CTLA4Ig (abatacept) is a fusion protein that acts by preventing the T cells from being fully stimulated. It is as effective as the TNF blockers (entanercept, infliximab, and adalimumab) in clinical trials. It is important to have these medications available

because 30–40 percent of people will not respond adequately to TNF blockers.

- Etoricoxib and Lumericoxib are two new selective non-steroidal anti-inflammatory drugs or COXIBs. They have been shown to be as effective as traditional NSAIDs, and they reduce the incidence of stomach ulcers and bleeds by up to 70 percent.
- An immunosuppressive medication that is used in transplantation is now being studied for use in rheumatoid arthritis. The medication, FK506, is produced from fungus and has similar effects to cyclosporine.

This chapter has attempted to review many of the medications used by patients with arthritis and related conditions. It is by no way complete. The common side effects of the medications that may be encountered have been discussed, but I have not provided a complete list. It is important to remember that all medications, including "natural" therapies, have potential adverse reactions. The prescription medications in this country undergo extensive reviews by Health Canada for their benefits and risks prior to ever being approved. It is important to understand why your physician has recommended a treatment and what benefit you should expect. You need to be aware of potential adverse effects and report them to your physician. It is your responsibility to take the medication as prescribed and, if you are not taking it, to let your physician know.

8 Complementary therapies

Alternative and complementary therapies have been defined as medical treatments not commonly taught or available at North American medical schools or hospitals, or treatments not prescribed by doctors. Some prefer the terms *mainstream* and *non-mainstream therapies*. Complementary therapies are used together with mainstream medical treatments, whereas alternative therapies are used instead of mainstream therapies. Alternative therapies often claim to cure disease, whereas complementary therapies are additions to conventional medical treatments and preventions.

Another more complex description of complementary therapies is "all health systems and practices other than those intrinsic to the politically dominant health system of a particular society or culture." They are defined by their users as preventing or treating illness or promoting health and well-being. This complex description is saying simply that what is a complementary therapy in one society may be mainstream in another. How a therapy is classified really depends on how it is perceived by the majority of people in the society. It is intriguing, from a Western viewpoint, that traditional Chinese medicine is mainstream in China, but Western medicine may be considered complementary there!

The classification of a therapy as alternative or conventional is arbitrary and can vary with time, person, and location. The most logical and least emotional classification of therapies is: those that work, those that may or may not work, and those that do not work as determined by rigorous testing. When complementary therapies are shown to work, they are usually brought into conventional practice; this process is called "integrative medicine." Conventional or complementary therapies proven not to work should be discarded.

Popularity of Complementary Therapies

In the United States, complementary therapies are being used commonly and with increasing frequency. In 1990, 33.8 percent of the general population had used at least one out of 16 different complementary therapies in the past year; in 1997, the figure had risen to 42.1 percent. Furthermore, at least US $34 billion was spent on complementary therapies in the United States in 1997. The popularity of these therapies is not confined to the United States, however, and it is estimated that four billion people worldwide (or about two-thirds of the world's population) use herbs for medicinal purposes.

Treating arthritis is one of the main reasons that people use complementary therapies. In a San Diego study, 84 percent of patients with arthritis or other musculoskeletal complaints used at least one of these therapies over a six-month period. In Montreal, usage for arthritis was 66 percent over 12 months, and in Edmonton, 55 percent at any time. In the Edmonton study, pain was greatly improved in 11 percent, mildly improved in 29 percent, and not improved in 59 percent. The amount of money spent on these treatments in Canada is more than $622 per patient per year.

In Canada, these therapies are most popular among females aged 45 to 64 years with a chronic disease. The use of these treatments is also associated with higher incomes and residency in western Canada.

Reasons for Use

There are many reasons that people use complementary therapies, and we will discuss them below. (Despite all these reasons, only

4–5 percent of the consumers of complementary medicine did not also use conventional medicine, however.) People say that complementary therapies are: convenient; "natural" and "safe"; beyond the limitations of conventional therapy; available despite the failure of the physician-patient relationship; useful for chronic disease; in line with their personal belief systems; simple; and convincingly promoted.

They're "convenient"

Convenience is an important factor. Complementary-therapy users do not have to wait to see a physician or specialist, but can self-prescribe a treatment that is easily available, and may be cheaper, less invasive, simpler, and easier to follow than what a doctor might have suggested.

They're "safe"

Safety is a major reason that many people use complementary therapies. It is felt that these therapies are benign compared to conventional treatments. Home remedies also sound harmless. Many of these treatments are touted as being "natural," which, to many, means no side effects, a superiority to "artificial" products, and a feeling of "returning to the earth." Organic products—on which no pesticides or herbicides are used—are appealing to many as well. The notion that these treatments are preventative is also attractive.

They "go beyond conventional medicine"

Conventional medicine has limitations. It provides some people with partial or minimal benefit, and others with no benefit at all. Some people cannot tolerate the treatments due to side effects, and others are too afraid to try the therapy because of the possibility of a side effect occurring. For some, conventional medicine has improved the disease but not eradicated it, and they would like to rid themselves of any residual symptoms. And there are those who are still suffering and are at a dead end: their physicians have nothing further to offer them. People expect conventional medicine to work miracles, and when it does not consistently overcome illness, their overblown expectations can lead to disillusionment.

They "avoid the physician"

Another reason that people turn to complementary therapies is a failed doctor–patient relationship. Perhaps the physician communicates poorly, lacks interest in the patient or the problem, is always rushing, or is paternalistic. The physician may scold the patient for trying complementary treatments when, in fact, the patient is trying to help himself or herself and be less of a bother to the doctor. Doctors often explain things using complicated and confusing ideas and terminology, or may prescribe too many drugs with little explanation. They may convey a sense of pessimism when hope is needed to treat the patient's despair as well as the signs and symptoms of the disease.

Physicians should listen to their patients with an open mind about complementary therapies, but the patients should expect honest and balanced replies that are in their best interests.

They "help chronic disease"

Having a chronic disease like arthritis increases the chances that complementary therapies will be tried. As the arthritis does not disappear spontaneously or get cured, anxiety, depression, desperation, discouragement, and frustration can lead patients to use complementary therapies, which can be associated with hope, optimism, and empowerment. These therapies allow the patients to participate in the healing process, and give them a chance to regain control of the situation.

They "work with my belief system"

Patients' personal belief systems will determine which treatments they prefer, and culture and religion play a role here. More modern movements like feminism, health consciousness, vegetarianism, environmentalism, and personal growth psychology are associated with the use of complementary treatments. There is more interest now in spiritualism, faith, and miracles. Many people are drawn to magic, mysticism, astrology, rituals, and the exotic or taboo. There are others who are anti-science: they do not believe that scientific breakthroughs will be relevant to their disease, they feel that science is rigid and rejects new ways of thinking, and they are sure that reason cannot solve all of the problems in the world. There are also people who have an antiestablishment bent: they feel that there is a class conflict between the rich, arrogant doctors and the average people seeking empowerment and democratization of the health care system. There are some who believe that there is a conspiracy by the medical community to keep effective treatments away from patients.

They're "simple and powerful"

Complementary medicine gives simple and easy-to-understand explanations, often using mystical-sounding words that imply tremendous power and benefit. The explanations may not be factual or specific, but they are appealing. Claims are made that "toxins will be removed, vital forces and energy will be restored, the immune system will be strengthened to let the body fight off the disease, and the body's yin and yang will be rebalanced." There is emphasis on a holistic approach.

They "must work ... look at the ad!"

Complementary therapies are also used because they are promoted so well. They are packaged as unequivocal cures and remedies, and wrapped in glowing optimism. They are marketed through the mass media, including newspapers, magazines, radio, television, books, and direct-mail promotions with unabashed enthusiasm. (Do you think that the interest of the media is in their profit or your welfare?)

This direct-to-customer-and-bypassing-the-medical-experts approach has been so successful that conventional pharmaceutical companies are now marketing their products the same way. Notice the use of "experts wearing white lab coats" endorsing the therapy. These products are stocked slickly on shelves of health food stores and pharmacies. People claiming to have been helped by a product may become salespeople, but are promoting the therapy for their own profit and not for patients' benefit. Some are involved in pyramid schemes. Friendly testimonials (statements of personal experience) of success with a therapy are seductive, and testimonials are even more effective when given by celebrities. Testimonials can be bought, and testimonials can be fabricated. Patients are urged to try products by well-meaning friends and relatives, and will try the complementary therapy so as not to offend or reject their friends and relatives. The most effective promoters are quacks who sell ineffective treatments or treatments containing unidentified active ingredients like cortisone. Most complementary therapies are not quackery, but they all need to be proven effective by scientific standards.

Quackery

Most complementary therapies are not quackery; however, in your search for these types of remedies, beware of the quack. A quack is someone who, for profit, promotes a medical scheme or remedy that is known to be false. The word "quack" is derived from the duck that makes a great deal of noise about nothing. Quackery is health fraud.

Quacks give the impression that they are independent thinkers, mavericks, or geniuses. They challenge traditional thinking, and will preach with absolute certainty simple explanations that contain only a grain of truth at most. They stress patient satisfaction over the safety and efficacy of their treatment in order to make money … patients feel satisfied while they are being taken for a ride! Even "legitimate" companies may promote a questionable therapy for profit. They will give you the pseudo-scientific jargon you want to hear, such as "channelling energy flows," "boosting the body's natural defences and immune system," "removing toxins," and "purifying the blood." (Centuries ago, "purifying the blood" meant "treating syphilis"!) Scare tactics are often used, such as, "the sunspots are ruining your joints." Only the quack has the solution to protect you from the sunspots and save your joints, and of course, the solutions tend to be secret. Their names alone could wipe out a plague … How could any disease stand up against Radon's Microbe Killer and Liquozone? How could you miss with Dr. Pierce's Favourite Prescription (21 percent alcohol), Lydia Pinkham's Vegetable Compound (21 percent ale), or Dr. Bull's Infant Cough Mixture (morphine base).

Charlatans, cranks, and health hucksters are different types of quacks. Charlatans are deliberate fakers. They are charming social predators who manipulate others without having any conscience, feelings, guilt, or regret. They are unusual human beings who can cause changes in your feelings and behaviour just by virtue of their magnetic and mesmerizing personalities. They are slick, fast-talking, double-talking, and persuasive individuals who are very confident and overly optimistic, and they often use false credentials and diplomas.

Cranks, on the other hand, truly believe in themselves and their remedies. They tend to be honest, selfless, and generous.

Health hucksters are business entrepreneurs and free enterprisers who are exploiting the public's interest in health. They are not concerned about the scientific validity of their products: they just want your business and your money.

Problems with Alternative Therapies

There are several problems and misconceptions about alternative therapies that you should consider before trying them. We will discuss in detail below how alternative therapies, in general: provide little or no evidence of efficacy; are promoted by unproven testimonials; underestimate or understate side effects; lack regulation; delay correct diagnosis and treatment; divert money away from care and research; exploit people; and delay needed lifestyle changes.

Not enough evidence

In many instances, there is not enough evidence that a treatment is effective. The proponents of the therapy should do controlled double-blind studies to make sure that the improvement attributed to a treatment is not a coincidence.

The natural course of some types of arthritis is that they can disappear spontaneously or come and go randomly. If, by chance, the treatment is taken at the same time that the arthritis was going to improve anyway, it will be assumed that the treatment was effective (whether it was conventional or alternative).

A placebo effect can also make it seem that a treatment is working (again, whether it is a conventional or alternative treatment). As many as 30–40 percent of people taking the placebo treatment in placebo-controlled trials will improve. This placebo effect may be due to the patient's expectations, faith, and hope that the new therapy will work. The ritual of receiving treatment and reassurance helps reduce suffering. A positive encounter with a health care worker who provides comfort, optimism, emotional support, attention, empathy, and caring will improve the patient, whether or not the new treatment being tried is effective. Also, patients who actively follow a treatment program (whether it is placebo, mainstream, or alternative) do better than those who do not follow a program.

Testimonials unproven

Testimonials should not be relied upon. If the testifier actually has arthritis, he may have improved because of a coincidence in the natural course of the arthritis or the placebo effect. Furthermore, you never hear the testimonials of those who received no benefit or had other problems with the treatment. In fact, the testimonials may be coming from the 1 percent of patients in whom the treatment worked, but not the 99 percent in whom it did not work.

Testimonials may be completely made up, and some people are paid to give testimonials that are not true. In addition, testimonials can be used to draw conclusions that the facts do not support. A testimonial may include the argument that many conventional drugs are derived from natural sources. Although this is true, it does not mean that all natural treatments work, and those that do work are usually incorporated into conventional medicine anyway. Another argument may be that a treatment has been around for hundreds of years. Again, while this may be true, it does not mean that the treatment is effective: it may mean only that nothing else was available to offer someone with arthritis.

Side effects understated

The frequency of side effects in complementary therapies is often underestimated. By and large the side effects of alternative treatments are less frequent and less severe than for mainstream therapies, but side effects do occur nonetheless. Do not be lulled into complacency by terms like "natural" and "organic": hemlock and arsenic are natural, but both are poisons. Interactions can occur between alternative and conventional medicines. It is not known whether these complementary treatments are safe during pregnancy, breastfeeding, and infancy, and the long-term effects of many of these treatments are also unknown. Allergic reactions can occur to these treatments just as they do to peanuts, dairy products, seafood, and pollens. Get reliable information about safety before starting something new, whether it is mainstream or not mainstream.

No regulations or standards

The lack of regulations and standards should be a bigger concern than it is when it comes to alternative therapies. There are two categories of ingested treatments: food and drugs. Many alternative treatments are marketed as foods, and are therefore neither rigorously inspected nor allowed to print health claims on their labels. Those that are marketed as drugs can make health claims on their labels, but they should have a Drug Identification Number (DIN) or a General Public number (GP) on the label, too. These numbers indicate that the Health Protection Branch of Health Canada has reviewed and approved the product, its formulation, labelling, and instructions for use.

Too often, the active ingredient is present in lower concentrations than labelled, if it is present at all! As an example, 50 commercial preparations of ginseng sold in 11 different countries were tested. The concentrations in 44 ranged from 1.9 percent to 9.9 percent, and 6 contained no ginseng at all. The concentrations of plant products can vary depending on the soil, sun, rain, and parts of the plant used (e.g., petals, seeds, leaves, roots).

In addition, the manufacturing process can vary. For example, l-tryptophan made by a company in Japan caused a serious side effect called eosinophilia-myalgia syndrome, whereas l-tryptophan from other manufacturers did not.

Alternative treatments can be adulterated with undeclared conventional drugs like corticosteroids, NSAIDs, tranquilizers, antibiotics, and ephedrine. When 2609 samples of traditional Chinese medicines were analyzed, 23 percent were found to be adulterated. Contamination with toxic substances like arsenic, mercury, lead, and bacteria was also found.

Delay diagnosis and treatment

Opting first for alternative therapies can result in the delay of making a correct diagnosis or instituting the proper treatment, and significant consequences could result. For instance, in rheumatoid arthritis, a great deal of the joint damage takes place during the first two years of the disease. If the proven treatments are begun early much joint damage can be prevented, but once the damage is done, no treatment known as yet can cause a complete reversal of the disease's progress.

Some alternative-medicine practitioners may actually advise a patient to stop taking conventional treatment, an action that can have disastrous consequences. In a Mexican study, 85 percent of patients with systemic lupus erythematosus who embarked on alternative therapy were told to discontinue their conventional treatment. Stopping conventional therapy under such circumstances was one of the main causes of death in the systemic lupus erythematosus patients in the study.

Divert funding

Money spent on unproven or ineffective therapies is diverted from the funding of proven and effective treatments. Pressure on medical coverage plans to pay for such treatments reduces the amount of money available for transplants, dialysis, heart surgery, and cancer treatments. Insurance premiums can also rise, making coverage unaffordable for poorer people. Furthermore, this money could be used for research to acquire new knowledge about arthritis and its management. The National Institutes of Health in the United States just spent US $50 million on research grants to investigate the efficacy of alternative therapies. Should the providers of the treatment pay for such research, or should the taxpayer?

Exploit people

Some alternative-care providers exploit people with illnesses like arthritis. They may do this by carrying on treatment for too long, or by selling you all kinds of unnecessary supplements, and it is a misconception that alternative therapies are cheap. Americans spent about US $34 billion for alternative medicine in 1997, and as these therapies become more popular, the costs rise. In 1997, the cost of care for low back pain by chiropractors exceeded that by orthopedic surgeons and general physicians, and the cost of alternative therapies for patients with systemic lupus erythematosus is currently nearly double the cost for those who use mainstream medicine. Regular pharmaceutical companies may also manufacture alternative drugs for profit.

Delay needed changes

Passive treatments (whether alternative or conventional) may appeal to patients because they are easier than making lifestyle changes that are more important and effective. It is better to control back pain with exercise and weight control than to take herbs, pills, or acupuncture, but which is easier and requires less personal effort? It should be noted, though, that sometimes alternative-care providers are more effective than mainstream caregivers in getting people to accept and follow lifestyle changes.

Buyer Beware

Most providers of complementary therapies are probably trying to help you, but some are not. Here are some danger signs that should alert you to the possibility of a fraud:

1. Treatment is a quick and effective cure! It promises that you will be cured—and not just of arthritis, but also of any other conditions. It works for almost everything! It is a miraculous breakthrough!

2. It is available from only one source and only for a limited time. It's an exclusive and secret formula. It's from an ancient or supernatural source.
3. There is no labelling. There are no directions for use, or list of ingredients or side effects.
4. There is a money angle. You are asked for payment in advance. Expensive treatments and tests are pushed. Visits seem too frequent. The practitioners insist that you only use their products.
5. There is an attempt to alienate you from your other caregivers. You are told to stop or reduce prescription medications. You are told to keep this therapy secret from everyone. This practitioner is paranoid about or belittles other health care providers. There are accusations that the medical community and research scientists are conspiring to suppress this therapy.
6. The practitioner has no authentic credentials. There is no licence to practise. There is no certificate from an approved school or organization in this specialty.
7. The practitioner suggests or asks for intimate sexual relations. There is no respect for your modesty.
8. Beware if the promotion of the therapy is too slick. Be careful of repeated publicity and advertisements in the mass media. Watch out for the personal testimonials, celebrity endorsements, unabashed enthusiasm, inaccuracies, exaggerations, and dramatizations. If it looks and smells like a snake-oil vendor, it probably is.

What to Do about Complementary Therapies

It is important to have as accurate a diagnosis of your condition as possible. You should be aware of the benefits and side effects of the mainstream therapies, and any harm that might occur if you delay starting them. If you want to use complementary therapies, make sure they are compatible with your present program of treatment. Discuss them with your physician.

Check the qualifications, training, licensure, and references of the complementary caregiver. Find out if the caregiver has any financial interest in the products that you are told to purchase. Do reliable companies make these products? Get a full description of the therapy in writing, including proof of efficacy, scientific references, safety profile, and the cost and length of treatment. Find out how and by whom the treatment will be supervised and monitored. Has the therapist asked about the rest of your health and made sure that this treatment does not interfere with any of your other conditions or therapies? If possible, speak to other clients. If there is no benefit by six to eight weeks, reevaluate the treatment or the practitioner.

Get information from independent sources like physicians, pharmacists, nurses, physiotherapists, or occupational therapists. Other sources include support groups, libraries, bookstores, medical journals, and books. Various organizations and agencies like the Arthritis Society (Canada), the Arthritis Foundation (USA), Health Canada, the Food and Drug Administration, the National Institutes of Health's Office of Alternative Medicine (USA), and the Better Business Bureau can provide you with more information. *Arthritis Today,* the magazine of the Arthritis Foundation, has had a series of articles on different complementary therapies. There are many reliable sources on the Internet, but you must be able to distinguish them from the less reliable websites. Please refer to Appendix II.

Classification of Complementary Therapies

Complementary therapies can be classified into different categories, including: alternative healing systems; mental, spiritual, and sensual; manual and moving bodyworks; electromagnetic and other radiations;

diet and nutrition; botanical therapies; zoological therapies; pharmaceuticals and nutraceuticals; and miscellaneous complementary treatments. Each category will be presented in more detail below as it applies to arthritis.

Alternative Healing Systems

In the group known as alternative healing systems are the following therapies: ayurveda, traditional Chinese medicine, naturopathy, osteopathy, chiropractic, homeopathy, Native North American healing, spa therapy, Tibetan traditional medicine, Latin American rural practices, past life therapy, folk medicine, and home remedies. At first glance, these seem like completely different therapies that should not be grouped together, but in actuality these treatments have several features in common. All of the alternative healing systems include spirituality, restoring a vital force, and holism.

The nature of the spirituality is related to the dominant religion or philosophical system in the originating culture (e.g., Taoism [traditional Chinese medicine], Hinduism [ayurveda], Buddhism [traditional Tibetan medicine], Native American healing, and Christianity [Christian Science]).

Many of these systems deal with restoring a vital force or energy that has gone awry to cause disease. These vital energies have been referred to as qi (China), Ki (Korea), prana (India), and Vital Force (Western).

Holism means that the illness must be considered in reference to the mind and body as a whole and their interaction with the environment. The emphasis is that the body can heal itself and stay healthy using mild remedies that correct imbalances in the vital forces, mind, body, and environment.

Below, we will discuss ayurveda, traditional Chinese medicine, naturopathy, osteopathy, chiropractic, homeopathy, Native American healing, and spa therapy.

Ayurveda

Ayurveda means "knowledge of life." It is a system of healing from India that dates back about 5000 years. Ayurveda tries to maintain harmony among the vital life energy (called prana) and the spiritual, mental, and physical forces of the body and the environment. Each individual has varying amounts of the three physiological energies called doshas (kapha, pitta, and vata). Each dosha consists of one or more of the five basic elements: earth, fire, water, air, and ether.

The harmony is maintained by a prescription of lifestyle changes, vegetarian diets, herbs, internal cleansing (panchakarma), exercises, yoga, meditation, breathing exercises (pranayama), and massages with herbal oils. The internal cleansing may involve bloodletting (with leeches), sweat baths, vomiting, laxatives, fasts, and enemas.

Herbs, yoga, breathing exercises, other exercises, meditation, and massage with oils may help arthritis to some degree. Herbs may, however, contain heavy metals like lead, mercury, and arsenic, and might interact with other medications. There also may be some risk from the internal cleansing techniques.

Traditional Chinese medicine

Traditional Chinese medicine (TCM) is about 3000 years old. In this philosophy, good health is due to the flow of qi (life force energy) through invisible channels in the body called meridians. Illness may result from a block or aberration in the flow of qi. Imbalances of the contrasting states of yin and yang (the dual nature of things) can also cause illness.

TCM uses acupuncture, acupressure, moxibustion, cupping, herbal therapy, qi gong, massage, manipulation, and diet to maintain and restore health. Moxibustion is the burning of the herb moxa or mugwort on an acupuncture point. Cupping creates suction above the part of the body needing treatment (the air inside a jar is warmed, the jar is then placed upside down on the skin, and as the air cools, a vacuum develops, causing suction). Qi gong includes meditation, relaxation training, visualization, breathing exercises, tai chi, and other movements and postures. The diet is linked to adding or omitting foods, which correspond to internal organs, channels, and various body parts.

TCM can enhance well-being, reduce anxiety, and promote relaxation, all of which can help arthritis symptoms. Arthritis symptoms may also be improved by acupuncture, qi gong, massage, and manipulation. Acupuncture needles should be sterile to prevent the transmission of infections. Some herbs can be poisonous if taken in large amounts. Some herbs may be contaminated with heavy metals or Western drugs.

Naturopathy

Naturopathy sees the development of illness in the same way that conventional medicine does, but it treats diseases by using "natural methods" rather than surgery and medicine. The goals of naturopathy are to prevent disease by encouraging healthy habits, and to alleviate illness by allowing the body to heal itself with natural therapies.

These therapies recruit the natural healing power of the body (equivalent to the vital force) to fight off disease. They include nutritional therapy and dietary supplements, promotion of healthy habits and exercise, botanical medicines, homeopathy, manipulation, hydrotherapy, counselling, acupuncture, and hypnotherapy.

Naturopathy reduces the risk factors for many diseases. The acupuncture, manipulation, hydrotherapy, diet, counselling, and hypnotherapy can provide some relief from the symptoms of arthritis. Naturopathy does not help severe diseases. Do not stop your prescribed medications.

Osteopathy

Osteopathy began after the US Civil War. Osteopaths are trained in orthodox medicine but they emphasize body alignment and manual therapy. It is felt that problems with the musculoskeletal system can affect one's health in many ways and that illness can upset the balance of the musculoskeletal system. Another principle is that manipulation can help most diseases by improving the circulation of blood (equivalent to vital energy).

The main tools used in this healing system are manipulation of soft tissues around the spine and joints, low amplitude manipulation of joints, gentle manipulation of the bone and tissues of the skull and spine (cranial manipulation), massage, relaxation therapy, exercises, and diet.

Osteopathy can discover and correct patterns of movement and alignment that may make arthritis worse. However, one must be cautious about the use of manipulation in certain instances.

Chiropractic

D. D. Palmer started chiropractic in Iowa in about 1895, but its origins probably date back to the ancient "bonesetters." The main idea is that the body can heal itself and that the nervous system influences all of the other systems in the body. The brain sends energy (equivalent to vital energy) to all parts of the body by way of the nerves contained in the spinal cord. Any misalignment of a vertebra (subluxation) could interrupt the flow of this energy, causing disease. Manual adjustments or manipulation of these subluxations is supposed to restore health.

These manual techniques include very brief, high-velocity, large-amplitude thrusts of the spine (adjustments), stretching, traction and the slow manipulation of joints. Some chiropractors may mix in herbs, vitamins, nutrition, homeopathy, and ultrasound. They will do X-rays for diagnostic purposes.

Chiropractic can help some types of mechanical musculoskeletal problems such as neck and back pain; however, there is no proof that it can cure conditions like heart disease or cancer. The treatments should not be painful. If there is no improvement by one month, other remedies should be sought. There have been rare reports of strokes and death as a result of neck manipulation injuring the vertebral arteries carrying blood to the brain. Avoid manipulation to inflamed joints and osteoporotic bones. Manipulation must not be done in the presence of unstable vertebrae (e.g., the cervical spine in rheumatoid arthritis) or brittle, fused vertebrae (e.g., ankylosing spondylitis). It probably should be avoided in people with a tendency to bleed, such as those taking anti-coagulants (blood thinners).

Homeopathy

A German physician developed homeopathy in the eighteenth century. The remedies used are based upon the identification of the patient's symptoms. A large compendium, *Homeopathic Pharmacopoeia,* is then consulted to determine which substances can cause the same symptoms. These substances can be plants, minerals, animal products, or chemicals.

The theory is that although a large dose of these substances will cause the same symptoms that the patient has, a very small dose will cure them. These remedies would displace the disease with a similar, but weaker illness that the body's vital energy could handle. These substances are diluted and shaken vigorously in water (or sometimes alcohol) repeatedly until less than one molecule of the original substance is left. It is claimed that the water retains a "trace memory" or "frequency" of the active ingredient in an electromagnetic form. This form supposedly contains the "healing life force" of the diluted substance.

The efficacy of homeopathy in arthritis has been nil to minimal. In a controlled study, homeopathy (Rhus Toxicum) was no better than placebo in treating osteoarthritis. The same treatment was tested in people with fibromyalgia but it was only slightly better than placebo. In two controlled studies of homeopathy, it was no better than placebo for the treatment of rheumatoid arthritis. In another study, it was somewhat better than placebo for treating rheumatoid arthritis, but many patients were excluded or dropped out, making the results questionable. Overall, benefit provided by homeopathy for arthritis is none to minimal, but it is very safe. The main danger of using it alone is that it may cause progression of the arthritis by delaying the institution of effective therapy. However, a trial of homeopathy in someone who has failed or cannot tolerate mainstream therapy is worthwhile.

Native North American healing

Native North American healing is a merger of medicine and religion. There is a belief in an integral relationship between the person, the environment, the cosmos, and spiritual forces in health and disease. Physical illness is attributed to spiritual causes. Not only living things but also inanimate objects like rocks contain spirits. Healing involves appeasing the spirits, ridding the ill of impurities, and restoring a healthful, spiritually pure state. There are variations in this system amongst the different Native nations.

The healing system involves purification or purging rituals, botanical medicines, shamans, and symbolic healing ceremonies. Purging rituals are performed in sweat lodges where heated rocks are doused with water. The steam causes profuse sweating. Prayers are also said. Some tribes use an herbal tea ("Black Drink") to induce vomiting. Herbs are used, such as willow bark to ease joint pain. (Willow bark contains salicin, the natural form of aspirin.) Shamans are trained spiritual leaders or medicine men (although many are women). They invoke the healing powers of the spiritual forces by prayers and ceremonies. Symbolic healing rituals may include chants, dances, drumming, medicine rattles, sand painting, masks, purification of the air, and sacred hoops or medicine wheels. Many healing rites are conducted in groups so that the family and the community are participating.

The major benefit of Native American healing is psychological and related to the mind–body connection. There is also a unique communal support system. Herbs like willow bark can reduce arthritic symptoms. This healing system can be used in conjunction with the orthodox treatments of arthritis.

Spa therapy

Spa therapy dates back to antiquity, but it became popular in Europe during the eighteenth century. The treatments revolve around the use of hot mineral waters and mud. The water usually comes from hot springs, and the buoyancy, heat, and chemical content of the mineral waters ease arthritic symptoms. The mud (peat, moor, or mud) contains varying amounts of organic material.

The mud is mixed with the hot mineral water and used as a bath or direct application to the skin (mud packs). It is a source of heat and minerals. Spa resorts are often located where the climate is also beneficial to the patient. Other therapies that may be offered are hot and cold applications, massage, underwater traction, ultrasound, electrotherapy, infrared and short wave radiation, exercise, diet, and relaxation.

Spa therapy can improve muscle tone, joint mobility, and pain. It can stimulate the body to produce more endorphins and cortisone. It can reduce the response of the immune system and the production of some of the mediators of inflammation. It can also improve the concentration of trace minerals in the body. Controlled studies show that spa therapy can help rheumatoid arthritis, ankylosing spondylitis, psoriatic arthritis, osteoarthritis, and chronic back pain for up to a few months afterwards.

Spa therapy complements mainstream treatments very well, but should not be used alone. It can be expensive and often involves travelling. The water can cause rashes or spread infection. A transient reaction to the heat (weakness, fatigue, and worse joint pains) can occur, and severe varicose veins may worsen. Care must be taken to reduce sun exposure in photosensitive people (such as those with systemic lupus erythematosus). Those who might lose consciousness from conditions like epilepsy, hypoglycemia, and heart problems should avoid the pools. High blood pressure can improve with spa therapy, but be careful that it does not drop too low or you will get dizzy and might fall or faint.

Mental, Spiritual, and Sensual Healing

The mental, spiritual, and sensual healing category includes such therapies as: placebo, relaxation and breathing exercises, stress reduction and relaxation, biofeedback, distraction techniques, visualization and guided imagery, meditation, hypnotherapy, yoga, prayer, spiritualism and religion, writing therapy, aromatherapy, music therapy, sound therapy, art therapy, dance therapy, and humour therapy. These methods involving the mind, spirit, and senses are totally compatible with the mainstream treatments of arthritis.

Many of these techniques are discussed in Chapter 5, "Pain and Fatigue" (relaxation and breathing exercises, stress reduction and relaxation, biofeedback, distraction therapy including guided imagery and visualization, meditation and hypnosis), and Chapter 12, "Exercises and Activities" (yoga). In this section, we will discuss prayer, writing therapy, and the sensual therapies (aromatherapy, and music, sound, art, dance, and humour therapies).

Stress, anxiety and depression can worsen the pain and other symptoms of arthritis and make you feel out of control. These techniques focus on the ways in which emotional, mental, social, and spiritual factors affect your health. They can reduce stress, depression, pain, and other symptoms associated with arthritis. They can give patients a sense of control and hope. These therapies are cheap, safe, and non-invasive. They do not involve the use of medications. However they do not help everyone and they require time, commitment, and lifestyle changes.

Prayer

Prayer is a tool used to appeal to a higher power in one's recognized religion or personal spirituality; prayer offers hope and promotes positive attitudes. Attending religious services provides social support and companionship. Participation in religion can enhance coping capabilities, quality of life, personal satisfaction, self-worth, self-esteem, and general well-being, and can reduce uncertainty, helplessness, dependency, and distress.

Studies show that religious people: have fewer physical and mental symptoms including pain; are less worried, depressed, and anxious; recover from surgery better; live longer; and use fewer medical resources. Some studies suggest that prayer and attendance at religious services may improve health. In one study of patients with various rheumatic diseases, the treatment group received five minutes of prayer by members of a church daily; this group did not fare any better than the placebo group. On the other hand, a study of intercessory prayer (individuals praying for the healing of other people) in long-standing, moderately severe rheumatoid arthritis showed significant short- and long-term physical improvement. Organized religion is not for everyone, however, and other spiritual pursuits should also be beneficial.

Writing therapy

Writing therapy can improve rheumatoid arthritis, although it may take up to four months to work. You have to write regularly about the most stressful events of your life and express your feelings about them. The writing should be in the form of a journal or letters that you never send to anyone.

Sensual therapies

Sensual therapies appeal to and engage at least one of the senses; they involve creating or experiencing art. Patients take an active role in their own care when applying these therapies. The sensual therapies do not cure diseases but they do reduce anxiety, promote relaxation, create distraction from pain and other symptoms, help one regain self-control, and improve wellness and quality of life. They are safe, non-invasive, and inexpensive. They include aromas, music, sound, art, dance, and humour.

Aromatherapy Aromatherapy delivers the fragrances of essential oils to the brain. They can be applied to the skin directly or by soaps, liniments, baths, and massages. They can be inhaled using steam, candles, or sprays. These essential oils are natural, high-quality, pure oils distilled from plants.

Music therapy Music therapy involves listening to or performing music under the guidance of a professional music therapist. It can involve listening to music, playing music, singing or chanting, or writing music. It can be done in a group or solo.

Sound therapy Sound therapy can be heard by the ear or felt as vibration by the body. Sound tapes or CDs of natural sounds (such as ocean waves or birds chirping) can reduce stress and promote relaxation. Sleeping can be made easier by masking other sounds with the help of a white-sound machine.

Sound can be focused on various areas of the body for therapy. It can also be applied to acupuncture points (sonopuncture). In conventional medicine, ultrasound is used for diagnostic imaging and for local pain relief. As lithotripsy (shock wave treatment), it is used to break down kidney stones and calcium deposits. Recently, it has been shown to help tennis elbow and plantar fasciitis in resistant cases.

Art therapy Art therapy uses the creation and appreciation of visual art to help ill people. The art could include painting, drawing, sculpting, mosaics, pottery, etc.

Art therapy can allow some people to express and communicate hidden feelings. It can provide insight, self-esteem, and distraction from the arthritis and pain. It can reduce stress, depression, anxiety, and loneliness, and facilitate rehabilitation. It was certainly of great benefit to Maud Lewis (see Introduction).

Dance therapy Dance therapy utilizes dance movements to help chronically ill people. Accomplished modern dancers teach it. It allows one to communicate feelings and release tension, anger, and frustration. It helps with relaxation, distraction, positive thoughts, and emotions. It can help loneliness, body image and confidence. It is also exercise that can improve muscle strength, conditioning, and coordination.

Humour therapy Humour therapy uses laughter to help people who are suffering from physical and emotional disorders. Funny people, books, videos, movies, toys, and CDs can bring on laughter. Humour can distract people from their pain and sickness, and can increase the production of endorphins, reduce muscle tension, stress, and depression, and improve communication and rapport with others.

Manual and Moving Bodyworks

The manual and moving bodyworks therapies include: manipulation, massage therapy, biofield therapeutics, reflexology, acupuncture, structural-functional (Alexander, Feldenkrais, Trager), yoga, qi gong, and tai chi. These therapies involve specific exercises and movements or manual manipulation done by others. Many of them are described in Chapter 12, "Exercises and Activities" (tai chi, qi gong, yoga, Alexander technique, Feldenkrais method, Trager approach, and Pilates system). There are few side effects but harm can occur from an incorrectly done action. They do not claim to cure disease, but do increase relaxation and reduce stress. Some claim to correct misalignments in the body, and others to augment or unblock the "energy flow" through the body.

Manipulation

Manipulation can be divided into three types: high velocity (popularized by chiropractic), low force, and craniosacral (both popularized by osteopathy). It is suggested that high-velocity manipulation improves the energy transmission through the nerves, that low-force manipulation improves the circulation of blood, and that craniosacral manipulation improves the movement of the cerebrospinal fluid around the brain and spinal cord. None of these theories is proven or even likely, however.

Manipulation appears to have a local effect on muscles and ligaments and a central effect on psychological relaxation. As a result, it is claimed that manipulation reduces pain, muscle spasm, and imbalances, and that it enhances function and range of movement. Studies of manipulation provide some proof that it can help mechanical neck and back pain, but not any better than conventional therapy or back education can. The benefits last up to several weeks. Manipulation may give some short-term relief from fibromyalgia and carpal tunnel syndrome, but symptoms can worsen in 1–2 percent of patients. Rarely, the vertebral arteries that supply blood to the brain can be injured by high-velocity neck manipulation, causing a stroke or sudden death. Unstable necks (as in rheumatoid arthritis) and stiff, brittle necks (as in ankylosing spondylitis) should not be manipulated.

Massage therapy

Massage is the manipulation of the muscles and soft tissues using pressure, stroking, etc. The philosophy of Eastern massage—which includes acupressure, shiatsu, and tuina—is to restore the healthy flow of the body's vital energy. The philosophy of Western massage is to relax muscles and tissues—included in this category are Swedish massage, deep tissue massage, trigger point therapy, myofascial release, skin-rolling massage, spray and stretch, and rolfing. Both the Eastern and Western types of massage result in relaxation, stress reduction, and easing of muscle tightness.

Massage can be done to different depths and with different pressures using fingers, thumbs, palms, elbows, and knees. Different movements can be used such as circular movements, gliding strokes, kneading, compressing, tapping, and vibration.

Massage can relax muscles, reduce stress and anxiety, loosen scar tissue or adhesions, and reduce edema and pain. An objective study showed that it does not increase the flow of blood to muscles, whereas light exercise does. There is no proof of long-term benefits, nor does it cure any diseases. It should not be used at sites of recent injury or phlebitis, and may have to be postponed in the presence of fever, infection, or acute inflammation. A registered massage therapist should be consulted for massage therapy.

Western massage Swedish massage uses stroking or kneading of the superficial layers of muscle over the whole body with lotions or oils. If done gently, it can be used in rheumatoid arthritis and fibromyalgia.

Deep tissue massage puts strong pressure on the deep muscles and tissues to reduce tension. It can cause soreness, but can be tried for muscle tightness and low back pain.

Trigger point therapy uses deep finger pressure on specific trigger points or muscle knots to relieve pain.

Myofascial release uses slow, gentle, steady pressure to stretch fascia (the connective tissue that surrounds muscle and organs and other tissues) to relieve tightness.

Skin-rolling massage may be painful at the start and may need anesthetic spray. It may help fibromyalgia.

Spray and stretch involves spraying a vapocoolant on the painful area to anesthetize it. The underlying muscle is then gently stretched. It can be used for myofascial syndromes and fibromyalgia.

Rolfing uses deep pressure to release the fascia so that body alignment, posture, and mobility improve. There are some other types of massage that include simultaneous psychotherapy and counselling.

Eastern massage Acupressure employs finger or hand pressure over acupuncture points to improve the flow of qi; it may help chronic backache. Shiatsu is a Japanese variant of acupressure that also incorporates stretching and massage; it is supposed to improve the flow of ki. Tuina is a traditional Chinese type of massage over pressure points.

Biofield therapeutics

Biofield or western energy therapies include polarity therapy, therapeutic touch, and reiki. The therapist uses the hands to restore the proper flow of the body's vital life energy; acupuncture points are not involved. These treatments are safe and gentle.

Polarity therapy Polarity therapy tries to balance the positive and negative currents of energy in the body to attain good health. The therapist touches key points on the body softly to balance and unblock the flow of energy. Sometimes gentle massage is added.

Therapeutic touch Therapeutic touch is based on the theory that there are energy fields that extend beyond the boundaries of our physical body. The therapist's hands enter these energy fields to smooth over any problem areas. Restoring these energy fields to normal can improve a person's health. One study suggested that this technique could reduce pain and improve function when applied to osteoarthritic knees. However, another study cast doubt on the concept of detecting energy fields around the body.

Reiki Reiki is Japanese for "spiritually guided universal life energy." Without touching the person being treated, the therapist channels spiritual energy into the patient to promote healing. An uncontrolled study showed that reiki could reduce pain.

Reflexology

Reflexology was derived from Zone therapy, which divided the body into 10 equal zones running from head to toe. In reflexology, organs and body parts are represented on the soles, sides, and tops of the feet. These areas in the feet are called reflexes. Gentle pressure on a specific reflex sends energy through these vertical zones to the corresponding organ or body part, causing it to heal. It has been suggested that it might lessen stiffness in rheumatoid arthritis and osteoarthritis and help Raynaud's phenomenon; however, so far, there is no proof of this. Reflexology may result in a sense of well-being and relaxation. It is safe and can be self-administered.

Acupuncture

Acupuncture is supposed to restore health and control pain by stimulating the acupuncture points that lie along the 14 meridians that run from head to toe. The qi (or vital life force) flows through these meridians, linking the external world to the inner body. There are over a thousand acupuncture points, each of which controls a particular body organ or function. The stimulation of these acupoints corrects problems affecting the flow of qi.

The Western explanation is that acupuncture releases endorphins and other chemical messengers in the body. To treat a condition, 10 to 12 acupoints need to be stimulated for about 20 minutes. An acute sprain or backache may take a few sessions to treat, but a chronic condition like arthritis may take one to two treatments per week for a few months.

Needle acupuncture uses fine, stainless steel needles that are twirled. Electroacupuncture sends a low current of electricity through the needle. Acupressure uses the pressure of a finger, roller, ball, or pointer over the acupoint. Moxibustion uses heat to stimulate the acupoint by burning the moxa herb over it. Magnets, low-frequency lasers, bee stings, and venom injections have also been used. Cupping uses heated jars that are put upside down over the acupoints. As they cool, a vacuum is created that suctions them to the skin. In aural acupuncture, the ear becomes a map of the body and needles are inserted into the appropriate areas of the ear for the condition being treated (e.g., drug addiction and neck pain). If the needles are inserted too deeply, they could injure nerves or other soft tissues. Sterile or disposable needles should be used to prevent the spread of infections such as hepatitis B.

Studies have shown that acupuncture can reduce the pain caused by surgery, fibromyalgia, osteoarthritis of the knee, rheumatoid arthritis, and arthritis of the back. Uncontrolled studies suggested that it could help depression and Raynaud's phenomenon. Other studies showed that it did not help psoriasis, Sjogren's syndrome, systemic lupus erythematosus, scleroderma, or the spondyloarthropathies.

Electromagnetic and Other Radiations

The electromagnetic and other radiations group of therapies use some form of energy to induce healing. This group includes magnets, pulsed electromagnetic therapy, electrotherapy (electro acupuncture and TENS), low-energy laser therapy, light therapy, and radon pads and inactive uranium mines. Electrical therapy delivered by acupuncture or transcutaneous nerve stimulation (TENS) is discussed in Chapter 5, "Pain and Fatigue," and in the section about acupuncture above.

Magnets

Magnets are applied to the painful areas. Stagnant magnets have a magnetic field but no electrical field. The strength of the magnets used for treatment ranges from 300 to 4000 G (Gauss). They can be applied to the skin as strips or discs, or can be incorporated into braces, splints, wraps, car seats or cushions, mattresses, insoles, and collars.

Studies have shown that magnets can reduce post-polio pain and pain due to diabetic nerve damage in the feet. Although magnets can reduce the inflammation in the joints of a rat model of arthritis, they have not been shown to help arthritis in humans. Magnets should be avoided if you have a pacemaker or other implanted electronic device. There is no harm in trying magnets otherwise, but be careful about the cost.

Pulsed electromagnetic therapy

This type of therapy supplies both an electrical and magnetic field to the area being treated. The painful area is put into a circular magnetic coil through which a low-level electric current is sent in pulses. The optimal strength applied to the area is less than 60 Hz for 6 to 10 hours per day.

This therapy stimulates bone cells (osteoblasts) to form bone, and cartilage cells (chondrocytes) to multiply and produce cartilage. It may also reduce inflammation and pain. This therapy is presently being used to stimulate the healing of fractured bones that fail to unite.

Three studies have shown that it can reduce pain and increase function in osteoarthritis of the knee and cervical spine and delay the need for knee replacements. However there is no evidence yet that it can stimulate the growth of new cartilage. There is no proof that it benefits rheumatoid arthritis or carpal tunnel syndrome. It should not be used in the presence of a pacemaker or other electrical implant, or in people who have cancer or are pregnant. Otherwise it appears to be safe, but it is costly.

Low-energy laser therapy or cold laser

This type of laser light penetrates deep into the tissues without causing damage or heat. It is applied to the skin over the targeted area for about five minutes during each of about 15 sessions. Benefits can last up to one year.

Mixed results were found in 36 studies. In the four studies that were controlled, there was no clinically relevant improvement in osteoarthritis or rheumatoid arthritis. Eye damage can occur if one stares directly into the instrument. It is expensive.

Light therapy

Light therapy uses different types of light—such as full-spectrum or natural sunlight, bright light, ultraviolet light, and coloured light—to treat different diseases. It can be used to light a room, or to shine on a patient or on a specific diseased part of the body. Light therapy is used in mainstream medicine to treat psoriasis and some other skin conditions, seasonal affective disorder (SAD—a form of depression related to the lack of light during the winter months), and jaundice in newborns. Sunlight stimulates the body to produce active Vitamin D for stronger bones. Bright lighting also reduces eyestrain and fatigue and can improve sleep. Unfortunately, sunlight can cause skin cancer and flare up disease in photosensitive individuals such as those with systemic lupus erythematosus. There is no evidence that light therapy can cure arthritis or autoimmune diseases or that it can regulate the immune system.

Radon pads and uranium mines

Radon is a radioactive gas produced by the atomic disintegration of radium. It is a health hazard. "Radon pads" that are supposed to emit radiation have not been found to be an effective therapy for arthritis. Sitting in an abandoned uranium mine—which is supposed to expose you and your arthritis to radon—has not proven useful as a treatment for rheumatoid arthritis.

Diet and Nutrition

Our health is affected by what we eat. As an example, eating a diet of fibre, fruits, and vegetables will reduce obesity and the incidence of heart disease and some types of cancer. Sometimes, fasting and enemas are used to "eliminate toxins." However, there is no evidence that these "toxins" exist: they have not been specifically identified. There are no miracle diets for arthritis. Mainstream and complementary dietary issues regarding arthritis are discussed in Chapter 11, "Diet and Nutrition."

Botanical Therapies

Botanical therapies or herbal medicines are plants or parts of plants (flowers, seeds, leaves, stems, roots, or bark) that are used to treat health problems. A true expert should have knowledge of botany, chemistry, and pharmacology. These agents are usually safe for minor ailments that would often be self-medicated, but they should not be used alone to treat serious medical problems. Pregnant women should probably avoid them.

Botanical therapies contain many chemicals. Some of them are the beneficial parts of the herb, and some may be toxic or inhibitory parts of the herb. The concentrations of the active ingredients can vary depending on the growing conditions (e.g., the soil and climate), the degree of maturity of the plant at the time of harvesting, the manner of preparation and drying, the species used, the parts of the plant used, the conditions of storage, and the age of the plant. As a result, standardization is difficult to achieve. Although they are natural, medicinal herbs can still cause side effects, allergic reactions, interactions with other drugs, and interference with lab tests.

Modern pharmacology will isolate the active ingredients from promising botanical treatments. About 25 percent of our conventional drugs are derived from plants. Some examples include aspirin (white willow bark), digitalis (foxglove plant), morphine (opium poppy), quinine (cinchona tree), vinblastine and vincristine (periwinkle), senna (leaves and pods of senna plant), taxol (yew tree), and ephedrine (ephedra or ma huang plant).

Because medicinal herbs are marketed as food supplements, they are not regulated. Although claims cannot be made that they treat, cure, prevent, or diagnose diseases, there are no purity standards or quality controls. Your purchase may contain impurities, foreign materials, conventional drugs, and animal and insect parts and feces. The amount of active ingredient will vary from container to container and from product to product; some products may not even contain the active ingredient. The labels rarely list the side effects or harmful interactions of the contents. The scientific name of the herb, its country of origin, and the parts of the plant used are also not shown. European (especially German) botanical therapies are regulated much better than elsewhere.

Herbs are available in many forms. Raw herbs are better if they are picked fresh or freeze-dried because the air-dried ones tend to lose their potency as they age. Herb extracts are concentrated forms of the plant sold as tablets, capsules, or powder. Tinctures are alcohol-based extracts of the herb. Infusions or teas are water-based extracts of the herb. Herbs can also be applied to the skin as poultices or salves.

It is worth obtaining reliable information about a botanical treatment before trying it. Refer to Appendix II for further information.

Alfalfa There have been suggestions but no proof that alfalfa can help arthritis. However, large amounts may cause systemic lupus erythematosus to flare up due to an ingredient called l-canavanine.

Aloe *(aloe vera)* There is no scientific proof that aloe gel taken orally will help arthritis. It may be soothing if applied to a sore joint as a gel or lotion.

Arnica When applied externally to sore areas as a tincture, it can diminish aches and pains.

Boswellia *(boswellia serrata)* This herb is also known as frankincense. It seems to have anti-inflammatory properties. A German study showed that it did not help rheumatoid arthritis. However, two other studies showed that it was effective for treating osteoarthritis and rheumatoid arthritis when combined with ginger, turmeric, and ashwagandha. Another study suggested that it reduced pain and stiffness in osteoarthritic patients when combined with turmeric and a zinc compound. It can cause nausea, diarrhea, and rash.

Devil's claw *(harpagophytum procumbens)* The active ingredient is thought to be harpagoside. It is taken from the roots of the plant for its presumed anti-inflammatory and painkilling properties. In French studies, it reduced pain and increased mobility in people with osteoarthritis. It relieved pain better than placebo in trials of low back pain. There is no evidence that it helps rheumatoid arthritis. It is well tolerated. However, because it stimulates stomach secretions, it should be avoided in people with peptic ulcers. It should not be used by pregnant women because it stimulates contractions of the uterus. It can interact with coumadin.

Echinacea *(echinacea purpurea, echinacea angustifolia)* This herb does not help arthritis. It is mentioned here because it is supposed to stimulate the immune system. Therefore it is not advisable to use it if you have rheumatoid arthritis, systemic lupus erythematosus, or another autoimmune disease.

Feverfew *(tanacetum parthenium)* This herb is used to treat migraines. Although it may have anti-inflammatory activity, a study showed that it did not help rheumatoid arthritis.

Ginkgo *(ginkgo biloba)* A German study showed that this herb increased the blood flow in the capillaries of the fingers. It was suggested that it could improve Raynaud's phenomenon, but so far there are no studies confirming this theory. It can cause mild headaches, stomach upset, and prolonged bleeding in those taking blood thinners.

Ginseng *(American, Asian, and Siberian)* Ginseng does not help arthritis but the Asian and Siberian varieties are touted to boost energy. This herb could increase the effects of steroids, estrogens, and blood thinners.

Marijuana *(cannabis sativa, cannabis indica)* Marijuana is made from the leaves, stems, and seeds of these hemp plants. It contains many different chemicals, but the cannabinoids are the ones most studied. They have analgesic and anti-inflammatory actions, and can enhance the effects of narcotics. Marijuana appears to be able to reduce the pain of muscle spasticity in multiple sclerosis and the chronic pain of cancer. There is only anecdotal evidence that it helps the pain of arthritis. The euphoria and relaxation it induces could also help the symptoms of arthritis. It is available in synthetic oral forms for controlling nausea and vomiting and stimulating the appetite. However, these oral forms have little analgesic effect compared to smoked marijuana. Attempts are being made to administer these compounds by nasal spray, inhaled aerosol, or skin patch to relieve pain.

Moducare *(pinus maritima, pinus pinaster)* This agent is made up of beta-sitosterol and beta-sitosterol glucoside from pine trees. They reduce the production of the cytokines IL-6 and tumour necrosis factor, which help produce autoimmune diseases. A pilot study suggests that this product might help rheumatoid arthritis. More studies are needed before it can be recommended. It is safe but should not be used during pregnancy or while breastfeeding, or in someone with organ transplants or multiple sclerosis.

Phytodolor (tincture of *populus tremula, fraxinus excelsior,* and *solidago virgaurea*) These plants are better known as aspen (leaf and bark), ash (bark), and goldenrod (aerial), respectively. This compound of herbs contains salicine, flavonoids, and isofraxidine. It proved to be better than placebo in several studies involving people with various arthritic conditions including rheumatoid arthritis, osteoarthritis, back pain, and epicondylitis of the elbow (tennis elbow). Some people experience gastrointestinal upset or allergic reactions.

St. John's wort *(hypericum perforatum)* This herb helps mild to moderate depression and insomnia. It needs to be taken for several weeks before an effect is noted. It may increase one's sensitivity to the sun, so people with systemic lupus erythematosus should be particularly careful when using it.

Stinging nettle *(urtica dioica)* Stewed nettle leaves might reduce the amount of anti-inflammatory drugs you take. The leaves can be taken orally or applied as a poultice. Stinging yourself with the nettles is painful and probably not therapeutic. In one study, stinging nettle led to a reduction in the dose of diclofenac used to treat osteoarthritis. There are no side effects, except for the possibility of allergy. Another study showed that a stew made from the aerial parts of this plant helped rheumatoid arthritis.

Thunder god vine *(tripterygium wilfordii hook F)* The active ingredients, triptolide and tripdiolide, are found in the roots. They interfere with the production of chemicals that mediate immune responses and inflammation. In studies of rheumatoid arthritis, this herb improved the symptoms and blood tests (such as the ESR and rheumatoid factor). It benefited the symptoms and lab tests and allowed the reduction of prednisone doses in uncontrolled studies of systemic lupus erythematosus. Further studies need to be done to substantiate its efficacy in psoriatic arthritis, ankylosing spondylitis, scleroderma, and other autoimmune diseases. The leaves and flowers of this plant are quite toxic. Side effects include rashes, skin pigmentation, gastrointestinal upset (especially diarrhea), loss of menstrual periods, suppression of sperm production, and low white blood cell counts. Treatment deaths are rare but have been reported to be due to heart and lung damage and shock.

Turmeric *(curcuma longa, curcuma domestica)* The active ingredient is curcumin. When combined with boswellia and zinc, turmeric inhibits inflammation and stimulates the production of cortisone. The combination of this herb with boswellia, ginger, and aswangandha improved the symptoms of rheumatoid arthritis and osteoarthritis in two studies. It is safe, but patients with gallstones or pregnancies are cautioned not to use it.

Wild yam (*dioscorea villosa*) Wild yam contains steroids, but not in a form that can be utilized by your body. There are no studies to prove that it is anti-inflammatory.

Willow bark Willow bark contains salicin, a source of aspirin. It can reduce pain in osteoarthritis of the knees and hips. A study showed that it also reduced the pain of cervical and lumbar arthritis. However, you would have to drink a lot of willow bark tea to equal two aspirins.

Zoological Therapies

This section deals with complementary therapies that are derived from animal sources. These therapies include shark cartilage, bovine cartilage, New Zealand green-lipped mussel, rattlesnake meat, snake venoms, ant venom, bee venoms, and other bee products. Fish oils, a source of omega-3 fatty acids, are discussed in Chapter 11, "Diet and Nutrition."

Shark cartilage

Shark cartilage is prepared from the skeletons of sharks. Unlike most animals, sharks' skeletons are made totally of cartilage and not bone. The cartilage is ground into powder and sterilized, and then distributed for use as a powder, capsule, or injection into muscle.

It has anti-inflammatory properties and prevents the growth of new blood vessels and tumours. It is promoted for the treatment of osteoarthritis, rheumatoid arthritis, psoriasis, and discoid lupus erythematosus, but there is no evidence to support its use in these conditions. It has no side effects but some varieties have an unpleasant odour or taste. If it is not white, then it contains impurities. It should be labelled "100 percent pure shark cartilage." Usage should be stopped if there is no improvement after six weeks.

Bovine cartilage

Bovine cartilage is obtained from the tracheas or noses of cows. It too may have anti-inflammatory and anti-cancer activities. There is no good evidence that it helps arthritis, however.

New Zealand green-lipped mussel

A secret extract of the New Zealand green-lipped mussel is being sold as a treatment for rheumatoid arthritis and osteoarthritis. It contains a viscous substance or mucus similar to the hyaluronic acid that is the main constituent of the fluid found in normal joints. There is no proof that it works.

Rattlesnake meat

Capsules of dried rattlesnake meat do not help arthritis. They should not be used because they can contain salmonella bacteria, a cause of food poisoning.

Snake venoms

Snake venoms have been used to treat arthritis. Cobra venom can transiently deplete the levels of complement, which is a series of proteins that help mediate immune reactions in the body. Two venom-based drugs (cobroxin and nyloxin), marketed for the treatment of pain, arthritis, and other disorders, were banned from the American market because they did not work. In animal experiments, cobra venom prevented or delayed the arthritis from starting, but failed to reduce the inflammation or alter the course of the arthritis once it had started. Another approach to reduce inflammation is to use venom from the Malaysian pit viper (arvin) to deplete fibrin. However, this approach failed as a treatment in an animal model of arthritis. Snake venom should be avoided because it is ineffective and could have serious side effects.

Ant venom

Ant venom from the South American tree ant (*Pseudomyrmex sp.*) was superior to placebo when used to treat rheumatoid arthritis. However, all patients receiving this product developed side effects, including painful skin lesions at the site of the injections, fever, chills, and anemia.

Bee venoms

Bee venom therapy began with bees actually stinging the patients. Treatment prescriptions varied from five stings per week to hundreds of stings over several months. Needless to say, this treatment is unpleasant, painful, and fear provoking. Allergic reactions can occur. Bee venom was then purified and given by injections under the skin of patients with rheumatoid arthritis, but it proved to be ineffective. Then, components of the bee venom were studied separately. Although some of them had anti-inflammatory properties, their performance in animal models of arthritis was not impressive. Furthermore, it is difficult and expensive to get the needed amounts of these substances to test in humans. So far, bee stings and purified bee venom have not proved useful for the treatment of arthritis in humans.

Other bee products

Other bee products have been promoted to increase endurance and energy. They are royal jelly, propolis, bee pollen, and raw honey. There is no medical evidence that these substances have any therapeutic value, however. Royal jelly has been reported to bring on acute attacks of asthma. Bee pollen is often contaminated with insect feces and eggs, rodent debris, fungi, and bacteria.

Pharmaceuticals and Nutraceuticals

Complementary pharmaceutical therapies are drugs that are being used for unproven reasons. Nutraceutical therapies are foods or food ingredients considered to have medical or health benefits. Because nutraceuticals are not classified as drugs, they bypass the need for expensive testing and vigorous efficacy trials. The pharmaceuticals often require prescriptions, but the nutraceuticals do not. Included in the pharmaceutical and nutraceutical category are vitamins, minerals, cartilage preparations, hormones, antimicrobials, vaccines, amino acids and DMSO (dimethylsulfoxide), and miscellaneous drugs.

Vitamins

The value of vitamins for the treatment of arthritis is discussed in Chapter 11, "Diet and Nutrition," in the sections dealing with antioxidants and with vitamins. In summary, Vitamins B3, B5, D, and E may have minimal beneficial effects on arthritis. Vitamin D is essential to prevent osteoporosis, but excess quantities of Vitamins A and D can be harmful. There is no evidence that huge doses of vitamins (megavitamins) help arthritis, even when combined with minerals and other nutrients (orthomolecular therapy).

Minerals

The use of minerals to treat arthritis is discussed in Chapter 11, "Diet and Nutrition." Minerals can be obtained from foods, and also from multivitamins. Unfortunately, mineral supplementation offers only minor improvement in arthritis apart from the use of conventional gold therapy.

Cartilage preparations

Cartilage is made up of collagen (mainly type II), proteoglycans (PGs), and water. Collagen and components of PGs like glucosamine and chondroitin sulfate are being studied for use in mainly osteoarthritis.

Glucosamine Glucosamine is needed to make and to repair cartilage. It stimulates the cartilage cells to produce the PGs and it has mild anti-inflammatory properties. Glucosamine supplements are extracted from crab, lobster, and shrimp shells. It is unlikely that reactions would occur in someone who is allergic to shellfish, but caution is advised.

Different forms of glucosamine are available, including sulfate, hydrochloride, and N-acetyl. There is no definite proof that one is more potent than another. The gastrointestinal tract absorbs 26–90 percent of the glucosamine.

Numerous studies have looked at glucosamine treatment in osteoarthritis, and although many of these studies were flawed, they suggested that glucosamine is beneficial. It can ease the stiffness, pain, tenderness, and swelling of joints affected by osteoarthritis and can lessen disability. It may perform just as well as NSAIDs such as ibuprofen and piroxicam, but with fewer side effects. There is no good evidence yet that glucosamine can restore the damaged cartilage. It is probably not as useful in joints with severe cartilage loss. It takes about two to eight weeks to work. The benefit may last for some weeks after the glucosamine is stopped. Nausea and indigestion seldom occur. Blood sugar levels should be monitored a little more closely in people with diabetes in case they rise.

Chondroitin sulfate Chondroitin sulfate is a component of cartilage. It is important for the normal metabolism of cartilage and it may have anti-inflammatory activity. Several studies have shown that it can reduce pain, disability, and the dose of NSAIDs needed in osteoarthritis, but there is no good proof yet that it restores the lost cartilage. It may not be as effective for joints with severe cartilage loss. Chondroitin sulfate takes at least two months to work, and its benefit may last for some time after it is discontinued. It is often used with glucosamine. Because it is a large molecule, absorption from the gastrointestinal tract is restricted (about 10 percent of the amount swallowed). It is safe but can prolong bleeding in those taking blood thinners. Sometimes nausea and indigestion occur. Chondroitin sulfate appears to be useful for osteoarthritis but more studies are needed.

Most preparations come from the tracheas of cows, and it is hoped that the cows were not infected with BSE (mad cow disease). Shark cartilage is a less common source of chondroitin sulfate because the ingredients are more variable and heavy metal contamination may occur.

Collagen, gelatin, and collagen hydrolysate Collagen (especially type II) is a major component of cartilage. This type of therapy was proposed because it might stimulate the cartilage cells to produce more collagen to heal the cartilage. Collagen supplements are obtained from the cartilage of sharks, cows, and chickens.

Gelatin products are another source of supplementary cartilage collagen. None of these have improved osteoarthritis.

An altered form of collagen, collagen hydrolysate, resulted in pain reduction in osteoarthritis of the hips and knees in one study carried out over 60 days. Another reason for using type II collagen is to suppress the immune reaction to joints in rheumatoid arthritis. Small doses of type II chicken collagen improved rheumatoid arthritis but larger doses did not. A study of type II cartilage from cattle did not help rheumatoid arthritis. Collagen is safe. However, the types and amounts of collagen can vary from preparation to preparation. Further research is needed in this area before recommendations can be made.

Hormones

Complementary hormone therapies that have been promoted for arthritis include melatonin, dehydroepiandrosterone (DHEA), and Liefcort.

Melatonin Melatonin is a hormone secreted by the pineal gland located in the brain. It regulates sleeping and waking times. Therapeutic doses of this hormone are supposed to boost the immune system and improve the quantity and quality of sleep one gets. In one study, fibromyalgia sufferers slept better using a nightly dose of melatonin. It may cause headaches and bad dreams, however, and it should not be used in people with autoimmune diseases because it is supposed to stimulate the immune system.

DHEA DHEA is a steroid hormone secreted by the adrenal gland. It is converted to male hormones (androgens) and female hormones (estrogens). When used as a treatment, it has predominantly male hormone effects, and androgens tend to suppress the immune system. Studies suggest that DHEA reduces pain, inflammation, fatigue, and prednisone doses in patients with systemic lupus erythmatosus. More studies are required, however.

DHEA is often manufactured from wild yams, but eating wild yams should not be relied upon as a source of DHEA because it is not in a form that can be utilized by the body. The products sold in stores can vary in amount and purity. The most reliable source of DHEA is a compounding pharmacy. Side effects include acne, hormonal effects on the breasts, uterus, and prostate gland, and liver abnormalities, especially in patients taking methotrexate or azathioprine. In women, it can cause balding, hair growth on the face and body, and a deeper voice. It may also raise estrogen levels and lower the beneficial HDL cholesterol.

Liefcort In the 1960s Dr. Liefmann, from Montreal, mixed prednisone, estradiol, and testosterone together in a potion that was called Liefcort and later Rheumatril. The female hormone, estradiol, and the male hormone, testosterone, were to prevent the side effects of the corticosteroid, prednisone. It was taken as a liquid under the tongue. Of course it was effective for the treatment of arthritis because of the prednisone (usual dose 15 mg per day). However, the patients still developed most of the side effects of the prednisone and then had difficulty weaning from the Liefcort.

Antimicrobials

Theories pop up about the cause of some types of arthritis being due to an infection. Although there may be absolutely no proof, someone will start promoting antibiotics as a cure.

In mainstream medicine, joints can be infected with bacteria, fungi, tuberculosis, and viruses. These organisms can be found in the joint and the infected joint can be treated with antimicrobials (this will not work for the viruses).

Lyme disease, rheumatic fever, and reactive arthritis are due to the body's reaction to an infection elsewhere in the body. Antibiotics do not cure these types of arthritis in the same way as they do an infected joint.

In other instances, antimicrobials have been used to treat arthritis successfully, but for the wrong reasons: the antibiotics were not acting by killing an infection, but instead had other properties that were beneficial. These properties include anti-inflammatory activity, immune suppression, and ability to block certain enzymes that play a role in arthritis. Examples include hydroxychloroquine, minocycline and doxycycline, gold, and sulfasalazine. However, metronidazole and clotrimazole were used to eradicate amoeba that were thought to cause rheumatoid arthritis, even though amoeba-like organisms have never been proven to cause it; these antimicrobials were not useful to treat rheumatoid arthritis.

Vaccines

Vaccine therapy for arthritis was popular in the 1930s and 1940s, when it was given to induce fever ("fever therapy"). This type of treatment was abandoned, however, because of the side effects and the failure to achieve sustained benefit. Vaccine therapy was resurrected in the 1970s using mixtures of influenza and bacterial vaccines, but its efficacy could not be confirmed.

Amino acids and DMSO

This group includes the amino acids (tryptophan, histidine, and S-adenosylmethionine [SAMe]) and the DMSO chemicals (DMSO [dimethylsulfoxide] and its derivative MSM [methylsulfonylmethane]).

L-tryptophan L-tryptophan is sold as a treatment for depression, anxiety, sleep disturbances, and premenstrual syndrome. However, a specific manufacturer in Japan produced a variant of this amino acid that led to a serious rheumatic condition called eosinophilia-myalgia syndrome.

Histidine Histidine is readily available from food. Because histidine levels are low in rheumatoid arthritis, treatment with histidine supplements has been promoted as a therapy, but there is no evidence that histidine helps rheumatoid arthritis.

SAMe SAMe is supposed to improve arthritis by reducing pain, improving joint mobility, and supporting cartilage production. It may act as an antidepressant and prevent liver damage. In studies of osteoarthritis, its therapeutic effect was better than placebo and equivalent to ibuprofen. In other studies, it was found to be better than placebo and as good as standard antidepressants in treating depression. It may occasionally cause nausea or indigestion. It is worth a trial for joint pain and depression, but more studies are needed especially in regard to the claims about protecting the cartilage. Do not use SAMe with methotrexate as there might be interference with the methotrexate.

DMSO DMSO is a by-product of the pulp and paper industry. It is a solvent and can penetrate and transport other chemicals through the skin internally. It can dilate blood vessels to increase the blood flow (vasodilatation) and alter collagen. Some of its other actions are analgesic and anti-inflammatory.

DMSO can be applied externally as a liquid or a gel to the skin over arthritic joints and other painful areas, and can be taken orally and by injection as well.

There is a great deal of experience with DMSO that indicates its efficacy in treating rheumatoid arthritis, osteoarthritis, tendonitis, bursitis, muscle pains, sprains, and strains, but the results from controlled trials are conflicting. It has been used to treat scleroderma (with possible benefit for healing the finger ulcers and improving the Raynaud's phenomenon), Sjogren's syndrome, and reflex sympathetic dystrophy, but again the evidence is not clear-cut. Better studies are needed. It can take six to eight weeks to work.

Do not use the industrial grades of DMSO. Your hands should be washed because it will dissolve anything on your hands and transport it through your skin to your mouth where you will taste it and breathe it out. It causes the taste of onions or garlic in your mouth and bad breath. Sometimes it can irritate the skin to which it is applied.

MSM MSM is derived from DMSO. It is found naturally in fresh fruits and vegetables, milk, fish, and grains, but the processing of food can destroy it. MSM is safe, and can be taken orally or applied as a lotion. It can reduce pain and inflammation and alter collagen. It has been promoted for the treatment of numerous conditions—including arthritis, lupus, back pain, bursitis, tendonitis, fibromyalgia, carpal tunnel syndrome, and temperomandibular joint syndrome—however, no well-controlled human studies have been done to substantiate these claims.

Miscellaneous drugs

Many other drugs have been touted as remedies for arthritis. Guaifenesin, gerovital, and the Mexicali cure have been selected for discussion here.

Guaifenesin Guaifenesin is an ingredient of many cough medicines and decongestants. Some people taking these agents noticed easing of their symptoms of fibromyalgia and rheumatoid arthritis. There is no proof that this drug can help these conditions, although one recent trial suggested that some people with fibromyalgia were helped. It is safe but because of its effect on uric acid, people with gout or kidney stones should avoid it.

Gerovital H3 Gerovital H3 contains procaine hydrochloride and was promoted in Romania as a fountain of youth and anti-arthritis therapy. Procaine hydrochloride is Novocaine, the local anesthetic, which can be given orally or by injection. Severe reactions are rare. There are no controlled studies to support its use as a therapy for arthritis.

Mexicali cure Many people with arthritis have been lured to Mexico, particularly Mexicali, to get treatment: each physician there sees about a hundred patients per day. The patients are sold a four-to-six-month supply of unlabelled wonder drugs, which, they are told, do not contain corticosteroids. The side effects of the drugs are not described, and there is no careful monitoring of the treatment. The arthritis improves. However, later, side effects appear and eventually the pills are analyzed. They turn out to contain various forms of corticosteroids, tranquilizers like diazepam (Valium), NSAIDs like indomethacin and phenylbutazone, antihistamines, and antibiotics. All these drugs are available in Canada. Do not fall for the Mexicali cure.

Miscellaneous Complementary Treatments

There is no end to the array of unproven remedies for arthritis. People have been buried in horse manure up to the neck, or have entered ultra-cold freezers in their bathing suits to do exercises, or, on a more pleasant note, have inhaled the gases emitted from apple brandy.

Copper bracelets and other jewellery have been used to stave off the symptoms of arthritis for eons. Research has shown that when copper is in contact with skin, it can dissolve in human sweat and permeate through the skin. Not everyone believes that this actually occurs with copper jewellery, however, as it is often finished with a coating that prevents the copper from touching the skin anyway. In one study, which compared copper bracelets to aluminum bracelets as a therapy for arthritis, a significant number of patients noted improvement in their arthritis symptoms after wearing a copper bracelet as opposed to an aluminum one. There is not enough proof to recommend copper bracelets, but they will not cause any harm. Just don't spend too much money for one.

Sticking with jewellery, it was noticed that the X-ray damage to the finger joints in rheumatoid arthritis was less in the fingers that bore a gold ring.

Myriad fluids and balms have been applied to arthritic joints. The list includes snake oil, cod liver oil, olive oil, peanut oil, motor oil, WD-40, turpentine, brake fluid, gasoline, kerosene, lighter fluid, silicone lubricant, and castor oil with myrrh. Some of these fluids are flammable. They can cause local skin irritation, allergic reactions, and chemical pneumonia from inhaling the fumes. Asian medicated oils and liniments may contain some of these agents, for example, turpentine oil in Hung Far and menthol and camphor in Tiger Balm. These skin rubs have not been tested for efficacy, but if you do pursue this avenue of therapy, at least choose the least toxic agent.

In summary, complementary therapies are becoming ever more popular in the treatment of arthritis and other chronic conditions, and some therapies may actually have some benefit. Others are nothing but a get-rich-quick scheme for their sellers, and may actually harm people with arthritis. You are urged to continue taking the medication your doctor has prescribed for you, and consult with your doctor about any complementary therapies you may want to try in addition to the mainstream medicine you are already using. Be sure that you become informed about any treatments that you are thinking about, that you are aware of expected effects and side effects, and that these treatments will not interact negatively with each other or with your other medications.

9 Research

Research has led to great advances in the treatment of arthritis in the last few years, and we now have a plethora of drugs that are used in its management. Methotrexate remains the gold standard for the treatment of rheumatoid arthritis, but several significant advances have recently been made, with the approval of leflunomide and the biological modifiers etanercept and infliximab.

None of these drugs would have been approved and available for use if patients with rheumatoid arthritis had not consented to be tested to see if the drugs were effective and safe. We now have sophisticated computer modelling, elaborate laboratory testing in which a drug's effects on tissues and cells can be analyzed, and extensive animal testing, but the only way to be sure that a drug works safely in humans is to test it on humans.

After being presented with some exciting beneficial effects of a drug in the mouse, an old sage once stated, "If a mouse comes to my office, I will use the drug." The implication is that we must have human data and cannot merely extrapolate from animal data. Clinical trials are carefully designed and monitored experiments that allow us to determine if drugs are effective and safe.

Why Do People Participate in Research Studies?

Patients' most common reason for participating in studies is that, despite trying all available therapies for their particular type of arthritis, they still do not have adequate control of their disease. So when a new drug comes along that shows promise, and the patients are offered the opportunity to try the new drug long before it becomes approved and available for general use, they take it.

Patients also agree to participate for purely altruistic reasons: they are aware that new drugs will not be released unless human trials take place, and even if they themselves may not directly benefit, their participation can help others.

It would be rare that a patient who enjoys complete remission with a current treatment would be asked to participate in a clinical trial.

What Is a Clinical Research Study?

A clinical research study (clinical trial) is a closely supervised evaluation of a medication or therapy to determine its safety and effectiveness for a specific disease. The patients receive medication, and physicians or other health professionals evaluate their responses to the medication.

All such trials must follow strict rules and stick to a detailed protocol, which is reviewed by a research and ethics committee. This committee is an independent group of medical and non-medical professionals and laypeople. They are entirely unconnected with the investigators and do not participate in the study, but do carefully monitor it. Their job is to ensure that the science of the study is sound, that the risk to the patients is acceptable, and, most importantly, that the participants in the study are completely informed about these risks and all of their options and rights.

Such trials generally fall into two groups: open-label and comparative. In an open-label study, the patient and the evaluator both know what treatment is being administered. The purpose of such a study is to determine if a drug works at all before embarking on a more rigorous comparative trial.

In a comparative (or controlled) trial, one group of patients receives the medication under study, while the other group (control group) receives either the traditional and approved drug or a placebo (an inert or inactive substance that looks exactly like the drug being tested). There may also be three groups, in which the new drug, the standard drug, and the placebo are compared. What a patient will receive is determined through randomization: the patient is chosen at random (like the toss of coin) to receive a particular numbered medication. Moreover, clinical trials are usually double-blind, which means that neither the patient nor the evaluator knows which drug the patient is receiving. Only at the end of the study is it revealed exactly what the patient was taking. All of these measures are crucial to avoid any bias on the evaluator's part.

How Do I Join a Clinical Research Study?

The first step in the process is to sign a consent form, which will be reviewed and approved by the ethics board. The form outlines in plain language the purpose of the study, the risks and potential side effects of the drug, the fact that you might be receiving a placebo, and that neither you nor the evaluators would be aware of this. The form itemizes the blood tests, X-rays, or other investigations that will be ordered and the risk, if any, of these tests. The number of tests and the number of visits over a specified period of time are clearly stated. The form also outlines the patient's rights, which include the right to decline to participate (the right to withdraw from the study at any time without in any way affecting future treatment). You can ask questions and expect immediate answers at any time before or during the study. You will receive treatment and compensation for any research-related side effect or injury, and you will immediately be informed of any new findings about the study drug that may influence your willingness to continue. This would include, for example, the occurrence of a side effect with the study medication that was not known at the start of the study.

Each drug you are taking or have taken in the past has gone through a rigorous development process, which included many steps and years of research before approval was given for human experimentation. The earliest phases of testing involve a very few patients who are given the drug in various doses and are very closely monitored with no blinding. The final step is a randomized double-blind controlled trial in a large group of patients who must meet rigid criteria. There are risks and these risks must be outlined in detail. Since the drug is new, once a large number of patients take the drug for a longer period of time, unexpected side effects can occur. This is why patients are so closely monitored and a phone call away from help. Patients who enter studies have an inadequate response to traditional therapy or have had unacceptable side effects with these drugs or they would not enter a study. Indeed they must exhibit disease activity to be allowed to enter according to the protocol. They enter in the hope they will benefit and accept the risk of being on placebo and the potential of side effects that have been outlined in the consent form. Even in this scenario there is altruism and a desire to contribute to knowledge in the hope of helping others as well as themselves. People could easily take the position of letting someone else try it and if it proves to be safe and effective then they take it, but, happily, there are always those who are willing to participate both for personal and altruistic reasons.

Diseases such as rheumatoid arthritis are devastating, and patients who have not experienced remission and who understand the nature of the disease are more than willing to try new therapies. They need to be assured that the greatest care is taken in monitoring the administration of these drugs and that their safety and rights are paramount. Until we have the ideal drug—one that is effective, safe, affordable, and easy to take—we will continue looking for better drugs and testing those that make it through the rigorous pre-clinical and open-label studies. The research process will go on, and until a cure for arthritis is found, we will continue to try and help patients to live well with arthritis.

10 Surgery

Many advances have been made in joint surgery over the last few decades, including improvements in: anesthesia; the design of joint replacements; the metals, plastics, and cements used for joint replacements; arthroscopic joint surgery; and post-surgical rehabilitation.

This chapter deals with the benefits and risks of surgery, the various types of anesthesia and joint operations, and the preferred surgical procedures available for each joint. In addition, it lists the things you should know before and after surgery.

Benefits of Joint Surgery

The purpose of surgery is to relieve pain, improve function, free trapped nerve tissue, and prevent further damage. Surgery should not be done to improve the appearance of a joint.

Pain is relieved by removing inflamed tissue (e.g., the synovium) and loose bodies (often made of bone and cartilage), and by removing the damaged ends of the bones in the joint (resection or excision arthroplasty). After the ends of the bones are removed, the new bone-ends can be fused (arthrodesis) or replaced with artificial joint surfaces (arthroplasty).

Pain and impairment are sometimes due to the arthritis causing a nerve to be compressed (e.g., a pinched nerve in the spine or in the carpal tunnel at the wrist). In this case, the surgeon relieves the pressure caused by any bone, cartilage, ligament, or tendon that is pressing on the nerve.

Surgery may also restore function by improving alignment and movement in a joint, and thus reducing the stress put on other joints that were compensating for it. Sometimes surgery is done to prevent or slow damage to a joint or adjacent tendon or nerve tissue, but surgery is rarely done to improve the looks of a joint. You may in fact be worse off with such cosmetic surgery if it results in a more painful joint with less function.

Because successful joint surgery reduces pain and makes activities easier to do, there are secondary gains. Independence and self-esteem improve. Activity levels, energy, and stamina increase. Conditioning, fitness, sleeping patterns, and general health get better.

When to Have Surgery

Surgery should be considered when non-surgical measures fail to control the pain and loss of function of an arthritic joint. It is a good idea to see a surgeon early when considering surgery to an arthritic joint so that you can get appropriate advice about managing the joint prior to surgery.

Joint surgery should not be delayed if compensating joints are worsening. If this is not an issue and the surgery is delayed, the surgeon should be sure to monitor the joint and the patient as time passes. Many things can happen to the joint and surrounding tissues over time, and if the joint is allowed to deteriorate too much then the surgery will not be as successful as it would have been earlier on. For instance, the joint can become too unstable or crooked for surgery to have much effect, or the bone can become too weak, too eroded away, or too full of cysts. The ligaments and joint capsule can become so tight that motion becomes restricted and contractures develop. The muscles can become too weak and wasted. The skin can become so fragile that wound healing is precarious. Furthermore, if surgery is delayed too long, the patient may become too old, too frail, too debilitated, or too unhealthy to undergo surgery at all.

Surgery must also be considered if nerve or vascular (blood-conducting) tissue in the brain stem, spinal cord, nerve roots, and peripheral nerves is being compressed. Releasing the nerve may restore sensation and muscle strength to the affected area, and will at least stop the further loss of sensation and strength. If the nerve compression is allowed to continue, than the loss of sensation and function will worsen, with less chance of recovery.

Drawbacks, Risks, and Complications of Surgery

Surgery can be complicated by: the rheumatic condition and its treatment; other pre-existing conditions and their treatment; the process of anesthesia; the surgical procedure itself; and mishaps that may occur during rehabilitation.

Drugs used to treat arthritis (such as corticosteroids, NSAIDs, and DMARDs) can pose risks for surgery. In addition, the arthritis may have caused the patient to have other conditions—anemia, prolonged bleeding, easy clotting, reduced heart, lung, and kidney function, neurological deficits, and muscle weakness—that would complicate the surgery further.

Some forms of arthritis can restrict the movement of the jaw and neck joints, making it more difficult for the anesthetist to insert a breathing tube (endotracheal tube). Some types of arthritis can destabilize the joints of the cervical spine so that excessive movement during anesthesia could damage the spinal cord. If many joints are affected by arthritis, the positioning of the patient during and after the surgery can be difficult.

Being elderly, having other health problems, and using certain other drugs are also risk factors for surgery. Conditions affecting the heart, lungs, hormone glands, kidneys, liver, stomach, esophagus, and neurological system can increase the risks of surgery. Psychological problems, blood disorders, and susceptibility to infection increase the dangers of surgery. Various medications can also contribute to problems at surgery. The table on pages 268 and 269 lists many risk factors that must be considered. Poor diet and nutritional status before surgery can delay recovery. Obesity can contribute to slower recovery from lower extremity joint surgery, to lung and wound infections, to blood clot formation in the legs, and to the technical difficulty of the surgical procedure itself.

Lower extremity blood clots (deep vein thrombosis or phlebitis) occur more frequently with knee and hip replacements. Infections can develop in the incision, in the joint itself, and in the bloodstream, which can spread the infection elsewhere in the body. Nerves and blood vessels near the surgical site can be damaged accidentally. Varying degrees of blood loss can occur with surgery. Because of the anesthesia, the blood pressure can drop too much, the pressure in the brain can rise too much, or the tissues can be deprived of oxygen and blood.

Anesthesia

As surgery is invasive to the body, it is important that the patient be as comfortable as possible and feel minimal stress or pain during the procedure. Anesthesia is used for this purpose.

Types of Anesthesia

There are three main categories of anesthesia: general, regional, and local. Regional and local anesthetics are preferred in certain clinical situations over general anesthesia because they are safer. Regional and local anesthetics provide excellent operating conditions, avoid the need to manipulate or insert a tube into the airway, and cause fewer breathing problems. The reduced response of the nerves and hormones to stress under these anesthetics can be better for the heart and blood pressure, and they provide a smoother transition into the recovery period.

Risk Factors for Surgery

Organ system	Condition	Drugs
Heart	Recent heart attack	Nitroglycerin
	Unstable or severe angina	Beta-blockers (e.g., propranalol)
	Heart failure	ACE inhibitors (e.g., captopril)
	Diastolic blood pressure above 110	
	Cardiomyopathy	
Lungs	Chronic bronchitis	Bronchodilators
	Emphysema	
	Asthma	
	Smoking	
	Reduced lung volumes	
	Reduced chest expansion as in ankylosing spondylitis	
Hormones	Diabetes mellitus	Insulin, pills for diabetes
	Adrenal insufficiency or suppression	Corticosteroids, Thyroid medications
Infection	Skin ulcers	
	Urinary tract infections	
	Dental problems	
	HIV	
Genito-urinary	Prostate disease	
	Kidney stones	
	Kidney failure	
	Dehydration and electrolyte problems	
	Pregnancy	

Risk Factors for Surgery (continued)

Organ system	Condition	Drugs
Blood	Bleeding disorders	Aspirin, NSAIDs
	Clotting tendencies	Anticoagulants
	Anemia	Immunosuppressants
	Low white blood cell count	
	Suppressed immune system	
Neurological and psychological	Elderly, confused, Parkinsonian	Anti-epilepsy drugs
	Withdrawal: alcohol, narcotics, tranquilizers, barbiturates, illicit drugs	MAO inhibitor antidepressants
	Depression, anxiety	
Miscellaneous	Peptic ulcer disease	
	Esophageal reflux	
	Liver disease	
	Dry eyes	

General anesthesia

With general anesthesia, the patient is unconscious as a result of medications given intravenously and inhaled through a mask. A tube is often placed in the airway (intubation) to maintain the flow of oxygen and to clear secretions. If the arthritis has caused restricted movement of the neck or jaws, instability of the neck, or swelling of the joints near the entrance to the trachea (cricoarytenoid joints), then intubation is more difficult. A fibre-optic scope may have to be inserted through the nose into the airway (trachea) to guide the breathing tube (endotracheal tube) into place. This may be done while the patient is awake, but the throat is "frozen" with an anesthetic spray.

Regional anesthesia

With regional anesthesia, the patient is awake and can hear what is going on. Liquid anesthetic is instilled into an area that will "freeze" a section of the body. This type of anesthesia is used to freeze the lower half of the body by injecting the anesthetic through a tube into the spinal canal in the lower back (spinal anesthesia), or into a space around the spinal cord (epidural anesthesia). It allows surgical procedures to be done on the legs (such as a total knee replacement). Sedatives can be given intravenously to "knock out" the patient if needed. The insertion of the catheter into the spine is more difficult when the lumbar spine anatomy has been altered by disease (e.g., the bone spurs that develop with ankylosing spondylitis) or by previous lumbar surgery (causing scar tissue).

Local anesthesia

With local anesthesia, the patient is also awake but the frozen area is smaller. Instead of freezing the spinal cord, a nerve or group of nerves is frozen. For example, anesthetic injected into the armpit can freeze the nerves innervating the arm and hand on that side so that surgery can be done on the hand or elbow.

Other Anesthetic Considerations

There are many other factors to be considered that relate to anesthesia, including positioning, body temperature, intravenous fluids, invasive monitoring, blood loss, and analgesia.

Positioning

Positioning of the patient during and after surgery is important when multiple joints are affected by arthritis. It is important to put the other joints and the spine into comfortable and safe positions. The anesthetist can also give more sedation and analgesia to treat the joints that are not anesthetized.

Body temperature

The anesthetist has to make sure that the body's temperature does not drop. Lower temperatures can worsen Raynaud's phenomenon and induce muscle tightness. Muscle tightness around the airway can lead to breathing being obstructed when the patient is waking up from general anesthetic.

Intravenous fluids

The quantity of intravenous fluids administered must be controlled. If too little fluid is given, the blood pressure could drop and the kidneys could deteriorate. If too much fluid is given, tissue swelling and fluid in the lungs could result. If the operation is being done on the neck or back, the patient is usually face down (prone); in this position, too much fluid could cause the upper airway to narrow with swelling.

Invasive monitoring

Sometimes, invasive monitoring is needed. For example, a catheter may be inserted into the radial artery at the wrist to measure blood pressure more accurately. Sometimes a catheter has to be inserted into the pulmonary artery (the artery that carries blood from the right side of the heart to the lungs) in order to measure the blood pressure in the lungs. A sudden change in the blood pressure in the lungs during the surgery can alert the doctors to such complications as reactions to the bone cement, or fat or air embolism (fat or air that has mistakenly entered the bloodstream and is carried to the lungs, where it can obstruct the circulation of blood). It is important to diagnose these problems as early as possible. Such problems are more likely to occur with complicated revisions of joint replacements.

Blood loss

It is important to minimize blood loss. To reduce blood loss, tourniquets can be used during surgery on the arm or leg being operated on, and the anesthetist can deliberately lower the blood pressure to reduce the loss of blood during surgery of the spine, pelvis, or hip (where bleeding tends to be greater). Blood can also be collected from the surgical site during the operation and then returned to the patient through a vein.

Analgesia

To make patients more comfortable after surgery, the anesthetist can arrange long-acting nerve blocks, or have painkillers flow (through the epidural, nerve blocks, or the intravenous tubing) either continuously or as needed by the patient.

Type of Anesthesia and Surgical Site

The type of anesthesia that is used in surgery will depend on the body part that is being operated upon. Below, we will discuss the anesthesia and some of the procedures that are common in surgery on the spine, shoulder, elbow and hand, hip, knee, ankle, and foot.

Spine

Surgery to the spine requires general anesthesia and intubation (insertion of a breathing tube). Intubation is riskier when neck arthritis and neurological dangers are involved. Blood loss is higher. The patient is placed in the prone position for spinal surgery, and as a result, the pressure in the eyes and on the joints and nerves can be greater. Furthermore, the breathing and blood circulation can be impaired and the upper airway obstructed. Invasive monitoring, controlled lowering of the blood pressure, and fibre-optic intubation may be needed.

Shoulder

Shoulder surgery can be done by freezing the network of nerves that travel from the neck to the arm behind the collarbone. In patients with advanced ankylosing spondylitis, care must be taken not to freeze the nerve going to the diaphragm. Because their rib joints are fused, these people cannot expand their chest wall to breathe, and must rely on their diaphragms for breathing.

Elbow and hand

Surgery of the elbow and hand or adjacent regions can be done with an axillary nerve block. The anesthetic is injected into the armpit around the nerves that enter the arm.

Hip, knee, ankle, and foot

Hip, knee, ankle, and foot surgery can be done with epidural and spinal anesthesia. If there is bony overgrowth due to diseases such as spondylitis or DISH in the lumbar spine, or if there is scarring from previous lumbar surgery, the needle for the anesthetic may have to be inserted lower down (caudal anesthesia) or higher up.

Surgery of the forefoot and toes can be done by blocking the two main nerves at the ankle.

Types of Surgery Available for Arthritic Joints

Several different types of operations can be performed on arthritic joints, including arthroscopy, synovectomy, soft tissue repairs, decompression, osteotomy, arthrodesis (joint fusion), joint resection (excision arthroplasty), joint replacement (arthroplasty), and experimental surgery (which includes cartilage transplants, stem cell transplants, and microsurgery). The type of procedure that will be done depends on the degree of damage to the joint and which joint is being operated upon.

Arthroscopy

In arthroscopy, a tube with a light source and video camera is inserted through a small hole into the joint. The view can be transmitted to a television monitor, and the doctors can use what they see to make diagnostic observations. Another tube may be inserted through a second hole to rinse the joint with saline solution (salt water) and cause the joint to swell out from the water pressure within. Flushing out the joint in this manner may clear it of debris, loose bodies, blood, and infection. Minor surgical procedures such as biopsies, synovectomy, removal of loose bodies, and repair of a meniscus (torn cartilage) can be done with special instruments inserted through a third hole.

Arthroscopy is done most often in the knee, but can also be done in other joints such as the shoulder, elbow, and hip. The surgery is often done on an outpatient basis. The advantages of arthroscopy include a quick recovery time, earlier weight bearing, no loss of joint movement, better wound healing, and less anesthesia. Pain, stiffness, and infection are possible complications.

Synovectomy

The removal of inflamed synovium from a joint or tendon sheath is referred to as a synovectomy. (For technical reasons, not all the synovium can be removed.) The synovectomy can be done through an arthroscope or through an incision (arthrotomy). The inflamed synovium will eventually grow back (within several months to a few years), but the procedure can be repeated. This procedure will control pain, fluid production, and inflammation in joints or tendon sheaths affected by such diseases as rheumatoid arthritis. It is uncertain whether this type of surgery can prevent further damage to the joint or tendon.

Soft Tissue Repairs

Tendons, ligaments, and muscles can be tightened, loosened, or reattached as needed. Nodules, tophi, and calcium deposits can be removed from around joints and tendons.

Decompression

Sometimes arthritis may lead to the compression of nerve tissue and blood vessels by bone spurs, discs between the vertebrae that are sticking out where they're not supposed to be, inflamed soft tissues (like synovium), and unstable joints. It is usually necessary to release the nerve tissue and blood vessels by surgically removing whatever is squashing them, and/or to stabilize the unstable joints by fusing them. The spinal cord and/or nerve roots exiting from the spine may need to be decompressed when bone spurs, discs, and ligaments (in spinal degenerative disc and joint disease) or inflamed synovium and unstable vertebrae (in rheumatoid arthritis) move in on these structures. The median nerve at the wrist is decompressed to treat carpal tunnel syndrome.

Osteotomy

In an osteotomy, a wedge is cut out from a bone in order to realign it. Because the bone is now in a different position, the forces through the adjacent joints are changed, and symptoms may be relieved. The realignment can also improve some types of joint deformity. This procedure is not done as often as it used to be, however, since the recovery time is so long and better procedures are available. It is mainly done for osteoarthritis (such as a bow-legged knee with arthritis in only the medial compartment) or for a bunion to straighten out the big toe.

Arthrodesis

In this type of surgery, the ends of the bones making up the joint are fused together using pins, wires, screws, plates, and bone grafts. Joint pain is eliminated and the alignment and stability of the joint are restored. However, the joint no longer moves, and the stresses that this joint used to absorb are now transferred to compensating joints that might begin to wear down faster. Arthrodesis is used for arthritis in the cervical and lumbar spine, wrists, thumb joints, ankles, and first MTP joints (main joint of the big toe).

Joint Resection

Removing the damaged end of a bone that is part of a joint, without replacing it with an artificial substitute, can relieve pain and improve joint mobility. However, the joint will become very unstable. This procedure is helpful when arthritis involves the balls of the feet (MTP joints) in the second to fifth toes; in this case, the heads or ends of the metatarsals (foot bones) are cut out. Similarly, in the arthritic elbow, pain and rotation can be improved by cutting out the head or end of the radius (the thicker and shorter of the two bones in the forearm).

Joint Replacement

In badly arthritic joints, the damaged areas are cut out and replaced with artificial components.

Great strides have been made in the area of joint replacement over the years. There have been improvements in the design of the replacements, in the materials and cements, and in the instrumentation. The components are made of metals like stainless steel, cobalt chrome, and titanium. The articulating surfaces are made from polyethylene, ceramics, and metal.

The components can be fixed in the joint with or without cement, which is methylmethacrylate (a dental glue). Cemented components heal quickly after surgery and allow for early weight bearing. If the bone stock is weak, cement is used to reinforce it, or bone can be used from a tissue bank (allograft bone). Uncemented components heal more slowly with delayed weight bearing because they have to allow for bone to grow into the roughened surface of the replacement. It is felt that uncemented components are less likely to loosen, however, so they are considered for people who will be much harder on their joints (usually younger people). Loosening of an implant depends on the type of components used, the underlying kind of arthritis, which joint is replaced, the degree of joint use, the age of the patient, and the condition of the bone.

Joint replacement is most commonly done in the hips and knees, followed by the shoulders, first row of knuckles in the hands (MCP joints), and then the elbows. There is marked relief of pain and improvement of the joint functions, but the joint will never be restored to normal. Long-term complications include loosening, infection, and wearing out of the components. Often the wearing out and the loosening occur together, but wearing out of the joint may occur without the patient knowing about it.

Experimental Surgery

Advances in joint surgery are continuing. Therapies that are currently showing potential good results are cartilage transplants, stem cell transplants, and microsurgery.

Cartilage transplants

Cartilage transplants are being perfected. Healthy cartilage cells (chondrocytes) are removed from a healthy part of the joint, put in cultures in the laboratory to multiply, and then reinjected into the joint in the hope that they will settle in the areas where the cartilage has been eroded and produce new cartilage. This technique is presently being targeted for small areas of cartilage loss in knees affected by osteoarthritis. It is not known yet whether these cells will produce cartilage that will stand up to all the stresses of weight bearing that our natural cartilage can, but the experiments are ongoing.

Stem cell transplants

Attempts are being made to obtain stem cells that can be implanted into damaged musculoskeletal tissue. Depending on where they are placed, these cells will become bone cells (which will produce more bone), cartilage cells (which will produce more cartilage), or fibroblasts (which will produce tendon or ligament). They will lead to healing by building up the bone, cartilage, or tendon or ligament that is needed.

Microsurgery

Microsurgery, or mini-incision surgery, uses high-tech instrumentation through much smaller incisions than are possible in conventional surgery. Even total hip and knee replacements can be done this way, with the aim that patients can be discharged from hospital the day after surgery. If this surgery is successful, patients experience less pain and fewer complications after surgery, and hospital costs per procedure drop considerably. However, it is not known how durable these joints will be in the long run.

Which Procedure Is Preferred for Which Joint

Once it has been decided to operate on an arthritic joint, the best procedure must be chosen. The choice will depend upon which joint is involved, the type and stage of the arthritis, the goals of the surgery, and the experience of the surgeon with all of the available procedures.

One should expect reduced pain and improved function but not a normal joint after surgery. The results of surgery are better if it is done before tendons rupture and before fixed contractures and dislocation occur. In children with arthritis, synovectomies and soft tissue surgery are often done early to try to prevent deformities and contractures in the growing child. However, surgery on the child's bones may be postponed until the bones' growth plates close.

Wrists and Hands

Surgery of the wrists and hands will relieve pain and realign the joints, but is not as successful at restoring function. Inflammatory types of arthritis are the main reason for joint surgery in the hands and wrists, as hand strength is dependent on a painless and stable wrist.

Wrists

In early wrist arthritis, the preferred surgery is a synovectomy done through an open incision or through an arthroscope. Sometimes, the synovium in the tendon sheaths crossing the wrist is removed as well. Tendons may have to be realigned and, if ruptured, repaired.

Advanced damage requires arthrodesis of the wrist (fusing the bones). This will relieve pain in 75–95 percent of cases and improve hand function. One wrist is usually fused in mild extension while the other wrist is fused in mild flexion so that each can perform different self-care activities.

Joint replacement has not been very successful in the wrist, as the silicone spacers break and cause a chronic inflammatory reaction. Total wrist joint replacement is done only rarely because of the high incidence of complications. These include loosening, infection, dislocation, and sinking of the implant into the bone. Management of these complications involves removing the replacement and fusing the wrist.

Hands

Early inflammatory arthritis of the MCP and PIP joints is treated by synovectomy, and sometimes soft tissue surgery to realign the finger and thumb joints is done as well.

With advanced damage in the MCP joints, sialastic implants are preferred. They are made of silicone and are referred to as Swanson arthroplasties. They act as joint spacers that reduce pain and straighten out the fingers, but they do not improve the range of movement because of their stiffness. They can fracture and dislocate.

Advanced damage in the PIP joints can also be treated with these Swanson implants, but the joint movement remains limited. Fusing these joints will relieve pain and improve stability and alignment, but the loss of movement will probably worsen the disability of the hand.

Advanced damage to the DIP joints can be treated by arthrodesis but not by implants.

Advanced damage in the three thumb joints (first CMC, MCP, and IP joints) is treated with a combination of arthrodesis and arthroplasty. Arthrodesis of all three joints should be avoided if possible because of the loss of thumb movement and function. The only alternative for the IP joint is fusion. The MCP joint can be fused or replaced with an implant. The first CMC joint can be fused or partially resected or cushioned with an implant.

In rheumatoid arthritis, systemic lupus erythematosus, and a few other inflammatory joint diseases, swan neck and Boutonniere's deformities can affect the fingers. If these deformities are reversible by manually straightening out the fingers, then they can be treated by soft tissue procedures with or without synovectomy. If these deformities become irreversible, a combination of soft tissue surgery, sialastic implants, and/or arthrodesis will be necessary.

Aggressive forms of rheumatoid arthritis and psoriatic arthritis can cause marked loss of bone in the finger joints (osteolysis); the fingers become shorter and the joints looser. Arthrodesis should be done without delay, to prevent further bone loss and the need for bone grafting. Unfortunately, the function of the hand will be greatly restricted due to the loss of joint movement. Implants may not hold in the rapidly eroding bone ends.

Elbows

In early inflammatory arthritis (like rheumatoid arthritis) of the elbow, an open or arthroscopic synovectomy can relieve pain and improve the range of movement. If there is a contracture of the joint, it can be released at the same operation. In early osteoarthritis, debris, loose bodies, bone spurs, and fragments can be removed by arthroscopy.

With advanced joint damage, arthroplasty should be considered, as it can result in marked pain relief, reasonable range of movement, and better function. However, the elbow will not be able to stand heavy lifting (lifting is limited to 2–5 kg). At surgery, the three nerves that cross the elbow can be injured. The components can loosen.

Excision arthroplasty is done only if necessary to relieve pain because it results in a weak, unstable elbow joint that functions poorly. Arthrodesis should be avoided. It will stop the pain, but there is no good functional position in which the elbow can be fused. Many tasks will be difficult or impossible to do.

Shoulders

In early arthritis of the shoulder, arthroscopic synovectomy and debridement (removal of damaged tissue) are of limited value. The capsule of the shoulder joint, which is made up of several tendons, is called the rotator cuff; only some of the time can tears in this structure be repaired to prevent degenerative arthritis. Chronic, resistant bursitis or tendonitis may be caused by the overlying bony extension from the shoulder blade (called the acromion) pressing on the bursae or tendons. Sometimes, part of this bone can be cut away (acromionectomy) to relieve the pressure and allow the shoulder to be elevated more easily.

For advanced shoulder arthritis, arthroplasty is often warranted. In this surgery, the head of the humerus (upper arm bone) is removed, and a metal ball with a stem is inserted into the remaining upper humerus. (Cement is used to fix it more often in rheumatoid arthritis than in osteoarthritis because of the weak bone stock.) The socket with which this ball forms a joint is called the glenoid; it is resurfaced with a polyethylene implant. Pain relief and improved function are fairly good. The joint mobility is dependent on the condition of the rotator cuff. In arthritis, it is often quite damaged and unrepairable. As a result, the active range of movement may not be much better than it was before surgery. Physiotherapy after surgery is very important to strengthen the muscles so that the active antigravity range of movement is maximized.

As a last resort, such as a failed or infected arthroplasty, the components are removed, leaving a humerus with a resected head. Pain is lessened, but the joint is unstable and limited in active movement.

Hips

Generally speaking, surgery is not done for early hip arthritis. However, if the socket of the hip joint (acetabulum) is underdeveloped from birth (acetabular dysplasia), osteoarthritis will eventually develop. To slow the onset of arthritis and to reduce pain, an osteotomy of the femur (the thick bone between the hip and the knee) or the pelvis can be done to realign the joint.

Total hip replacement is the surgery of choice for advanced hip arthritis. It relieves pain and improves activities like walking and standing in over 90 percent of patients. The upper femur is removed (including the ball and neck), a hole is drilled into the shaft of the femur, and a metal ball and stem are then implanted into the bone. The socket is reshaped to fit a metal cup into which different types of liners can be placed. Cement may or may not be used to fix these implants. Usually a hybrid procedure is done in which the ball and stem are cemented but the cup is uncemented and fixed in place with screws.

In inflammatory types of arthritis like rheumatoid arthritis, the bony socket can get very thin and worn, and the femoral head could break through it into the pelvis (this is called protrusio), making surgery more difficult. To prevent this, bone grafts are needed to reinforce the socket before the artificial cup is implanted. Recovery and weight bearing take longer. It is important to operate on the hip before this occurs.

Early complications occur in less than 5 percent of people having total hip replacement. These complications include damage to the sciatic nerve, infection, dislocation, and poor positioning of the implant. Blood loss during this type of surgery has been reduced due to improved techniques, and although anemia may result, patients can recover without the need for transfusions. Blood clots can develop in the leg veins (deep vein thrombosis or phlebitis), and occasionally the clot can break off and lodge in the lung (pulmonary embolism). Blood thinners (anticoagulants) can prevent these blood clots from developing. Infections can be prevented by giving antibiotics at the time of surgery and, sometimes, by using cement mixed with an antibiotic. The leg that has had the surgery may become longer or shorter than the other leg, and a lift may be needed for the shoe worn on the shorter leg.

As time passes, other problems may develop, such as loosening or wear and tear of the implants, stress fractures, infection, dislocation, and bone formation in the muscle around the hip. Hip replacements can last for 10 to 20 years or more. Some complications necessitate another operation to repair or replace the arthroplasty, but the results may not be as good as the original. Rarely, it happens that a failed replacement cannot be changed and so the implant is removed and muscle is put between the ends of the bone (girdlestone arthroplasty). Pain is relieved but the joint is very unstable and weak, so aids are needed for walking.

It takes about three months to recover fully from the first hip arthroplasty, and during this time it is important to keep the hip muscles strong with exercises. Sitting on raised seats and avoiding positions that increase the risk of dislocation will protect the new hip. High impact work and sports should be avoided. Activities like golf, swimming, cycling, and walking are fine. Ask your surgeon about the advisability of doing other types of activities. Your surgeon may want you to take antibiotics before any medical procedures that might cause bacteria to enter the bloodstream and then infect the artificial joint. Such procedures include some types of dental work and instrumentation of the bowel or bladder (colonoscopy, sigmoidoscopy, and cystoscopy).

Knees

Arthroscopic synovectomy can improve the pain, swelling, movement, and function of a chronically inflamed knee whose cartilage is fairly well preserved. In early non-inflammatory arthritis of the knee, arthroscopic debridement and irrigation, loose body removal, and cartilage repairs can be helpful.

If osteoarthritis involves only the medial or lateral compartment of the knee with angulation of the shin (e.g., bow-leg), then an osteotomy of the tibia (the inner and larger of the two bones of the lower leg) can be done to alter the weight bearing forces through the joint. This procedure is not as effective as a replacement and its recovery takes longer, but it definitely has its uses. People who use their knees a great deal, such as those who do a lot of physical labour, are much harder on those joints than less physical people might be, and so would likely find that a joint replacement would not withstand the rigours of their work and would loosen quickly. The osteotomy would allow them to continue their work, buying them a few more years of work time until they need a joint replacement, and perhaps allowing them time to find a job that is easier on the knees. However this procedure is done for heavy labourers will require a careful assessment of the patient's expectations.

In advanced knee arthritis, total knee replacements are successful in over 90 percent of cases. Pain and mobility are greatly improved. The range of movement of the knee after surgery is dependent on the range of motion before surgery and also on the type of prosthesis that is used. In total knee replacement surgery, the knee is cleaned out and the surgeon prepares the back of the kneecap (patella) and the ends of the bones—the tibia (the shinbone) and the femur (the thigh bone). A metal implant replaces the surface of the end of the femur, and a metal implant with a plastic surface is cemented into the end of the tibia. A plastic component is implanted into the back of the patella. Weight bearing and range of movement exercises are started the day after surgery. Full cooperation in physiotherapy immediately after surgery is crucial to obtain the maximum range of movement. Building up the muscle strength in the leg is important for walking to progress from a walker to crutches to a cane to unaided. Full recovery takes three to six months.

Immediate post-operative complications include deep vein thrombosis and delayed healing and infection of the incision. In the long term, joint infection, loosening, and wearing away of the polyethylene can occur. High-impact loading activities should be avoided.

Ankles

There is little to be done surgically for early arthritis of the ankle. In rheumatoid arthritis, the posterior tibial tendon (which runs down the inner aspect of the ankle to the arch) can get inflamed and damaged. This tendon maintains the arch of the foot and prevents the ankle from turning inwards. Synovectomy of the tendon sheath and tendon repair can help maintain alignment and reduce pain.

Advanced ankle arthritis is managed by arthrodesis. It will control the pain and improve the alignment of the ankle, making walking easier, but the flexion-extension movement of the ankle will be lost. During surgery, the ends of the tibia and talus (ankle bone, with which the tibia forms the ankle joint) are exposed to raw bone. The ankle is realigned and then held together with screws and bone graft. Newer techniques include arthroscopic ankle fusion. Casts, splints, and limited weight bearing are required for three months. It may take another three months to recover fully. Complications are common, and include delayed healing of the incision, infection, stress fractures, and failure of the joint to fuse.

Total ankle arthroplasty is done only rarely, due to the high failure rate, but new developments are occurring. Complications include migration and loosening of the components, infection, poor healing of the incision, and stress fractures.

Feet

There are no procedures for early arthritis of the foot. Advanced arthritis of the midfoot is treated by arthrodesis of the joints involved, and metal staples and bone grafts are used. Sometimes an osteotomy is done at the same time to improve the alignment of the foot. Although movement is lost, pain is relieved and walking is improved. Sometimes a triple arthrodesis is needed, in which three joints are fused: between the calcaneus and talus (which move the foot inwards and outwards), the talus and navicular (instep and arch), and the calcaneus and cuboid (outstep). Complications include infection, residual deformity, and failure of the fusion to take. Sometimes in rheumatoid arthritis a triple arthrodesis and ankle fusion are necessary. Although pain is relieved, walking is then very awkward due to the overall lack of movement. A rocker sole can be added to the shoe to make walking easier.

Toes

The aims of forefoot surgery are to relieve pain, reduce deformities, improve walking, and allow for better-fitting shoes. Forefoot surgery leads to satisfaction in 80–90 percent of cases.

There is little to be done for early arthritis. Advanced arthritis in the big toe usually involves the ball or bunion joint (first MTP). The treatment of choice is arthrodesis with realignment if needed. It relieves pain and improves weight bearing but results in less ability to move the big toe. Silicone implants have been unsuccessful because of residual pain, recurrent deformity, weakness of toe flexion, inflammatory reactions to the silicone, and progressive wearing away of the surrounding bone.

The major problems in the second to fifth toes are pain in the balls (second to fifth MTP joints) of the feet, dislocation of the MTPs and deformities of the toes with secondary corns, calluses, blisters, and skin ulcers. Excision arthroplasties of the MTPs are done through an incision on the top of the foot, although sometimes the incision is made on the sole of the foot. Usually the heads of the metatarsals (long bones between the midfoot and toes) are cut away, but sometimes the bases of the proximal phalanges (toe bones) are cut away instead. Tendons may be cut to correct the toe deformities. In addition the PIP joints of the toes may be straightened out and fused. Pins are used to hold the fusion in the corrected position, and are removed a few weeks later.

Spine

The main concern in the spine is damage to nerve tissue by the arthritis, and this can happen anywhere along the length of the spine, from the base of the brain right down to the tailbone. Arteries supplying blood to the brain and spinal cord can also be compressed by the arthritis.

Various neurological problems can arise depending on the location of the pressure. There can be nerve pain, numbness and tingling, loss of sensation, and loss of muscle power or paralysis. There can also be significant pain at the site of the arthritis. In degenerative forms of arthritis (like osteoarthritis, disc disease, and spinal stenosis), bone spurs, protruded discs, and thickened ligaments can compress the spinal cord and nerve roots. In inflammatory forms of arthritis (like rheumatoid arthritis), the inflamed synovium and the unstable vertebrae will press on the nerve and vascular (blood-conveying) tissues in the brain stem, cervical spinal cord, and nerve roots. In ankylosing spondylitis and other types of spondylitis, the vertebrae fuse together, making them susceptible to unstable fractures. If the vertebrae do fracture, dislocation or a vertebra slipping forward at the level of the fracture could compress the spinal cord and nerve roots at that level.

Surgery is aimed at relieving the pressure on the nerve tissue and stabilizing the unstable vertebra by fusing them. Decompression of the spinal cord can be done from the back by removing the spinous processes and bony vertebral plates (called laminae); this procedure is called a laminectomy. The spinal cord can be decompressed from the front as well. The nerve roots can be decompressed by enlarging the canals between the vertebrae that house the nerve roots (foraminotomy). The surgeon will also remove inflamed synovium, disc and ligament protrusions, bony spurs, and calcifications, depending on the type of arthritis. If parts of the spine are unstable, the vertebrae are realigned and fused. Depending on the location, wires, plates, screws, and bone grafts are used to fuse these areas. For several weeks after the surgery, the patient would need to keep the area motionless by wearing a collar and halo.

Possible complications are damage to the nerve and vascular tissues, infection, fractures, and anesthetic problems. Halos and collars can be uncomfortable, make opening the mouth difficult, and can cause rashes at pressure points. Some movement will be lost due to the fusion. The joints above and below the fusion will assume more stress, making them prone to accelerated arthritis.

Severe flexion or forward stoop deformities of the spine (kyphosis) may result from such conditions as ankylosing spondylitis. Because of pain, trouble functioning due to the deformity, or a nerve being threatened by compression, surgery may be needed. A spinal osteotomy is done at a predetermined level. In this surgery, a "wedge" of bone is removed from the posterior of the spine, and the spine is then arched backwards into this wedge and fused in this new extended position. Similarly, major side-to-side curvatures of the spine (scoliosis) can be straightened by a combination of osteotomies and fusions that are maintained by long metal rods. These are complicated procedures that should only be done by an experienced spine surgeon.

Pre-Operation Considerations

You will need to do a lot of research before making a decision about surgery, and the first step in this process will be to get an opinion from a surgeon or surgeons.

Consult a Surgeon

Consulting with a surgeon does not commit you to having surgery. You are simply getting an opinion about the options available for handling your joint problem. You may in fact need a second opinion to make a decision with which you are comfortable.

With the help of your physician, rheumatologist, physiotherapist, support group and other patients who have had similar surgery, choose a surgeon. The surgeon should be qualified and experienced in the type of surgery that concerns you, and should be doing this type of surgery frequently. Choose a surgeon carefully and do not feel ashamed to contact the surgeon's office to ask more questions. Make sure you understand what you are getting into. Once the surgery has been done, you are at the point of no return, and there are no guarantees. Among the questions you might want to ask at this stage are the following:

- What are the surgical and non-surgical options?
- What, if any, problems are there in delaying the surgery?
- Can I picture exactly what will be done to the joint?
- How much improvement can I expect in my pain, joint movement, and function?
- Will there be things I cannot do or am not allowed to do?
- What kind of anesthesia can I choose?
- What complications could I face with this surgery?
- How long will the procedure benefit me, and what problems can occur down the line?
- If this procedure eventually fails, what can be done to salvage it?

Reduce Risks Before Surgery

You must take an active role in making the surgery as successful as possible. Consider some of these suggestions:

- Get assessed by a physiotherapist and occupational therapist before surgery so that you can learn to do the exercises required after surgery. They can show you pictures, videos, and pamphlets regarding your type of surgery, and can introduce you to others who have had similar surgery. They will identify and address potential post-operative problems and plan for appropriate discharge assistance.

- Get dental work done to prevent problems with loose teeth and infected gums that could be a source of infection. Make sure any other infections or sites of possible infection are treated.
- Make sure other health problems are stable and that necessary blood tests, X-rays, electrocardiograms, and lung function tests, etc., have been done.
- Make sure your doctors are aware of potential arthritis-related problems, such as cervical spine arthritis and the use of corticosteroids, aspirin, NSAIDs, and immunosuppressants. The corticosteroid dose has to be boosted during surgery. Also, people taking corticosteroids may have fragile skin, so warn staff about using a minimal amount of adhesive tape. Aspirin and NSAIDs can prolong bleeding. Immunosuppressants and corticosteroids can slow healing and increase the chances of infection.
- Exercise to improve your conditioning.
- Improve your diet and nutrition. If you are overweight, lose weight. If you are underweight, gain weight.
- Stop smoking (all surgical outcomes are worse in smokers).
- Wean off alcohol and other addictive substances so withdrawal problems do not occur during your hospitalization.
- Make sure that high blood pressure and diabetes are controlled.
- Donate one or two units of your own blood before the surgery if the surgeon feels that transfusions might be necessary.

Make Financial Arrangements

Having made financial arrangements before the surgery will ease your mind during your recovery time. You might want to do the following:

- Pay your bills before hospitalization.
- Make sure you have a will and power of attorney.
- If you have extended care health insurance, see what it will cover.
- Make sure that your life and disability insurance are up to date.
- Find out if you are eligible for any other financial aid.

Prepare Your Home and Yourself

If you know before the operation that everything is in place for your return home, you will be able to set aside those details and concentrate on preparing yourself for the surgery.

- It is natural to have some fears and anxiety before surgery, but try to minimize them. Reduce anxiety by learning as much about the surgery as you can. Speak to others who have had surgery. Most hospitals now have preoperative clinics where patients are prepared for surgery and assessed so that they know what to do and bring.
- Learn relaxation techniques.
- Provide a living will if this will make you more comfortable.
- Rearrange your home in preparation for your return after surgery.
- Do your grocery shopping and prepare frozen meals before entering the hospital.
- Arrange for any home care providers that you might need after surgery.

Prepare for Hospitalization

Make sure you have everything you need for the hospital and any rehabilitation facility you may have to attend afterwards, and understand your timeline and last-minute preparations.

- Know what time to arrive at the hospital and the location of the admitting department.
- Know when you are allowed your last food, liquid, and pills.
- Do any needed at-home preparation and cleansing of the surgical site.
- Take a list of your medications, allergies, and medical history, and pack your medications.
- Take your comfortable shoes, splints and assistive devices, glasses, dental needs, hearing aids, and walking aids.
- Take pajamas, robe, non-slip slippers, and bathing suit (if you will be doing pool therapy later).
- Take a list of phone numbers, some photos, a Walkman, a cheap watch or clock, and reading material. Leave jewellery and valuables at home, however, as things are often misplaced or stolen in the hospital.
- Have the visiting hours and hospital phone numbers handy for your relatives and friends.

Post-Operation Considerations

We will next discuss what will happen after the operation: while you're in the hospital, in rehab, at home, and what to expect over the long term.

In Hospital

After the surgery, you will be transferred to the recovery room for monitoring and recovery from the anesthesia. Painkilling medications will be given to keep you comfortable. You will be made to breathe deeply and cough to rid your body of the anesthesia and prevent pneumonia and lung collapse. You will be asked to move your toes, fingers, and eyes, etc., to show how your nervous system is doing; you will be asked to move your ankles, if possible, to prevent clotting in your leg veins. Your blood pressure and pulse and other vital signs will be followed to make sure there are no problems. When all is stable, you will be transferred to a bed on the ward (or discharged home if your operation is an outpatient procedure).

Once in your room, you should have adequate medication to control your pain. At first, you will receive a narcotic such as morphine through your intravenous connection (or through tubing connected to your spinal canal if epidural anesthesia was given). You might be able to administer it yourself by pushing a button on a portable pump (PCA—patient-controlled analgesia). Let the nurses know if you cannot use the PCA because of arthritis in your hands. You will gradually be switched to oral painkillers. If you had been taking narcotics such as codeine before surgery, you may have built up a tolerance and may require more than the average amount of narcotics after surgery. You may need analgesia before physiotherapy too so that you can get the most out of the physiotherapy.

Within one to two days of surgery, the physiotherapist will start to mobilize you and initiate passive exercises. If there were bone grafts, protrusio of the femur through the pelvis, fractures, osteotomies, or fusions, mobilization will be slower and gentler to allow for the bones to heal. Mobilization will be slower for uncemented joint replacements as well. The goals of rehab are to attain the maximum range of movement and muscle strength, and optimum functioning of the joint and patient. Ice packs will be used to reduce pain and inflammation. Various cast changes and splinting may be needed. Assistive devices will be given to protect your joints and make activities easier. For example, with hip or knee surgery you will progress from wheelchair to walker to crutches to cane to no walking aids.

You will be able to resume eating and taking your pills within one to two days of the surgery. You will receive antibiotics for about two days to prevent infection. You may be given blood thinners by mouth or by injection for a few days to prevent blood clots from forming in your legs. Within a few days, all your intravenous lines, drains, and catheters will be removed.

The dressings will be changed to less bulky ones and then removed when the drainage stops. You should find out when the stitches or staples are to be removed from the incision. There may also be casts and splints to deal with.

You must ask the surgeon for a follow-up office appointment and a discharge prescription. Questions you might want to ask at that visit are as follows:

- Will further surgery on this joint or another joint be needed in the future, and will the surgeon make the necessary arrangements?
- What symptoms might indicate a problem with the surgery?
- Will you need preventative antibiotics for certain situations?
- Will you trigger the metal detectors at the airport?

In Rehab

Rehabilitation may be carried out while you are still in the hospital, or you may do it as an outpatient. Depending on the procedure, you should be feeling much better after one to four weeks, and back to full activities by three to six months after the operation.

The goal is to make you as independent and as safe as possible. You will learn techniques to control pain and to protect your joints, and exercises for flexibility, strength, balance, and conditioning. Activities will be made easier by assistive devices, home modifications, and education. You should know which activities are to be avoided or limited. Ask about sports, work, driving, lifting, sex, ambulation, stairs, and sitting heights.

After surgery of a lower limb joint, the therapists will check the lengths of your legs. If there is a discrepancy, a lift may be added to the shoe of the shorter leg.

At Home

At home, you may need help with preparing meals, doing housework, moving around, and taking care of personal grooming. You may need a raised chair and toilet seat, a bathtub bench, and grips. Scatter rugs should be removed to avoid tripping. A pillow may be needed between the legs after a hip replacement to prevent dislocation. You will need advice about getting into and driving the car, resuming sexual activity, and when and how you should proceed in returning to work.

In the Long Term

It will be necessary to continue the exercises for range of movement and muscle strength. Only do those activities you are allowed to do with your repaired joint.

If you have any joint implants, ask about using preventative antibiotics whenever there is a possibility of bacteria entering your bloodstream. Learn the symptoms of an implant becoming infected, loose, worn out, or fractured, and seek help if excess stress is being shifted to a joint replacement to compensate for a problem in another joint.

Joint surgery is called for to relieve pain and restore function when non-operative measures are inadequate. Expect a good outcome but not a normal joint. The type of anesthesia (general, regional, or local) depends on the type of surgery and patient risk factors. The type of surgery needed depends on which joint is to be done and how advanced the arthritis is. The surgical procedures include arthroscopy, synovectomy, soft tissue repairs, nerve tissue decompression, osteotomy, and joint fusion, resection, and replacements. Get all the information you need to make the decision to have surgery. Rehabilitation after the surgery is very important to the success of the operation. Make sure all your health problems are dealt with before surgery. Prepare yourself and your home for before and after the surgery, and take care of the joint as advised for good long-term results.

11 Diet and nutrition

There are no miracle or wonder diets. If there were, would so many different dietary remedies exist? While there are some individuals whose arthritis seems to improve after certain changes in their diet, the majority of people are not so fortunate. This chapter will discuss the benefits and components of a healthy diet, and will take a look at several conditions—obesity, gout, and osteoporosis—that can be related to diet. Finally, we will look at several foods and practices that have been popularly associated with arthritis, and see whether current research actually shows any connection with the disease.

A Healthy Diet

It is important to maintain a healthy diet for your general health and for preventing your arthritis from progressing faster. However, the pain and fatigue of the arthritis and the adverse effects of the drugs may reduce your appetite and affect your ability to shop for and prepare nourishing food. Feeding yourself and chewing may be problematic if the hand, arm, shoulder, or jaw joints are involved. Consultation with a dietitian or occupational therapist may overcome some of these problems.

A healthy daily diet includes two litres of water and various vitamins and minerals obtained from eating vegetables, fruit, and grains. Good sources of carbohydrate are whole-grain foods in the form of pasta, bread and cereal, rice, fruit, and vegetables. Fortified bran cereal and brown rice contain fibre, which helps the bowel excrete wastes, eases constipation, and benefits heart disease, raised blood sugar, and diverticular disease of the large bowel. You should avoid high cholesterol, saturated fats, and trans-saturated fats, but eat fish and seed oils. Meat, fish, eggs, milk, cheese, yogurt, and soy products provide protein.

Diet-Related Conditions

Your diet can have a direct effect on several physical conditions, including obesity, gout, and osteoporosis.

Obesity

Obesity puts you more at risk for osteoarthritis of the knees and hands. Excess weight increases the forces put through the lower extremity joints and low back. Overweight individuals can also develop sleep apnea syndrome, in which the excess weight around the neck can obstruct breathing during sleep, leading to snoring, non-refreshing sleep, and non-breathing spells. Fatigue and even fibromyalgia can follow. Other hazards of obesity include heart disease, strokes, high blood pressure, raised blood sugar, and cancer of the breast, uterus, colon, and kidney. Losing weight improves your mobility, lessens the pain and rate of progression of damage in the joints of the lower extremities already affected by arthritis, and can lead to improved sleep, energy, and well-being. Losing just two to four kilograms could help.

The only ways to lose weight are to eat less and to exercise more. Reduce your food intake gradually without depriving yourself or going on fad diets. The types of food you eat are important. To be healthy, you should eat less fat and sugar, but more fruit, vegetables, whole grain products, fibre, and water.

Gout

In the condition known as gout, there is too much uric acid in the blood and so uric acid crystals form in the joints. These crystals cause recurrent attacks of acute inflammation and chronic damage of the joints. This excess of uric acid accumulates because the body is making too much uric acid from purines and/or the kidneys are not removing enough uric acid. Purines are released from the cells of certain foods we eat and from the breakdown of cells within our bodies.

Many foods contain high concentrations of purines, and if you eat less of such foods, less uric acid will form in your body (see table below). Dehydration, starvation, and certain foods and drugs can raise the body's level of uric acid by interfering with the kidneys' uric acid excretion (see also table below). By avoiding alcohol, low-dose aspirin, diuretics, and starvation, and by drinking at least two litres of water per day, you will help your kidneys to excrete uric acid more efficiently. As a result of these dietary measures, the body's uric acid level will diminish by a small degree and the uric acid crystals may stop forming in the joints. These dietary measures may then help

Foods and Drugs That Raise Uric Acid Levels in the Body

By increasing the purine load	By reducing uric acid excretion by the kidney
Meat: liver, kidneys, pancreas	Alcohol
Fish: anchovies, herring, scallops, mackerel,sardines	Diuretics
Vegetables: dried beans and peas, asparagus, cauliflower, mushrooms, spinach	Low doses of aspirin (ASA)
Alcohol	Cyclosporin
Chemotherapy destroying cancer cells	Lead intoxication
	Starvation
	Dehydration

prevent acute attacks of gout, but they will not control an acute attack of gout that is already in progress.

Osteoporosis

Getting enough calcium from childhood to early adulthood will help you to attain a good peak bone density. Maximum bone density is reached at about the age of 35, after which bone density will gradually lessen. Therefore the greater your bone density is at its peak, the longer you will take to develop osteoporosis, a condition in which the bones become thin, brittle, and prone to fracturing.

Getting 1000–1500 mg of calcium and 400–800 IU of Vitamin D per day is recommended for healthy bone. Vitamin D supplements may help fractures heal. If you are unable to obtain adequate amounts from your food (see table on page 302), then supplements will be necessary. To activate Vitamin D, about 15 minutes' daily exposure to sunlight (for the ultraviolet rays) is required, which can be a problem for photosensitive people such as those with systemic lupus erythematosus.

The dietary intake of calcium can be calculated by multiplying the number of dairy servings in a day by 300 mg. Examples of one dairy serving are 250 mL (8 oz) of milk or yogurt, 500 mL (16 oz) of cottage cheese, or 30 g (1 oz) of hard cheese.

The amount of elemental calcium in a supplement tablet will depend on whether it is made of calcium carbonate or calcium citrate. A 500 mg tablet of calcium carbonate contains 40 percent (200 mg) calcium. A 500 mg tablet of calcium citrate contains 21 percent (105 mg) calcium. Calcium carbonate will reduce the amount of iron your body can absorb, so it should not be taken with meals or iron supplements. Calcium citrate will not interfere with iron absorption from food. Some calcium carbonate products are not very soluble, so chewing Tums or Rolaids or using calcium citrate may be better. Avoid taking more than 500 mg of calcium at one time

Foods for Osteoporosis

Foods containing calcium	Foods containing Vitamin D
Milk and dairy products	Fortified milk and dairy products
Canned salmon and sardines	Tuna and fish oils
Oysters	Egg yolks
Broccoli and dark green leafy vegetables	Green leafy vegetables (collard greens, kale)
Tofu	
Almonds	
Calcium-fortified orange juice and soy drinks	

as your body can only absorb so much at a time, no matter how much you take. Split the dose over the day to maximize its absorption. Calcium supplements may cause stomach irritation and constipation, but a high calcium diet does not increase the risk of forming kidney stones.

Those who are lactose intolerant will not be able to digest dairy products, and will need calcium supplementation. People with other gastrointestinal conditions in which nutrients are not absorbed well will need calcium and Vitamin D replacement. Vitamin D deficiency results in reduced calcium absorption and loss of bone mass. Vegetarians have higher bone mass on average than non-vegetarians.

Chronic alcohol use leads to fractures by reducing the bone density and increasing the chances of falls and other trauma. Although caffeine and antacids containing aluminum cause a negative calcium balance, they may not contribute to osteoporosis and fractures. It is also uncertain that eating too much protein or phosphorus (as in soda pop) is associated with osteoporosis. Fluoride in high doses may protect against fractures, but doses that are too high can lead to brittle bones (fluorosis). The amounts of fluoride in tap water are too small to benefit bone. Corticosteroids and excess thyroid replacement are associated with osteoporosis and fractures.

Isoflavones are a group of compounds (found in foods like soy) that have estrogen and anti-estrogen effects. Taking 100 mg of soy isoflavone per day can reduce menopausal symptoms. Early studies suggest that soy isoflavone increases bone density in menopausal women, but its effect on preventing or promoting breast cancer is unknown.

Do They Really Affect Arthritis?

Arthritis is a chronic disease for which people would love to find a cure. Unfortunately, this has led to some confusion around the ability of different foods and practices to help or worsen arthritis. In this section, we will look at some of the things more commonly linked with arthritis, and explain what is known to date about their actual effect on the disease.

Food Sensitivity

The relationship of certain foods to the worsening of arthritis symptoms is mainly anecdotal, and surveys suggest that less than 5 percent of people will have their arthritis actually improve if they avoid specific foods or food additives. The most frequent culprits are cow's milk and dairy products, red meats, corn, wheat, and tartrazine dyes. You may wish to eliminate one of these foods from your diet for one to two weeks as a test. If the arthritis does not improve, then begin eating these foods again. If it does improve, then restart the food to see if the arthritis worsens. If it worsens, then eliminate this food from your diet. If the arthritis does not worsen, then continue eating this food.

There have been stories of people who have improved their arthritis by avoiding "nightshades" (potatoes, tomatoes, eggplant, bell peppers), but no good studies have been done to support this strategy. However, there is certainly no harm in trying this approach for a few weeks to see if it helps.

Celiac disease (or sprue) is an intestinal disease caused by an inherited sensitivity to gluten, and up to 25 percent of people with this condition have recurrent attacks of a non-destructive form of arthritis. Following a gluten-free diet will alleviate the symptoms of the disease (including the arthritis).

There is some suggestion but no definite proof that an amino acid (called l-canavanine) found in alfalfa seeds and sprouts might aggravate systemic lupus erythematosus.

A recent study showed that middle-aged women who drank four or more cups of decaffeinated coffee per day had a greater chance of developing rheumatoid arthritis. However, drinking more than three cups of tea per day in this same group was associated with a lower risk of developing rheumatoid arthritis, and caffeine and caffeinated coffee were not associated with rheumatoid arthritis.

Fasting

Fasting does not cure any medical conditions and can actually be dangerous to your health, especially if you are already thin. However, eating no food other than water frequently improves rheumatoid arthritis (including the joint swelling and the sedimentation rate [ESR]) after about three days. This improvement occurs because fasting suppresses the immune system. Obviously, prolonged fasting is not practical, however. The benefit is lost by one week after stopping the fast, but some people have prolonged the benefit by reintroducing foods one at a time. Some people prolong fasting by consuming water, tea, and vegetable and fruit juices.

Vegetarian Diets

In a study of 27 patients with rheumatoid arthritis, 12 had improved pain and stiffness after four weeks of a vegan diet that also included reduced amounts of coffee, tea, spices, and sugar. The improvement continued for at least two years in those who stuck to the diet. If you decide to eat a restricted diet, make sure you take supplements to replace any missing nutritional elements. Deficiencies of Vitamins B12 and D are not uncommon with vegetarian diets. Diets higher in vegetable protein are associated with less bone loss and fewer hip fractures than diets higher in animal protein. A vegetarian diet may also help you improve your general health and lose weight.

Dong Diet

This diet was a fad for arthritis some years ago, but a study has shown that this diet does not help arthritis. The diet includes vegetables (except tomatoes) and chicken, but eliminates fruit, dairy products, egg yolks, vinegar, pepper, chocolate, alcohol, soft drinks, and all additives and preservatives.

Fish Oils

Prostaglandins and leukotrienes are two families of chemicals that the body makes from fatty acids. Some of these chemicals contribute to the inflammatory process. Fish oils containing omega-3 fatty acids can reduce inflammation by causing the body to make less of the inflammatory and more of the non-inflammatory prostaglandins and leukotrienes. Fish oils can reduce the morning stiffness and the joint tenderness and swelling in rheumatoid arthritis by a small amount, and may improve Raynaud's phenomenon and the skin and joints of psoriatic arthritis patients. The dose of NSAIDs might also be reduced. Fish oils do not seem to help osteoarthritis. The results of studies in systemic lupus erythematosus are inconsistent, although one study suggested that high doses of fish oils might reduce the amount of corticosteroids required.

Fish oils must be taken in large quantities for a period of at least three months to be effective. Omega-3 fatty acids are found in cold-water fish, such as salmon, mackerel, herring, tuna, sardines, bluefish, halibut, swordfish, trout, and cod. A more practical way to obtain enough omega-3 fatty acids is to take supplements containing 1.7–2.7 g/day of eicosapentaenoic acid (EPA) and 1.1 g/day of docosahexaenoic acid (DHA). They should be introduced gradually in order to reduce such side effects as nausea, bloating, belching, and loose stools. They may interfere with blood thinners. Avoid using them with cod liver oil as Vitamins A and D may accumulate to toxic levels. They are particularly worth trying if non-steroidal anti-inflammatory drugs cannot be used.

Plant Seed Oils

Plant seed oils work in a similar fashion to the fish oils. Flax seed oil contains omega-3 fatty acids, whereas evening primrose, borage seed, and black currant seed oils contain the omega-6 fatty acid gamma linolenic acid (GLA) in addition to some omega-3 fatty acids. The recommended dose of GLA, about 1800 mg/day, may help rheumatoid arthritis to a small degree. Other foods that contain omega-3 and GLA fatty acids are canola, soybeans, tofu, beans, walnuts, pecans, collards, kale, and spinach. GLA can cause mild gastrointestinal side effects and interact with blood thinners. Evening primrose oil may not be safe for people with seizure disorders.

Other types of omega-6 fatty acids may actually worsen inflammation and pain by being converted to inflammatory prostaglandins and leukotrienes. Eating less of these foods (e.g., safflower, corn, sunflower, and cottonseed oils) may help reduce inflammation. They are often found in processed foods, some of the fat in meat, and foods fried in cooking oils.

Avocado and Soybean Unsaponifiables (ASU)

ASU, which contains one-third avocado oil and two-thirds soybean oil, is available as Plascledine 300 in Europe. Studies indicate that it reduces pain and disability in osteoarthritis. The dose is 300 mg/day.

Antioxidants

Small, oxygen-containing chemicals called oxygen radicals contribute to tissue damage and inflammation. In joints, they can damage the hyaluronic acid in the joint fluid, and the collagen, proteoglycans, and cells in the cartilage. Antioxidants counteract the oxygen radicals. Antioxidants are made in the body naturally but can also be obtained from external sources, including Vitamin A (retinol and beta-carotene), Vitamin C (ascorbic acid) and Vitamin E (alpha-tocopherol).

Vitamin E at a dose of 600 mg/day can reduce the pain of osteoarthritis but if it doesn't by eight weeks, stop taking it. At a dose of 600 mg twice daily, it can reduce the pain but not the inflammation of rheumatoid arthritis. Sometimes doses greater than 1000 mg/day may prolong bleeding. There is no evidence that Vitamin C helps rheumatoid arthritis, but one study suggests that it may slow the progression of osteoarthritis of the knee at a dose of 200 mg/day. There is no evidence that Vitamin A benefits arthritis except for one study that suggests but does not prove that it might help osteoarthritis of the knees. It has recently been shown that chronic high doses of Vitamin A (more than 3000 g/day), particularly in the form of retinol, contribute to the development of osteoporosis and hip fractures in post-menopausal women.

Other Vitamins and Minerals

Vitamin B3 (niacin) may lessen the pain of osteoarthritis and may improve Raynaud's phenomenon (because it can dilate blood vessels), but it also causes the skin to flush and the blood pressure to drop. Vitamin B5 (pantothenic acid) may reduce pain and improve mobility in rheumatoid arthritis. Vitamin B9 (folic acid) contributes to cartilage nutrition, but there are no studies to indicate that folic acid helps arthritis (except that it can reduce some of the side effects of methotrexate, a drug used to treat several types of inflammatory arthritis). Osteoarthritis of the knees progresses faster in those who have low blood levels of Vitamin D and ingest less than 200 IU per day.

Calcium has already been discussed in this chapter regarding its role in osteoporosis; it may also prevent muscle cramps, but does not help arthritis.

Boron helps the body use calcium and magnesium, and causes some anti-inflammatory activity. One study suggested that it benefits osteoarthritis. Boron is found in fruits and vegetables. Too much boron from supplements could raise estrogen levels, which could be a problem for some women.

Copper is needed for healthy bones, has some anti-inflammatory properties, and can increase the potency of the non-steroidal anti-inflammatories (NSAIDs). Copper compounds were given by injection a few decades ago to treat rheumatoid arthritis, and seemed to help but there were many side effects. There is no proof that oral copper helps arthritis. Copper is found in seafood, organ meats, nuts, cocoa, seeds, dried beans, and water from copper pipes.

Magnesium is important for bone health, muscle function, and energy. One study showed that magnesium combined with malic acid reduced pain and fatigue in fibromyalgia when compared with a placebo. Magnesium is present in nuts, grains, fish, milk, and leafy green vegetables. Too much magnesium can cause diarrhea, muscle weakness, and fatigue. If you are using medications to treat high blood pressure or if you have reduced kidney function, you should consult your doctor before taking extra magnesium.

Selenium is an antioxidant. Studies of its efficacy in the treatment of rheumatoid arthritis are contradictory: some studies indicate that it does not help at all, while others show that it helps somewhat but that it takes up to eight months to get the desired effect. Mushrooms, eggs, garlic, lean meats, and seafood contain selenium. Large doses can be toxic, however, and can cause hair loss, tooth decay, and swelling of the legs.

Zinc is needed for collagen production and normal functioning of the immune system, and may cause anti-inflammatory activity. One study showed that it helped rheumatoid arthritis, but subsequent studies did not show this. Lean meat, seafood, soybeans, peanuts, eggs, cheese, wheat, and bran contain zinc. Too much zinc can cause vomiting, headaches, and fatigue. It can interfere with corticosteroids and immunosuppressants.

Single Food Fads

There is no proof that the following foods or food substances help arthritis: Brewer's yeast, garlic, cod liver oil, alfalfa, gin-soaked raisins, apple cider vinegar, molasses, honey, or bromaline (an enzyme from the pineapple plant, which has mild anti-inflammatory properties).

Ginger, on the other hand, may cause the body to make fewer prostaglandins and leukotrienes. Derivatives of ginger may block pain at the nerve receptors, possibly improving the pain and swelling of osteoarthritis and rheumatoid arthritis to a minor degree. Ginger may also help muscular discomfort. It can be taken as a powdered ginger supplement, an extract, or a tea (1 g/day). It may interact with blood thinners.

Bowel Cleansing

Overgrowth of normal bowel bacteria in blinded loops of intestine (as may occur in the intestinal bypass procedure that used to be done to treat obesity) can cause an inflammatory arthritis. It is treated with antibiotics or removal of the blind loops. Infections of the bowel with external microbes such as salmonella in genetically susceptible people (having HLA-B27) may lead to reactive arthritis but it does not respond to antibiotic treatment.

Some people believe that waste builds up in the folds of their large intestine (colon) and is then absorbed into the bloodstream ("auto-intoxication"), causing illnesses such as arthritis. However, diets and enemas (colon therapy, colonic irrigation, high colonic) to "detoxify the bowel" have not proved useful for treating arthritis. Complications such as infection, perforation of the bowel, and electrolyte disturbances are possible. This type of therapy should be avoided if you have bowel diseases like ulcerative colitis or Crohn's disease.

The bottom line regarding diet and arthritis is that a healthy diet is of utmost importance. Eat nutritious foods that will give your body what it needs, and take supplements as your doctor advises to fill in any nutritional gaps. Diet has a direct effect on obesity, gout, and osteoporosis. Some vitamins and minerals may have a minor beneficial effect on arthritis. Eating more omega-3 (EPA and DHA) and GLA fatty acids and ASU, and less omega-6 fatty acids, may benefit some types of arthritis. Only a small minority of patients with arthritis are affected by food sensitivities. Beware of fad diets and the "therapy of the week"; instead, educate yourself, and consult your doctor or dietitian about the most beneficial diet-related measures you can take to help your arthritis.

12 Exercises and activities

Exercise is important for joint mobility, stretching muscles and tendons for flexibility, strengthening muscles for power and endurance, and improving general fitness and conditioning.

A physiotherapist will assess your musculoskeletal system and general health, design a therapeutic exercise program with you, and teach you the exercise program and how to self-manage it. You will learn to exercise independently at home and in your community, and exercise videotapes, pamphlets, and worksheets will help you to remember your program. You can consult the physiotherapist for advice, or talk to kinesiologists, personal trainers, and instructors of special exercises like yoga and tai chi. Local resources such as exercise and aquafit classes at community centres and Arthritis Society centres can be utilized.

These exercise programs must be followed regularly in order to improve your arthritis and general health. Do not substitute routine home or work tasks for your exercises. Routine tasks do not put joints through a full range of movement, nor do they strengthen the weakest muscles. These exercises are designed to correct specific joint problems.

The variables that make up an exercise program are intensity, duration, and frequency. *Intensity* refers to the amount of effort or exertion that is used during the activity. *Duration* refers to the length of time that an exercise is done. It may be measured in minutes or by the number of times (repetitions, or "reps") that a certain manoeuvre is repeated in a row (a set) and the number of sets to be done during an exercise session. *Frequency* refers to the number of exercise sessions that you do per day and per week.

Benefits of Exercise

Inactivity is harmful to people with arthritis, as exercise benefits the joints, cartilage, bone, muscles, ligaments, tendons, fitness level, mood, general health, and ability to perform one's daily activities. Exercise improves or maintains the range of movement of your joints, prevents joint contractures, and reduces joint pain, stiffness, and inflammation. Joint movement aids the nutrition of cartilage and the removal of waste from cartilage; as cartilage has no blood supply, it relies on movement to move fluid in and out.

By increasing the density of bone, exercise becomes an important factor in treating and preventing osteoporosis. Exercise stretches muscles, ligaments, and tendons to reduce stiffness and to increase flexibility. Muscles will become stronger and bulkier. As a result, joint stability will improve, more shock will be absorbed by the muscles, and less energy will be expended while carrying out an action. Joints will be less prone to injury and fatigue will lessen.

Aerobic exercise enables the heart to pump blood more efficiently and the lungs to increase their breathing capacity. Stamina and endurance improve significantly, and there is a reduction in pain and stiffness. Fewer medications may be needed. Disability lessens: the ability to perform daily activities becomes greater, and balance, coordination, posture, and breathing mechanics improve. One's degree of independence increases. Self-esteem and confidence grow. The feelings of depression, tension, anger, and helplessness diminish, and a sense of well-being begins to develop. Exercise makes one sleep better, too.

Exercise increases the production of endorphins and proteins and reduces the blood sugar and cholesterol levels. As a result of exercise, the body will make less of the "bad" cytokines (like tumour necrosis factor) that worsen arthritis. Exercise also improves one's general health by reducing excess weight, lowering the mortality from coronary artery disease, reducing high blood pressure, and preventing or delaying the onset of non-insulin-dependent diabetes mellitus. Blood is less likely to clot in the blood vessels and strokes occur less frequently. The risk of developing cancer of the breast and colon is reduced. Even constipation improves with exercise.

The longest follow-up study of the effect of exercise on rheumatoid arthritis was five years. People in the study exercised for five hours or more each week, and showed a reduction in the progression of joint damage, in the occurrence of work disability, and in the need for hospitalization.

Types of Exercise for Arthritis

The main types of exercise that are prescribed for managing arthritis are range of movement, stretching, strengthening, aerobics, and body awareness. Each one is described below.

Range of Movement

Arthritis usually limits the mobility of a joint. Range of movement exercises are done to improve this limitation of mobility in all the directions that a joint can move and to prevent contractures of the joint. In addition, they reduce stiffness and pain and increase your ability to perform activities.

All joints should be put through a complete range of movement at least once daily to preserve the range of movement that you have. This principle applies not only to the joints of the arms and legs, but to your neck, back, jaws, and ribs (the rib joints are used to expand your chest when breathing).

Each joint should go through a full range of movement 5 to 10 times per session in order to improve the joint mobility; two sessions should be done daily. Hold each movement for two to three seconds. If a joint is particularly sore, then reduce the reps to three to five times per session. If the joints are very inflamed, then reduce the reps to one to two times per session, but do not stop exercising the joint entirely.

Stretching

These exercises are designed to improve your flexibility by stretching your muscles and tendons. Tight, short muscles increase joint pain. Muscle groups should be stretched slowly and gently. Large amounts of fluid in a joint may loosen the capsule and ligaments with repeated, forceful stretches. Very unstable joints may dislocate if forcefully stretched. The key muscle groups for stretching are the elbow extensors, wrist flexors, small hand muscles, hip flexors and extensors, knee flexors, and ankle downward flexors. Each stretch should be held for 15 to 20 seconds and repeated two or three times. If the joints are inflamed, avoid stretching that part of the body temporarily.

Strengthening

Resistance exercises will increase the power, endurance, and size of your muscles, and will strengthen your bone and cartilage. There will be better stability, support, and shock absorption to protect your joints from injury. Tasks will become more effortless and less fatiguing. The two types of resistance exercises recommended for arthritis are isometric and isotonic.

Isometric exercises contract your muscles without moving your joints: the force exerted by the muscles increases without any change in the length of the muscle fibres. The main muscle groups that should be strengthened are the shoulder abductors, elbow flexors, wrist extensors, small muscles of the hands and feet, hip extensors and abductors, knee extensors, and ankle upward flexors. The contractions should be held for six seconds and repeated 5 to 10 times with 10-second rest periods between contractions. These exercises are the first step in preparing you for more vigorous activities, including the isotonic exercises.

Isotonic exercises use weights or elastic fitness bands (e.g., Thera-Band) to provide steady resistance while the joint is moved through a partial range of movement. The amount of resistance remains constant, while the speed of the joint movement against the resistance varies. Do not extend the joint to the end of its range or injury may result. Light weights can also be strapped to the ankles and wrists when walking. With pool therapy, the water can provide resistance as well. Exercise machines can also be used. These exercises should be started slowly with small, padded hand weights (0.5–1 kg) or light elastic fitness bands. Do not overdo it: contract the muscle slowly, and then relax to the starting position.

For both types of strengthening, start with just a few repetitions per set and then gradually build up to 10 per set. Do two sets if there is no pain, but take a break between sets. Do these exercises three times per week but one to two days apart to allow the muscles to recover. Do half as many if the joints are mildly sore or swollen, and stop temporarily if the joints are flared up. Breathe in with relaxation and breathe out with exertion. Avoid overexertion and tensing up the muscles.

Aerobic

Aerobic exercise involves the rhythmic, continuous motion of large muscles, as in walking, swimming, dancing, or cycling. It builds up your endurance, stamina, conditioning, and heart, lung, and muscle efficiency so that you can do more tasks and activities for longer each day. It also reduces joint pain and inflammation, depression, and excess weight.

These exercises should be done for 5 to 10 minutes three times per week to start, then gradually increase over a few months to 20 to 30 minutes four to five times per week. Do not do aerobics when your joints are too inflamed. Try to get your pulse rate to rise to a target level above your resting rate. Your maximum pulse rate is (220 minus your age) beats per minute. Your target level should be 60 to 80 percent of your maximum pulse rate. For example, the maximum pulse rate for a 40-year-old is 180 beats per minute ($220 - 40 = 180$). The target level is 108 to 144 beats per minute ($180 \times 0.6 = 108$ and $180 \times 0.8 = 144$).

Body Awareness

Exercises such as yoga and tai chi can improve your balance, posture, breathing, and coordination. As a result, you will be less prone to injuries and accidents such as falls. There will be less stress on vulnerable joints, and back and neck deformities will be prevented.

Exercise Routine

You should develop your routine over several weeks to a few months. Begin with range of movement and stretching exercises. Isometric exercises can then be added. Once these are mastered, isotonic exercises can be started, followed by aerobics. After that, add in recreational activities.

Exercise should be done regularly each day, at times during the day when you have the least fatigue, pain, and stiffness. Set aside 20 to 60 minutes twice daily, and balance exercise with rest. Wear comfortable, loose-fitting clothes and cushioned supportive shoes. Make sure you are warm in cool weather and cool in warm weather. Drink water or other fluids often—before, during, and after exercise. Take a hot shower or bath before exercising if you are stiff and sore. Ice any inflamed joints before exercising.

Warm up by doing the range of movement and stretching exercises or by mild walking or cycling. Your body will become warmer and more limber. The temperature of your muscles and joints will increase so that they can work more efficiently with less chance of injuries like pulled muscles. Exercise your worst joints first.

After you have warmed up with the range and stretching exercises, start the strengthening exercises and aerobics.

Cool down by doing gentle stretches over about 5 to 10 minutes. By doing so, your heart and blood vessels will safely adjust to the reduced demand and your muscles will be less sore and tight the next day.

If you are fairly stiff on awakening, start the day by doing your range of movement and stretching exercises in bed. If your work is sedentary, get up and move around at least every hour. Do some of your exercises in the chair or when you get up to move around.

Precautions

Reduce or avoid exercise for an inflamed joint, and protect it with a splint during your exercise routine.

Avoid bouncing or high-impact-loading exercises such as running, racquet sports, basketball, and high-impact aerobics: they will put too much strain on your joints. Also avoid stairs, standing on one leg for too long, and carrying loads greater than 10 percent of your body weight if your lower extremity joints are involved. Walking too fast increases the stress put on your knees. In addition, exercise on soft, level surfaces with cushioned shoes to absorb the impact before it hits your joints. Wear good shoes: they should have low, wide heels, good support for the arches and ankles, and room for the toes. Orthotics may be needed.

Aerobic exercise may be limited by some of the non-joint features of the rheumatic diseases, such as pericarditis (inflammation around the heart), pleurisy (inflammation around the lung), vasculitis (inflamed blood vessels), lung fibrosis or scarring, heart valve lesions, blocks in the heart rhythm, and kidney complications.

Don't overdo the exercises. Overuse can make your joints more painful, hot, and swollen. Ice, elevation, rest, and modifying the exercises will help. If the exercises cause fatigue, stop, rest, and scale back your program. Exercise should be done at a moderate, not strenuous, level. You should feel as if your body is working but you should be able to talk normally and carry on at a comfortable pace. If you have not exercised for a while, start back slowly or else you will have sore joints, stiff muscles, and fatigue.

Protect your back. When doing standing exercises, hold on to the back of a chair or other support. Use a chair with a backrest when you are doing exercises in the sitting position. Avoid sit-ups and other flexion exercises of the back if osteoporosis is present, as the sudden rise in pressure with such exercises is transmitted to the bodies of the vertebrae in the back, increasing the chance of fracturing one or more of them.

Warning Signs

The most common reason for stopping exercise is not pain, but exercise intolerance, which includes fatigue, shortness of breath, dizziness, nausea, tired legs, very red face or pallor, profuse sweating, and uncomfortable heat. Some people feel chest pain, tightness, or pressure. If you are feeling these symptoms, it is best to stop the exercise, but resume it later at an easier pace—do not give up. If these symptoms recur, check with your doctor.

Muscle pain or cramps can occur during exercise. Stop the exercise and stretch the muscle until the pain eases up, then restart the exercise carefully. If the exercise worsens joint pain, heat, or swelling, stop the exercise then rest and ice the joint. When the problem settles down, restart the exercise program, but modify it to protect the joint that was aggravated. Differentiate these overuse problems from muscles that become sore several hours after exercising. This type of pain lasts 24 to 36 hours. It is handled by doing more stretching in the warm-up and cool-down periods and scaling back the intensity of the exercises. As you become more fit, it becomes less of a problem.

You probably did too much too fast if muscle or joint pain lasts for more than two hours after exercising, if fatigue lasts until the next day, or soreness lasts for one to two days afterwards. When you restart the exercises, reduce their intensity and frequency and then slowly build them up again.

Commitment

Many people find it difficult to stick to a regular exercise program. Have a vested interest in the program by being involved with the physiotherapist in designing it. Learn to manage the exercise program yourself. The plan should be realistic and easy to accomplish so that you do not get discouraged. Write down the specifics and use a calendar or organizer. Keep a diary or chart listing the exercises done and their duration and frequency. If it would be helpful, make a contract with yourself or bet a friend or family member that you will stay the course.

Make exercise a routine or habit in your life: it takes a few months to make the plan part of your lifestyle. Have confidence in your ability to become fit. Setbacks and lapses are common—just get back to exercising as soon as possible. Even if you are tired, walk for five minutes.

Listen to music, use a Walkman, watch television, or talk on your cell phone while you exercise. Exercising with a friend or relative or in a group or class may motivate you. Vary your exercises and incorporate enjoyable activities so that you do not get bored. Combine your walk with a task such as exercising your dog, going to the bank, or doing your shopping. Having a coach, personal trainer, or instructor will encourage you to continue exercising.

Exercise Activities

There are several physical activities that will provide you with a pleasurable workout. They include walking, hiking, bicycling, swimming, water exercises, water walking, dancing, low-impact aerobics, rowing, using a cross-country ski machine, ice-skating, and skiing. You can interchange these activities for variety, aiming to do one of them daily. Walking, bicycling, and pool exercises will now be discussed in more detail.

Walking

Walking is worth doing when your arthritis is not in an acute phase; it will increase your fitness level, leg strength, and bone density. Dress for the weather, wear good shoes, and walk on flat surfaces. If the weather is bad, walk in a mall. Use a walking stick if it makes walking easier. Avoid leaning forward from the waist, slumping, or whipping your elbows. Keep your chest up, abdominal muscles in, and shoulders down and relaxed. On the other hand, you may prefer to use a treadmill, where it is easy to measure your progress and pulse, and regulate the speed, incline, and duration of your walk. Start by walking for 5 to 10 minutes at a slow pace three times per week. Gradually increase the pace and the length of time that you are walking, with the goal of eventually walking five to seven days per week. Scale back on a bad day, but keep the routine going.

Bicycling

Bicycling can be done outdoors on a regular bicycle during good weather, or indoors on a stationary bicycle all year round. The equipment can be adjusted for your needs regarding height of the seat, padding of the seat, and height of the handlebars; there is even back support on some stationary bicycles. Pedal with the balls of your feet and keep your knees only slightly bent. Avoid high gears. Wear shorts or pants that will not get caught in the chain, and wear bike gloves and a helmet when using a moving bike.

Bicycling allows you to do aerobic exercise while reducing the weight bearing on your lower extremity joints. It does not jolt or injure your joints. In fact, it will decrease joint swelling. Your functional capacity and muscle strength will increase. It is simple, relatively inexpensive, and enjoyable, and can be done individually or in a group, and for a lifetime.

Start slowly with minimal resistance for 5 to 10 minutes three times per week. Gradually increase the intensity, duration, and frequency, with the aim of cycling five to seven times per week.

Pool Exercises

A swimming pool allows for a wide variety of exercise strategies. Range of movement and stretching exercises can be done with the aid of the heat and buoyancy of the water. Upper and lower limbs and the trunk can be isolated for strengthening and range of movement exercises. Lap swimming and water walking can improve your general conditioning. Walking and standing drills can be started in the pool to re-educate the body for weight bearing skills, and positioning techniques for reducing pain can be taught more easily in the pool. Exercises can also be done to improve balance, agility, and coordination, and to simulate athletic or work skills.

You don't need to know how to swim. You can exercise in the shallow water, hold on to the side, or use a flotation device. Water exercise is safe (it is difficult to fall or injure yourself in the water). The water provides heat, buoyancy, fun, support, assistance, and resistance. The pool temperature ranges between 28 and 30 degrees

Celsius and the air temperature is about 27 degrees Celsius. The buoyancy reduces your body weight by 90 percent! Movement is easy and smooth, and the heart rate is reduced so that a greater level of exercise is tolerated. Resistance can be increased by speeding up movements and by using devices like water wings or large mitts. Certain activities or tasks that would normally be done "on land" can be started with less trouble in the water before progressing to land. Weight bearing and joint impact can be avoided in the pool. Furthermore, the pool can be used during a flare-up of the arthritis.

Pool therapy can result in a reduction of pain and stiffness and an improvement in strength, stamina, mobility, coordination, flexibility, posture, cardiovascular endurance, and gait. It is pleasurable, relaxing, and allows for socializing. There is no sweating while exercising in the water.

In patients with low back pain due to mechanical stresses or degenerative disc or joint disease, or back pain due to vertebral fractures from osteoporosis, pool therapy is very helpful. By reducing the effects of gravity, there is less pain with active exercises, more trunk mobility, and less chance of stressing the discs, joints, ligaments, and vertebrae while strengthening the muscles.

In ankylosing spondylitis, the reduction of gravity leads to a less flexed posture. Diaphragmatic breathing is improved. Extension exercises are more easily done in the water.

With lower limb arthritis, water makes it easier to practise walking normally. It allows you to return to work sooner and to do more activities of daily living earlier. With upper limb arthritis, water makes it easier to do exercises in many different directions so that the strength, range of movement, and posture of these joints improve faster.

There are situations in which pool therapy should not be chosen, however, such as when you have fever, infections, or skin wounds or ulcers. It is not safe to do pool exercises if you have uncontrolled seizures, severe cardiovascular disease, or severely high or low blood pressure. The pool should also be avoided if there is incontinence of the bowel or bladder, a colostomy bag or urinary catheter, or a tracheotomy or stomach tubes.

Additional Forms of Exercise

Other forms of exercise can be included in your program, but you will need a specially trained instructor to teach you any one of the exercise systems discussed in this section.

Tai Chi

Tai chi provides both exercise and relaxation. It evolved from the martial arts as a way for qi, the life force, to flow through the body. The movements and their names are derived from nature and animals. Each movement involves a series of slow, controlled motions that flow into a long graceful gesture. It is performed with relaxed breathing from the diaphragm, meditation, quiet, and concentration. It is often done outside, surrounded by nature. All joints, muscles, and tendons are exercised.

Tai chi is safe for persons of all ages with arthritis. One should aim to do it for 10 to 40 minutes daily. It improves balance, flexibility, mobility, pain, muscle strength, stress, and depression, and it prevents falls in elderly people. More information can be found at www.taichiforarthritis.com.

Qi Gong

Qi gong (chee gong) is similar to but older than tai chi. It has fewer movements, and the movements are held for a few seconds with pauses between them. It is easy for people with arthritis to do, and can even be done in a wheelchair or bed. It can reduce pain and depression and improve mobility and function.

Yoga

Yoga (or "union") is an exercise and meditation system developed in India for uniting the body, mind, and spirit. Its main components are proper breathing, movement, and posture. There are several branches of yoga, but all involve gentle movements that you can perform at your own pace in positions called asanas that are named after animals and nature. The asanas can be done while sitting, standing, or lying. In these positions, various stretches and breathing techniques (pranayama) are employed. Yoga is usually done barefoot on a mat, and it can be done individually or in a group.

Yoga can improve strength, energy, flexibility and balance, and can reduce stress and depression. Studies have shown yoga to be superior to splints for treating carpal tunnel syndrome. It can improve the pain, tenderness, and restricted movement caused by osteoarthritis of the hands, and yoga can also help rheumatoid arthritis.

Alexander Technique

An actor named F. Matthias Alexander developed this method, which teaches you how to move and hold your body differently in order to reduce pain and stress on joints. It is useful for changing bad postures, positions, and body use in order to ease or prevent pain. Some of these bad habits may have been originally adopted to avoid pain from another region. (For instance, your right knee may become painful as a result of it compensating for osteoarthritis in your left hip.) It teaches you better ways to use arthritic joints and painful muscles. Movement, activities, and balance will take less effort. A study showed that the Alexander technique improved balance and reaching in older women, and it also reduced chronic pain more than some other techniques.

Feldenkrais Method

Moshe Feldenkrais, a Russian Jew who had injured his left knee while playing soccer, developed this method while recuperating. It makes you aware of how you move and carry yourself. Through a series of range of movement and flexibility motions, you learn better postures and ways to lessen stress on joints.

Trager Approach

Milton Trager, a physician and boxer, developed this approach, which has a passive and an active component. The passive component is referred to as "tablework." A practitioner moves the subject in ways that he or she naturally moves, and with a quality of touch and movement that cause the recipient to feel that the movements are effortless and free. The active component is called "mentastics"; it is the way the feeling of effortless movement is maintained and reinforced. Simple self-induced movements that you can do on your own during your daily activities release deep-seated physical and mental patterns, which result from your responses to prior physical and emotional trauma. Deep relaxation, better physical mobility, and mental clarity will follow. No specific number of repetitions, length of sessions, or frequency are recorded.

Pilates System

Joseph Pilates (pronounced pill-AH-teeze) was a nurse who designed exercise devices for immobilized patients by attaching springs to their beds. The Pilates system calls for a series of controlled movements to be performed on specially designed exercise equipment with the supervision of a trained teacher. Many dancers use Pilates, as it improves flexibility and strength for the entire body without building up muscle mass.

The abdomen, lower back, and buttocks are supported and strengthened, enabling the rest of the body to move freely. Weak muscles are strengthened, and bulky muscles are elongated. The emphasis is on stretching and strengthening to improve strength, flexibility, posture, and coordination. The Pilates system works the body as a whole, coordinating the upper and lower musculature with the body's centre.

Leisure Activities

Leisure activities can exercise your mind, spirit, and body. They are relaxing and fun to do, but make sure that you do not get so carried away that you do not move around from time to time to loosen up and that you do not tire yourself out. These activities should not aggravate the arthritis. Explore community resources, newspapers, universities, colleges, schools, and the Internet for leisure activities.

Children with Arthritis

Children with arthritis should be encouraged to play and exercise. Not only will their pain, muscle bulk, bone strength, and disability improve, but they will feel more like the other kids. Their sense of helplessness will be lessened or avoided.

Children should be able to do isometric exercises by age four years. They enjoy pool therapy, and range of movement, aerobics, and strengthening exercises can be done in the water. Extension exercises of the neck are important to combat the tendency of juvenile onset rheumatoid arthritis to cause flexion deformities of the neck. Also, knee and hip flexion contractures occur quickly, so range of movement and flexibility exercises and lying prone should be emphasized. Flexion contractures of the PIP joints of the fingers need exercise therapy as well.

Aerobic exercises could include activities like bicycling, tricycling, swimming, skating, hiking, dancing, and walking. However, high-impact and contact sports like hockey, football, rugby, and trampoline should be avoided.

Seniors with Arthritis

With aging comes a reduction of cardiovascular fitness, muscle mass and power, bone density, joint mobility, energy, good posture, and balance. As a result, the functional capabilities of seniors decline progressively. The presence of arthritis in older adults will complicate this situation further. Inactivity will lead to worse exercise tolerance and fitness, stiffer joints, weaker and more wasted muscles, and worse balance and coordination. Their activities of daily living will become even more limited. Light to moderate intensity exercises can counteract these changes as well as reduce the risk factors associated with chronic diseases. Exercise can also improve seniors' psychological well-being.

Because older persons with arthritis have reduced physical reserves, it will take them two to three months to adapt to the work of exercising. Their physical performance and disease activity will vary from day to day. Their commitment to exercise will be affected by reduced motivation and energy, slowness, and less time to dedicate to the activity. Their goals should be realistic: they should start by exercising for 20 minutes twice weekly. They should warm up for 5 to 10 minutes with stretching and cool down with five minutes of stretching.

Studies have shown that regular aerobic and strengthening exercises improved the walking speed, transfers (e.g., getting out of a bed or chair), and disability in elderly patients with osteoarthritis or rheumatoid arthritis. Exercise did not worsen the pain or disease activity in the rheumatoid arthritis patients, or the pain or joint damage in the osteoarthritis patients. It resulted in better functional capacity, fitness, strength, and mobility. Tai chi reduced the risk of falls in the older population.

Older people with arthritis should do the range of movement and stretching exercises in the morning and evenings. Doing these exercises in the evenings lessens the next day's morning stiffness in those with rheumatoid arthritis. They should start with one stretch per muscle group per session three times weekly, and then gradually increase to 4 to 10 per muscle group per session daily.

Isometric exercises should begin at one contraction per muscle group. The contraction should be held for about six seconds, as holding a contraction for more than 10 seconds can raise the blood pressure. Slowly increase the number of reps to 8 to 10. Rest for 20 seconds between contractions. Gradually add in isotonic exercises to strengthen 8 to 10 muscle groups. Eventually do one set of four to six reps. All these muscle-strengthening exercises can be done just twice weekly. Allow two days between strengthening sessions for the muscles to recover.

Aerobic exercises should also begin at low intensity, and the starting duration should be 20 to 30 minutes a day in divided periods of no less than five minutes. Then, slowly consolidate the duration into one 20-to-30-minute continuous session per day, and increase the frequency to three to four days per week.

Exercise should not be done if the person has uncontrolled problems with heart rhythm, third-degree heart block, recent changes in an electrocardiogram (ECG or EKG), unstable angina, acute congestive heart failure, or a recent heart attack. If there are any problems with the heart muscle or valves, high blood pressure, the control of a metabolic disease like diabetes mellitus, kidney failure, or abnormal thyroid function, then hold off exercising until the doctor gives the okay.

13 Arthritis and sexuality

Sex is a very important part of healthy living and, certainly, of our relationships with partners. Not only that, but sex provides several physical benefits that can really help someone with arthritis, including improved sleep, reduced pain and anxiety, and relaxation of the muscles. It is, however, something that many of us feel embarrassed to talk about, even with our physicians, so people with arthritis and their partners may be without some information that could potentially improve their sex lives. The purpose of this chapter is to discuss some of the common problems that people with arthritis face and to offer some solutions.

Studies suggest that a significant number of people do not have a change in their sex lives after the onset of arthritis. People with arthritis can have a satisfying sex life. However, it is not hard to imagine that fatigue, pain, and joints that just don't move could pose some problems.

Fatigue

Fatigue is a common problem for people with arthritis and other chronic illnesses. Most do not allow the fatigue to keep them from having a life, however. They plan their activities to make the most of their energy and work around the fatigue, and making love may require some forward planning also.

- Plan for the time of day that you feel the best.
- Pace your activities so you are not exhausted

- Plan a weekend away, when you don't have to cook, clean, or take care of other responsibilities.

As your arthritis is better controlled, the fatigue also improves. Exercise is certainly beneficial in the long term to improve your energy level and stamina, and sex can be a pleasant workout!

Pain

Pain is a big problem. You may not be in the mood for sex because the pain is all-consuming; your partner may be afraid of making the pain worse. Some forward planning can help here as well. Preparing yourself for lovemaking in the ways suggested below will have the effect of reducing or relieving your pain, and can actually be a pleasurable part of the sexual experience itself.

- Take your medication such that it will have its maximum effect at the time when you are planning to make love. You should take it 30 minutes ahead of time.
- Take a warm bath or shower beforehand. If you do this with your partner, it is more fun.
- Have your partner give you a massage. This will relieve muscle tension and pain, and will help you relax and get in the mood. You can give your partner a massage as well.
- Make yourself comfortable, and have a pillow to support your neck or low back. Have a comfortable bed or even a waterbed as this may help if repetitive movements cause pain.

You and your partner need to be able to communicate well so that if you are experiencing pain, you can give a signal that would mean "try something else but do not give up completely." Good communication is the key to pleasurable sex for people without arthritis, and it is even more important where arthritis is involved.

Depression and Self-Image

Depression is common with chronic diseases. Its symptoms include poor sleep, early-morning awakening, and loss of libido (sex drive).

The treatment of depression with arthritis is the same as if depression were the primary problem, and sometimes medications can make a big difference to how you feel. Not all of the effects can be good where sex is concerned, however. Some medications for depression can cause you to have a decreased interest in sex, and some can make your mouth and vagina dry. If you are concerned about depression or these side effects of antidepressant medication, be sure to discuss your concerns with your physician.

When patients have arthritis, they often feel unattractive. They feel older because they are stiff and sore, and may feel that their hands or feet are ugly. They may feel unattractive to their partner, even though they are still the same person that the partner was attracted to in the first place.

On the other hand, your partner may communicate that he or she is not in fact attracted to you, and this needs to be explored fully. Your partner may feel that way because of being afraid of physically hurting you, or may be having trouble accepting any physical changes. Whatever the reason, it needs to be discussed openly and sensitively. Often, discussing issues like these will bring you closer together.

What are the solutions to this type of problem?

- Feel good about yourself. This may mean dressing in a style or colour that looks good and makes you feel better. It may mean having your hair done, or getting a manicure. If you are confident and feel good, then you will be more attractive.
- Communicate with your partner, who needs to know that in fact you still have an interest in sex. Your partner needs to know that you will not be hurt and if you are, you will let her or him

know. Together you will try and figure out something else that would work better.

- Nourish your relationship. If you are not interested in sex, you need to let your partner know this as well. When your disease is very active, the fatigue can be profound and you feel ill. Often at times like these, you may not feel up to having sex, but you can still express feelings of affection and appreciation for your partner.

Medications

Some arthritis medications will decrease your libido, and some will also cause impotence (making a man unable to get an erection). Most of the medications used to treat arthritis do not cause these problems, but some common medications that might work in this way would include corticosteroids (prednisone), muscle relaxants, narcotics, and antidepressants. If you are concerned about these issues, you should talk with your pharmacist or physician.

Physical Barriers

Rheumatoid arthritis, Sjogren's syndrome, and lupus may be associated with dryness of the eyes, mouth, and vagina. The vaginal dryness may cause intercourse to be painful, and the best solution for this problem is to use a lubricant. K-Y jelly, Replens, Astroglide, and Mukogel, all of which you can purchase in the pharmacy, are recommended.

If you have arthritis affecting the hips and/or knees, then the physical act of making love can be painful. See the illustrations on pages 333 and 334 for some positions that you may find more comfortable.

If the woman has hip or knee flexion contractions, then the positions illustrated on pages 334 and 335 may be helpful.

Other Solutions

For some people with severe arthritis, the physical act of intercourse is not possible. For others who have had hip replacement surgery, intercourse is not recommended for six weeks afterward (but you should ask your orthopedic surgeon this question specifically).

This position can be used if the man's back is affected by arthritis.

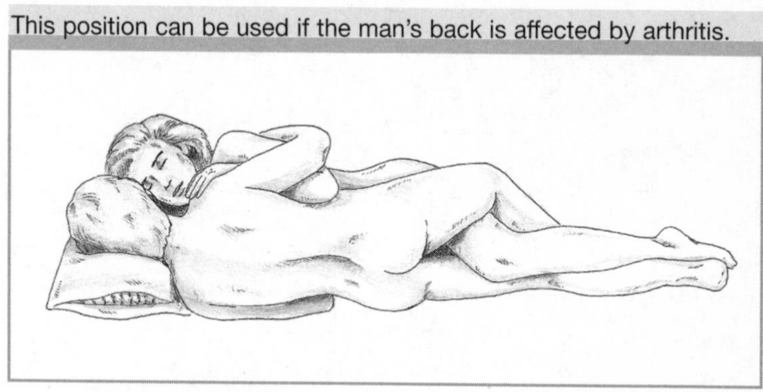

The man supports his weight on his arms to avoid pressure on the joints. The woman has her hips and knees bent with a pillow supporting the knees. This position can be used if the woman is unable to move her legs apart.

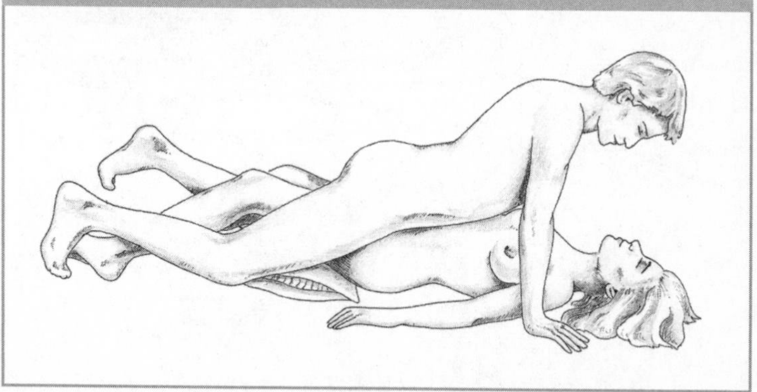

This position can be used if the man's back, hips, or knees are affected by arthritis.

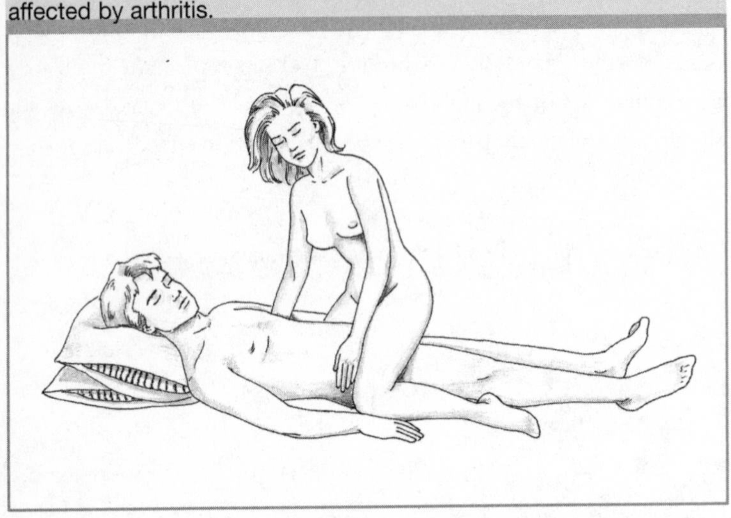

This position can be used if the woman has hip or knee flexion contractions, or many painful joints (it will avoid pressure being put on the joints).

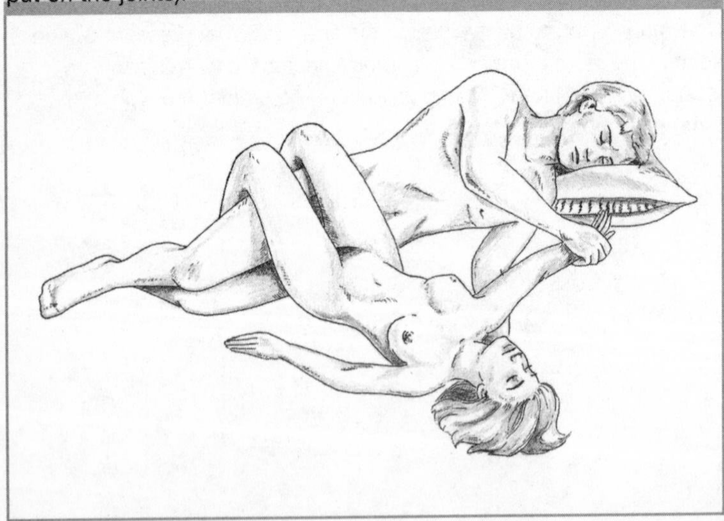

This position can be used if the woman's hips are affected.

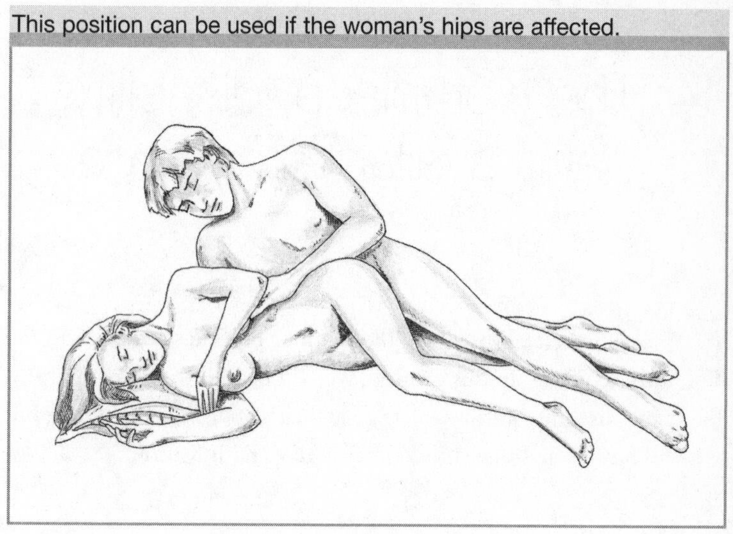

That is not to say that these people cannot still have a satisfying sex life, though, because there are other means of enjoying lovemaking, including caressing, cuddling, and stroking. Both partners can reach orgasm if sensitive areas of the body are stimulated. Having oral sex is also another approach to finding sexual fulfillment (some people may not be comfortable with this, and certainly, as with any act of lovemaking, mutual consent is mandatory). When the hands are severely affected by arthritis a vibrator could be tried, but it may irritate the genitals if used frequently or for too long, and it should be avoided if the skin is thin and dry.

With planning, imagination, and sensitivity, people with arthritis can make pleasurable sex a part of life: arthritis in itself does not have to be a barrier to a fulfilling sex life. Appendix II lists many books, organizations, websites, and other resources that offer help to people with arthritis, and you are encouraged to use these resources for more information regarding arthritis and sexuality.

14 The workplace, disability, and available resources

Musculoskeletal disease is the number one cause of disability in this country. In this chapter, we will discuss the work environment and disability as they relate to arthritis and similar diseases, but we will not discuss musculoskeletal injury and litigation.

Dealing with Disability

If an individual is no longer able to meet occupational requirements as a result of arthritis, what steps need to be taken? First, and foremost, is to diagnose and treat the underlying disease. Then, modifications to the workplace may be able to be made. If the modifications are not enough, the person might need to switch jobs, take a retraining course, or undergo vocational rehabilitation. Disability should only be considered when all of the previous steps have failed. There are many positive aspects to remaining employed: financial stability, improved self-esteem, feelings of usefulness, improved control of the disease, a drug plan, a pension plan, and social interaction. Thus, it is in most patients' best interests to return to work. Taking a period of short-term disability is often effective for newly diagnosed disease or disease flares and, after adjustments to therapy and an integrated exercise program, many patients can return to the workforce.

Understanding Disability

The first step in accommodating for chronic arthritis is to have the disease diagnosed and treated. There may still be a gap between what a person can do and what she wants or needs to do, however, and this is disability. Disability is a change in an individual's ability to meet personal, social, or occupational demands as a result of impairment.

A physical impairment does not necessarily translate into a disability, however, as many things influence disability besides the impairment. Two people may have the same impairment but their disabilities may be different. For example, if a pianist breaks his wrist, he cannot play or rehearse: his impairment results in a disability from his occupation. I am a physician who looks after patients with arthritis, and if I break my right wrist, I can still work. The fact that I am left-handed also affects the degree of disability resulting from the impairment. I can play the piano, but I was never very good at it and only play for my own enjoyment; my impairment may disable me from a recreational activity, but it is not disabling me from my occupation. Factors that have been shown to affect musculoskeletal disability include the disease, the severity of the disease, age, sex, education, personality, social support, peer support, work experience, the occupation, and the amount of freedom to direct one's own activities in the occupation.

Functional disability, impairment, and handicap

If a person needs or wants to perform a task and cannot do it, this is called a *functional disability*. Insurance companies (including Workers' Compensation and the Canada Pension Plan) have different definitions of disability, but they are all specifically looking at the work environment. The Canada Pension Plan provides that an individual is disabled if he or she is unable to work at any job for which he or she is reasonably qualified, and the disability must be prolonged and severe for the person to qualify for benefits. Although individual insurance policies differ in wording, generally speaking, they consider you disabled if you are unable to perform your own occupation for a period of two years. To continue to qualify after two years, you must be disabled from any occupation.

Impairment is a physical or mental limitation to normal function as a result of a disease. Impairment is objectively determinable by a physician, and impairment does not necessarily mean the person has a disability. Examples of impairment would include loss of range of motion to a joint, or muscle weakness.

Another term that is used in a disability setting is *handicap.* A handicap is a barrier or a disadvantage to accomplishing a task. A handicap can be overcome by compensating for the barrier or disadvantage. Some examples of devices used to overcome handicaps include wheelchairs, prostheses, and crutches.

In his book, *Rehabilitation Medicine: Principles and Practice,* Dr. Lee Kirby has described impairment, disability, and handicap as follows: "An impairment represents a problem at the tissue level, a disability represents a problem at the whole person level, and a handicap represents the problem at the environmental and societal level."

Disability assessment

A disability assessment can only be completed when the doctor knows how the ability of the individual compares to previous function or accepted normal standards for age and sex. Activities of daily living, or ADLs, are behaviours that are observable and measurable, and are frequently used in an assessment of disability. ADLs are used to measure the ability to do a task. Some examples of ADLs are locomotion (walking, wheeling, climbing stairs) or work (lifting, equipment operation). In assessing ADLs, the required level of function, the severity of the limitation, and the limiting factors must be considered.

Adjustments within the Workplace

The second step in accommodating for your chronic arthritis is to make adjustments for your disability within the workplace. Among the considerations you might make at this stage are whether to tell your current or potential employer about your condition, and potential changes to the workplace that might make it easier for you to continue with your job.

Do you tell your employer about your condition?

As a rule, if your disease is interfering with (or has the potential of interfering with) your ability to do your job, or if your job is affecting your disease, then it is reasonable to discuss your disease with your employer. If there is no effect on your work, then it is not necessary to inform your employer.

If your disease is interfering with your job, your employer may have already come to her own conclusions as to why you are not performing. A frank discussion with your employer gives her the opportunity to make adjustments in your work to accommodate your disease, and gives you the opportunity to make suggestions.

If work is affecting your disease, then you cannot continue all your employment responsibilities without making some changes to the work environment. Failure to make changes will inevitably lead to your going off work.

Employment law says that an employer is not allowed to dismiss you from your employment because of disability unless your disability prevents you from performing a bona fide occupational requirement—a task that absolutely must be able to be performed by anyone doing that job. (For example, it is a bona fide occupational requirement for a fireman to be able to carry heavy hoses in an emergency situation.) Employers will usually make accommodations for disability; however, if you find yourself in a situation where you feel you were discriminated against as a result of your disability, you should consult with the individual responsible for human resources in your organization. This could be your supervisor, personnel manager, or union representative. If you cannot identify an individual, then you should consult a lawyer or human rights official.

Do you mention your condition when applying for a job?

If you are asked a question directly, you should answer truthfully. It is always best not to lie. If you do not believe the disease will affect your ability to do the job and the question is not asked directly, then it may not be necessary to disclose your condition. If you will require time off work for treatments or medical appointments that can interfere with your work, you should advise your potential employer. If you are able to meet the demands of the job and have the requirements, you cannot be discriminated against because of disability.

Potential adjustments to the workplace

There are many potential adjustments to the workplace. These may be physical changes, changes in scheduling, or changes in your number of hours worked.

Physical changes might include something as simple as having your workstation assessed, changing the screen on the computer, or adjusting the height of your computer to help a sore neck. A good chair with a lumbar support may help with back pain. It is often worthwhile both to you and your employer to have an occupational therapist visit the workplace.

You might make changes to your work schedule in order to better work around your arthritis. Shift workers who are diagnosed with arthritis must often reconsider their ability to cope with shifts that are at odds with the body's natural sleep–wake pattern, as fatigue is already a problem. Constantly changing between day and night shifts is very difficult, as the body needs to maintain a steady sleep–wake pattern in order to function at its best. Regular sleep is important to all of us, but especially to those who have pain and a chronic disease. Regular daytime hours are preferable, although some nurses or personal care workers find that regular night shifts are easier as the physical workload is less. Therefore, choose the shift that is better in your situation, and then stick with it as much as possible.

Switching Jobs

If physical and scheduling modifications do not make a difference, then maybe another position would be more suitable to your abilities. If you are a nurse, then a clinic job that has regular hours and few physical demands may be more appropriate than hospital work. If you are a truck driver, short-haul jobs or a job that doesn't require unloading may accommodate your abilities. If you are self-employed as a carpenter, then maybe you can explore alternative employment that would use your experience, such as a foreman's position.

Vocational Rehabilitation

Vocational rehabilitation should always be considered but, unfortunately, it is often only considered after you are receiving disability payments. If you are receiving disability, then most insurance companies will pay for vocational rehabilitation. Vocational rehabilitation can be combined with a physical assessment done by a physiotherapist. A vocational assessment should look at your interests or skills, your education and your disabilities, and help you to find new employment. If you require retraining, the Canada Pension Disability Plan makes provisions so that you will continue to receive your monthly payment while retraining. Please see the section on the Canada Pension Plan.

Career choices

Education gives you alternatives. As a rule, a good education is important if you have chronic arthritis, as it is unlikely that you will be able to remain in a job requiring a lot of physical labour for a prolonged period of time. For example, a job as a plumber is not a good choice for a young man with ankylosing spondylitis, since he would need to do a lot of physical labour, and might often be bent under a sink or into other awkward positions.

There are several other considerations besides the job itself. If he were self-employed or worked for a small company (as many plumbers do), then our young plumber may not have access to a drug plan or disability insurance. If he didn't have a drug plan or disability insurance, he would be unable to obtain benefits because he already has a disease. If he were to work for a large firm or become a member of a large union, then he would probably be covered under the firm or union's group benefit plan.

An example of a job that might be more suitable to our young man with ankylosing spondylitis would be a position as a schoolteacher. Teachers' daily activities are varied, so he would not be sitting (or working in awkward positions) for prolonged periods and becoming stiff. He would not be expected to do heavy physical labour, and teachers generally have a drug plan and disability plan. I am not suggesting that these are his only options, but only highlight these factors for people with chronic arthritis to consider when making a career choice.

Disability

If all possible efforts at modifying the workplace, switching jobs, retraining, and vocational rehabilitation have failed, then going on disability is an option. In order to qualify for disability payments, you must have first paid into a disability plan, whether this is a private plan or the Canada Pension Plan. The policies vary in their requirements for disability. Some will require you to be disabled from your own job; others will require you to be disabled from any occupation. You need to review your disability policy to understand the requirements. Sometimes, your employer's personnel office can help.

Often, an assessment from your physician is all that is required, but you may need an assessment from a specialist: it depends on the nature of the disability and the insurance plan. If you are off on short-term disability, then qualifying for benefits is usually fairly straightforward. However, if the disability is prolonged or permanent, then you may be asked to see a specialist (retained by the insurance company) who will assess your disability. Or, you may be asked to see a physiotherapist who is trained to do assessments in the workplace.

If there is potential to return to the workplace, then your insurance company may require you to do a work-hardening program with a physiotherapist. This is to build strength and endurance so you may effectively return to work. Another alternative is to return to work on a part-time basis with a schedule of progressively increasing hours approved by your physician. Sometimes it may be most beneficial for individuals to continue permanently on a part-time basis.

Another alternative that the insurance companies offer is job retraining, which is very useful to many people. As I outlined in the beginning, there are many benefits to remaining employed. We know that as a rule, people on disability are more likely to suffer from depression and their lifespan is shorter, no matter what initially caused the disability. A continuation of employment can assist in alleviating some of these potential complicating factors.

What is the physician's role?

The role of the physician is to diagnose the underlying condition and to make recommendations for management. It is to provide education about the disorder and to help set realistic goals for the patient and his or her family. A physician should help the patient to accept the condition and to adapt and achieve despite any loss.

The physician should act as an advocate to provide the decision makers with all the appropriate information necessary to make a decision on disability.

Disability Benefits

Disability benefits may come from a variety of sources, including the Canada Pension Plan, the Disability Tax Credit, Employment Insurance, and drug plans and formularies. We will discuss these next.

Canada Pension Plan

The Canada Pension Plan (CPP) offers coverage to Canadians for disability benefits, benefits for children of disabled contributors, retirement pensions, and survivor benefits.

In order to be eligible for CPP disability benefits, you must be under 65 years of age and have contributed to the plan for a minimum number of years. Since January 1, 1998, you must have contributed for four out of the last six years. Exceptions to this include a late-applicant provision if your contributions were made too long ago to meet the minimum qualifying period. You may qualify provided that: you meet the rules that were in place at the time your disability began; you have been continuously disabled; and you were incapable of applying earlier. The provision also applies if you stopped contributing to raise your children and they were under age seven.

The CPP legislation reads that a disability must be severe and prolonged. You must be unable to carry out on a regular basis any occupation for which you are reasonably qualified. CPP does not take into consideration socioeconomic factors or the availability of work in a particular region. CPP does not issue partial disability.

CPP will pay for a vocational rehabilitation program if you are on CPP disability, if your condition is stable, and if your doctor agrees that you can participate. Also, with a rehabilitation program, you would be likely to return to work. The vocational rehabilitation program allows you to retrain, and you will be allowed a three-month trial period of work to determine if you are able to continue.

If you want an application form for CPP, you may call 1-800-277-9914. A separate application is needed to obtain benefits for children of disabled contributors. For further information, you may go to the CPP website: www.hrdc-drhc.gc.ca/isp/cpp/disabi_e.shtml.

Disability Tax Credit

The Disability Tax Credit is available to some Canadians who are disabled. Although you may be considered disabled from work (either by CPP, the Workers' Compensation Board, or an insurance company), this does not mean that you are disabled according to the Disability Tax Credit criteria. These criteria are very specific and are intended to compensate people who require assistance with activities of daily living, including dressing, feeding, bathing, and ambulation. You should check with your physician to determine if you are eligible.

Employment Insurance

Employment Insurance disability benefits are available for people who have paid into Employment Insurance (EI). This will provide short-term disability benefits. It is best to contact your local authorities for further information.

Drug Plans and Formularies

There are several issues that you need to be aware of regarding drug plans and formularies. The drug plans administered through private insurance plans all vary, but they usually have a formulary of medications that they will cover, and other medications may be covered under a special exemption policy (which will require a form filled out by your physician). The policies also vary as to the amount of co-payment for medications. If you already have a disease when you apply for a drug plan, then the company may not cover medications for that disease: it is important to understand this prior to starting the policy. If you are employed by a large company, or are part of a large plan through a union, then they may not require a medical before insuring you and will therefore cover the costs of medications for pre-existing disease. If you retire or are given a retirement package and have a pre-existing disease, then it is important to try and keep the policy even if it means paying for it yourself, as it is very difficult to become insured after you are diagnosed with a disease. The same would apply for disability insurance and life insurance.

Each province has a formulary of medications that it will provide under its pharmacare program. In some provinces, the program applies only to seniors and people on social assistance; in other provinces, it includes everyone. The medications that will be covered are different in each province, and there is a special access policy for some medications. To be eligible for a medication under a special access program, you must have a specific disease or condition and must have not received benefit from other, less expensive medications. Many of the new medications for arthritis are insured under the special access program, but some of the new medications are not covered at all.

This chapter has attempted to discuss some of the common questions and problems around work, insurance, and disability that I see in clinical practice. Appendix II lists further resources that you might want to try.

There is no question that chronic arthritis will have an impact upon all aspects of your life, including your life in the workplace. A positive attitude, acceptance of the disease, taking responsibility for yourself, and a desire to move forward are essential components not only of a successful work environment, but of a more fulfilling life.

Appendix I:
heredity and environment

The definitive cause of most types of arthritis is not known: the causes vary from one type of arthritis to the other, and most types of arthritis are a result of more than one factor (they are multifactorial). Some of these factors we inherit in the genetic material received from our parents, and others are acquired from the environment. Often, there is an interaction between inherited factors and things in our surroundings.

Hereditary Factors

Human beings have 23 pairs of chromosomes, and each chromosome contains the genes that we receive from our parents. These genes are what determines our eye colour, hair texture, whether we'll have our mother's nose or our grandfather's ears, and also whether we will be likely to develop certain types of arthritis. Each gene is a code or blueprint for a different protein, and the genes that we receive from each of our parents determine what inherited factors we are given that may make us more or less likely to develop arthritis. A minor chemical change in a gene can lead to a protein not being produced or to a protein being made with a changed structure that causes it not to work properly.

Many genes determine the make-up of our immune system. Some of these immune genes code for proteins that become receptors on the surfaces of cells. These receptors can distinguish between our own proteins and proteins that are foreign to us (antigens). These receptors are called human leukocyte (white blood cell) antigens (HLA), and there are four main groups: A, B, C, and D. In each group, there are many inherited types and subtypes of receptors—they determine an individual's own unique immune response to foreign chemicals.

Many forms of arthritis are associated with certain HLA types, as will be discussed below. For instance, a person who inherited the HLA-B27 surface receptor might develop reactive arthritis following a bout of food poisoning with the salmonella bacteria. Most people would just get diarrhea, but 20 percent of those with HLA-B27 would bind an antigen from the salmonella differently than those who do not have HLA-B27, causing the immune system to respond with arthritis.

Some genes code for the proteins that form our organs and tissues. For instance, type II collagen makes up the supporting structure of cartilage. A small chemical change in its gene can cause the body to make an inferior form of type II collagen that would lead to a weaker supporting structure for the cartilage. This substandard cartilage would then wear out much more easily, resulting in osteoarthritis.

Many genes code for enzymes. Enzymes are proteins that control the rates of chemical reactions in our body. A person could inherit a defective gene for an enzyme instead of the proper gene for that enzyme. The defective gene might result in a deficiency of the enzyme, or it might result in an abnormally functioning enzyme. For instance, a small percentage of people with gout have inherited a partial or complete deficiency of the HGPRT enzyme. As a result, their metabolism of purines will be altered so that their bodies produce excessive amounts of uric acid while processing the purines. As a result of this excess, uric acid will deposit in joints as crystals, causing gout.

The inheritance of the X- and Y-chromosomes determines our gender (XX for females and XY for males). Gender is another factor that plays a role in arthritis. Most people with systemic lupus erythematosus and rheumatoid arthritis are female, whereas most people with ankylosing spondylitis and gout are male.

Gene types are studied in various diseases to determine the role of heredity. The actual genes can be studied by analyzing their DNA chemical structures or by analyzing their protein products, such as HLA types, enzymes, and collagen.

Studying the frequency of the different types of arthritis in identical and non-identical twins, in family members, and in different genders and races also helps to identify the importance of heredity. Identical twins are genetically exactly the same, whereas non-identical twins have only about 50 percent of the same genes. If the frequency of a disease is higher in identical twins than in non-identical twins, then a genetic factor is involved. If a disease is more frequent in blood relations than in other family and household members (such as spouses), then a genetic factor is involved. A link with one of the genders suggests an association with the X- or Y-chromosomes or with the sex hormones.

Environmental Factors

Environmental factors can be divided into several groups: physical/mechanical, infection, chemicals and drugs, weather, diet, and psychological factors. Some play a role in causing the arthritis, and others play a role in modifying the arthritis that already exists. Some environmental factors do both.

Physical/Mechanical Factors

Mechanical factors include trauma to joints, such as a fracture or a torn meniscus (torn cartilage). The structure of the joint becomes altered and subsequent use wears out the cartilage faster than normal, resulting in osteoarthritis. Repetitive use of joints (such as moving up and down while squatting) can lead to osteoarthritis of the knees. Wearing high-heeled shoes causes abnormal stresses to go through the lower back, hips, and inner knees. The abnormal usage and positioning of the ankles and joints of the feet in ballet can lead to osteoarthritis.

Infection

Infection of a joint is called septic arthritis. Intravenous drug users can introduce bacteria such as Staphylococcus aureus into their bloodstream. The bacteria are carried to and then deposited in one or more joints, and these infected joints will be damaged rapidly unless antibiotics are given. Sometimes, infections occurring elsewhere in the body react with the immune system to cause a reactive arthritis. In these cases, the microorganism is not actually infecting the joint, as it is in a septic joint. Antibiotics do not cure this type of arthritis. Examples of reactive arthritis include rheumatic fever following a "strep" (Streptococcus pyogenes) infection of the throat, or post-dysenteric arthritis following food poisoning with salmonella.

Chemicals and Drugs

Sometimes, exposure to a chemical can lead to arthritis. Drugs such as procainamide can induce a reversible form of systemic lupus erythematosus. Factory workers handling vinyl chloride can develop a form of scleroderma. Too much lead in the system can contribute to gout.

Weather

Climate may play a role in aggravating arthritic symptoms but not in causing them. Cold weather can cause muscles to tense so that a cold draft can make arthritis in the neck more painful. Cold can also aggravate Raynaud's phenomenon. Hot weather can make inflamed joints more swollen and painful. A drop in the barometric pressure or an increase in the humidity can worsen arthritic joint pain and fibromyalgia. Reduced gravity in space can accelerate osteoporosis and cause backache due to the expansion of the vertebral discs. The ultraviolet light from the sun (or fluorescent lights) can aggravate systemic lupus erythematosus.

Diet and Psychological Factors

Dietary factors are discussed in Chapter 11, "Diet and Nutrition."

Psychological factors such as distress, depression, and anxiety do not usually cause arthritis, but they can worsen the pain, fatigue, disability, sleeping pattern, ability to cope, and immunity.

Inherited Factors in Specific Types of Arthritis

In studies and examination of patients with specific types of arthritis, it has been noted that these types of arthritis are often found in people with the same inherited factors. We will discuss these below.

Osteoarthritis

In a very small number of patients with generalized or multiple joint osteoarthritis, there is a defect in a gene on chromosome 12 that codes for type II procollagen, a component of cartilage. There is also a group of inherited diseases, which cause loose joints (hyperlaxity); such conditions include Marfan's syndrome and Ehlers–Danlos syndromes (the most common type is related to an abnormal form of type V collagen). With the everyday use of these unstable joints, premature osteoarthritis can develop. Premature osteoarthritis of the hip joint can be due to congenital hip dysplasia. In this condition, the "socket" part of this ball-and-socket joint is underdeveloped and cannot properly absorb the forces of weight bearing transmitted to it from the "ball."

Twin studies have shown that osteoarthritis of the distal finger joints, Heberden's nodes, and osteoarthritis of the knees are twice as common in identical twins as in non-identical twins. Osteoarthritis of the hips and cervical and lumbar spine is more frequent in identical twins than in non-identical twins, and osteoarthritis of the hands and lumbar spine are more common in non-identical twins than in siblings who are non-twins.

Other family studies show that the risk of getting osteoarthritis is greater if an immediate family member has it, such as a grandparent, parent, or sibling. Heberden's nodes are twice as common in mothers and daughters and three times more common in sisters. Having a slipped or prolapsed disc in the spine as a teenager is associated with a history of having a first-degree relative (parent, sibling, or child) with a prolapsed disc.

Diffuse Idiopathic Skeletal Hyperostosis (DISH)

There is a higher prevalence of DISH in Pima Indians in Arizona, but a lower prevalence in the American black population. It affects males more than females.

Rheumatoid Arthritis

The HLA-DRB1 gene marker has been associated with rheumatoid arthritis. This marker has several subtypes. In various studies, rheumatoid arthritis was found to be associated with the 0401 and 0404 subtypes in white populations, the 0405 subtype in oriental populations, and the 0901 subtype in Japanese populations. These genes more strongly influence the *severity* of the rheumatoid arthritis than they do the *susceptibility* to rheumatoid arthritis. Having two of these markers is worse than having only one. Patients with these subtypes have more progressive joint damage and extra-articular features such as nodules.

The chances of both identical twins having rheumatoid arthritis is 10–30 percent; the chances are less for brothers and sisters. If one member of a family has rheumatoid arthritis, then another family member is three to four times more likely to get rheumatoid arthritis than a non-relative is. The rates of rheumatoid arthritis are higher in Native North Americans (e.g., Yakima and Chippewa) and in white Finns and West Germans. On the other hand, the rates are lower in China, Japan, and Africa. The rates are lower in rural black populations compared to urban black populations, which makes an argument for the role of an environmental factor as well. Females have a two to four time greater prevalence than males.

Juvenile Onset Arthritis

Rheumatoid arthritis beginning in people under the age of 16 years is associated with HLA-DR4. Juvenile chronic polyarthritis without the rheumatoid factor is linked to HLA-DRw8. The type of juvenile arthritis that involves only a few joints but is associated with inflammation of the eye (iritis) occurs with HLA-DR5 and HLA-DRw8.

Gout

Inherited enzyme defects, which lead to an overproduction of uric acid, have been identified in a minority of patients with gout. Two of these are located on the sex-linked chromosomes (the X- and Y-chromosomes). They are HGPRT (partial and complete deficiencies) and PRPP (overactive). Two others are not sex-linked: glucose-6-phosphatase deficiency and fructose-1-phosphate aldolase deficiency.

It is estimated that probably 20–40 percent of persons with gout have a family history of gout. Also, about one-quarter of the first-degree relatives of a person with gout have elevated levels of uric acid in their blood. About 90–95 percent of those with gout are male.

Pseudogout

No specific gene is associated with pseudogout, and most cases occur sporadically in older people. However, about 100 families have been found around the world in which there are many affected relatives with the disease, often starting at a younger age. The first families described were Hungarians living in Czechoslovakia, and families in the Chiloe Islands of Chile and in Spain. Genes peculiar to each family that was studied have been found on either chromosome 5 or chromosome 8. A defect in an enzyme that transports pyrophosphate has been found in some of these families.

Ankylosing Spondylitis

HLA-B27 is present in about 90 percent of white patients with ankylosing spondylitis, compared to only 6 percent of unaffected white persons. If HLA-B60 is also present, the susceptibility to ankylosing spondylitis increases by about three to six times. HLA-B7 and its associated HLA types B38, B39, DR1, and DR8 are associated with ankylosing spondylitis, too. Other partially inherited risk factors for ankylosing spondylitis include Crohn's disease (chromosome 16) and psoriasis (chromosome 17).

Both identical twins have ankylosing spondylitis in 60–75 percent of cases, compared to 12.5 percent of non-identical twins. The chance that a sibling of a person with ankylosing spondylitis will have ankylosing spondylitis as well is about 10 percent. First-degree relatives of white ankylosing spondylitis patients have a 20 percent chance of having ankylosing spondylitis if they are HLA-B27 positive. Ankylosing spondylitis is more common in white than in black people, and three to 10 times more men than women have ankylosing spondylitis.

Psoriatic Arthritis

Psoriatic arthritis is associated with HLA-B16 (made up of B38 and B39) and HLA-Cw0602. When spondylitis is associated with psoriasis, it too is associated with HLA-B27. In addition to determining susceptibility to psoriatic arthritis, HLA also predicts its severity. HLA-B39, B27, and DQw3 are associated with the development of more joint deformities.

Family studies show that psoriatic arthritis is 100 times more likely to occur in family members of someone with psoriatic arthritis than in non-relatives.

Reactive Arthritis

HLA-B27 is present in 90 percent of persons with reactive arthritis compared to 6 percent of the white population at large. Reactive arthritis is more common in arctic and subarctic populations (such as the Haida, Chuckchi, Inuit, Navajos, Pimas, and Finns) because they have a greater frequency of HLA-B27 (18–50 percent of their people). On the other hand, reactive arthritis is uncommon amongst the Chinese, Thais, Japanese, and Africans because they have a low incidence of HLA-B27 (0.5–6 percent of the population at large).

Rheumatic Fever

Rheumatic fever is associated with a genetically determined coiled structure on the surface of B-lymphocytes called D8/17. It is present in 90–100 percent of patients with rheumatic fever, but in only 10 percent of the population at large. HLA-DR7 and Dw53 have been associated with rheumatic fever in Brazil. Rheumatic heart disease is a complication of rheumatic fever. It is linked to

HLA-DR4 and DR2 in caucasian and black populations, and to HLA-DR1 and DRw6 in black South Africans.

Lyme Disease

Chronic arthritis can be a result of Lyme disease. Unlike other features of Lyme disease, it occurs with HLA-DR4 (subtype DRB1*0404 and *0408).

Systemic Lupus Erythematosus

Systemic lupus erythematosus has a complex genetic pattern, and is associated with several different inherited markers. It is associated with HLA types as follows: HLA-DR2 and HLA-DR3 in white populations, HLA-DR2 in Japanese and southern Chinese, and HLA-DR3 in American black populations. In addition, systemic lupus is associated with inherited deficiencies of complement (complement proteins help antibodies clear antigens from the body). There are 11 components of complement (C). Genetically determined deficiencies of C1, C2, C4, and C4A are associated with a high incidence of mild forms of systemic lupus erythematosus.

Both males and females with systemic lupus erythematosus have abnormalities in the metabolism of estrogens (female hormones) and androgens (male hormones). The inactivation of testosterone (one of the androgens) is accelerated. Also, the conversion of estrone (one of the estrogens) to a more potent form of estrogen is increased in patients with systemic lupus erythematosus and their first-degree relatives (parents, siblings, or children). This relative increase in estrogen and decrease in androgen augment the body's immune responses. Between puberty and menopause, the incidence of systemic lupus erythematosus is 10 times more common in women than men.

The chances of both identical twins having systemic lupus erythematosus are 23–69 percent compared to 2–9 percent in non-identical twins. The chance of a first-degree relative having systemic lupus erythematosus is 1–4 percent. If both first- and second-degree relatives (grandparents, aunts/uncles, nieces/nephews, grandchildren) are considered, then the chances of another family member having systemic lupus may be as high as 10–16 percent. In the United States, the prevalence of systemic lupus erythematosus is greater in black and Hispanic groups, and in Great Britain it is more common in black people from the Caribbean. It also appears to be more common in the Chinese and in North American natives (such as Sioux, Arapahoe, and Crow).

Scleroderma

HLA associations in scleroderma are complicated. There is an association between HLA-DR1 and limited scleroderma, and HLA-DR5 and diffuse scleroderma. HLA-DR3 and the complement C4A deficiency gene are also linked to scleroderma.

Both identical twins will have scleroderma 5.9 percent of the time; this is a 300 times greater chance than of someone in the population at large having it. More than one family member with scleroderma is otherwise rare. There is a greater incidence of Raynaud's phenomenon and of antinuclear antibodies in the first-degree relatives of people with scleroderma. Of scleroderma patients, 99 percent have no first-degree relatives with scleroderma, and 98 percent have no relatives at all with scleroderma.

Scleroderma is three to four times more common in women than in men. It appears to be more common in the Choctaw Indians in southwest Oklahoma and in the Japanese. The disease is more widespread in black people, Thais, and the Choctaw than it is in Europeans, white Americans, and Australians.

Polymyositis and Dermatomyositis

These diseases are associated with HLA-B8/DR3 and DRw52 in white children and adults. In black populations, HLA-DR3 is not associated. Polymyositis alone is linked to HLA-B14 in white people and HLA-B7 and DRw6 in black people. Inclusion body myositis occurs with HLA-DR1, DR6, and DQ1.

Fibromyalgia

There is very little evidence that fibromyalgia has a hereditary component. There is a higher incidence of mood disorders such as depression in family members. Also, 85 percent of sufferers are female.

Polymyalgia Rheumatica and Giant Cell Arteritis

These diseases are associated with HLA-DR4. They tend to occur in white individuals whose background is northern European (especially Scandinavian). Four times as many women than men are affected.

Hemochromatosis

In hemochromatosis, there is a defect in the gene that codes for the protein that controls the absorption of iron from the intestine. As a result, toxic levels of iron accumulate in various tissues, including cartilage. The iron causes the cartilage to deteriorate, leading to the development of arthritis in many joints. Hemochromatosis is also associated with HLA-A3.

Hemophilia

Hemophilia is a bleeding disease caused by an inherited deficiency of a clotting factor—either factor VIII or factor IX. The defective gene is carried on the X-chromosome. In females, the other X-chromosome can compensate for the missing clotting factor, so females do not get the bleeding disorder but do become carriers of the disease (with a 50 percent chance of passing on the affected X-chromosome to any male child). In males, there is only one X-chromosome, so they cannot compensate for the deficiency and will become bleeders. Bleeding into a joint causes an acute arthritis. If the bleeding recurs in the same joint, the arthritis will become chronic and the joint will become damaged.

Environmental Factors in Specific Types of Arthritis

Common environmental factors have also been found in patients with specific types of arthritis. We will discuss these below.

Osteoarthritis

Injuries affecting the mechanics of a joint can result in osteoarthritis. Such injuries include: a fracture through a joint or a bone adjacent to a joint causing a misalignment; a torn or surgically removed meniscus ("cartilage"); a torn ligament causing instability of a joint; and a dislocation of a joint. A joint that has been damaged by another type of arthritis (such as septic arthritis) is also susceptible to developing osteoarthritis.

As you get older, it becomes more likely that you will have osteoarthritis. About half of the population over the age of 65 years has X-ray evidence of osteoarthritis.

Overuse of a joint in a physically demanding and repetitive way can result in osteoarthritis. Certain types of work, hobbies, and sports have been implicated (see table below). Knees subjected to repetitive bending (such as in doing 30 or more squats or kneels or climbing 10 or more flights of stairs per day) are prone to osteoarthritis. Someone who has worked as a farmer for more than one year has a greater chance of developing osteoarthritis of the hips. A construction worker or labourer who stands for more than two hours per day or works for at least 20 years doing heavy lifting or walking more than three kilometres daily is at risk for developing osteoarthritis of the hips.

However, reasonable recreational exercise, done within the limits of comfort without putting the joints through abnormal motions and without any underlying joint abnormalities, should not lead to any joint damage even over many years. Running or jogging is probably not a risk factor for developing osteoarthritis in the absence of any other risk factors.

Excess weight is a risk factor for osteoarthritis of the knees and hands. Its association with osteoarthritis of the hips is not certain. Furthermore, once osteoarthritis of the knees is established, obesity worsens the pain and disability. For every kilogram of excess weight, the pressure on the knees and hips increases by three kilograms while walking. Weak muscles around joints may contribute to osteoarthritis. Muscles stabilize joints and absorb shock before it impacts the joint cartilage. The best example is weakness of the quadriceps muscles (the muscles in the front of the thighs), which can cause osteoarthritis of

Repetitive Use Activities Implicated in Osteoarthritis

Persons	Location of osteoarthritis
Miners	Elbows, knees
Pneumatic drill operators	Shoulders, elbows
Cotton pickers	Hands
Diamond cutters	Hands
Seamstresses	Hands
Wrestlers	Knees, elbows
Ballet dancers	Ankles, feet
Boxers	Knuckles
Baseball pitchers	Shoulders, elbows
Cyclists	Joint between kneecap and knee

the knee to begin and, once begun, to progress. Poor posturing of the ankles and arches of the feet and bad footwear can contribute to the development of osteoarthritis of the feet and toes. Wearing high-heeled shoes frequently can contribute to the onset and progression of osteoarthritis of the knees (the medial or inner compartment and behind the kneecap). The jaw joints can develop osteoarthritis as a result of dental misalignments, clenching of the jaws, and grinding of the teeth. The clenching and grinding are often due to tension and stress. Stress can also cause muscles to tighten elsewhere with pain, for example, around the shoulder girdle and neck. Cracking the knuckles, however, does not predispose to osteoarthritis.

Hormone replacement therapy may protect against the onset of osteoarthritis in menopausal women, but the results of studies are not consistent. Changes in the weather (such as a drop in barometric pressure or a cold draft) may be associated with more aching in the joints. Frostbite of the hands and feet in youngsters can lead to osteoarthritis of the finger and toe joints.

Poor posture of the neck and back can cause and worsen osteoarthritis and disc problems in the spine. The worst neck positions occur while sitting or lying. Some of the worst positions for the neck are lying on your side with the neck tilted or on your front with your neck twisted and without proper pillows supporting your neck in a straight line. Others occur while doing deskwork, reading books, operating computers, using a handset phone for long periods, watching television and movies, and doing other close work (especially if reading glasses are needed). Wrestlers and football and rugby players experience a lot of punishment to their neck.

The major risk factors for low back pain and disc disease are repetitive lifting, vibration of the whole body, and cigarette smoking. Lifting is a factor when objects weighing more than 10 kilograms are lifted frequently, especially if they are held away from the body and the body is twisted and the knees are not bent. Vibration to the body occurs chronically in truck and tractor drivers and forklift and crane operators. Weak trunk and pelvic muscles contribute to back problems as well. Standing without one foot on a stool or bar, sitting with your knees below your waist, and lying on a poor mattress will increase your low back pain.

Diffuse Idiopathic Skeletal Hyperostosis (DISH)

Obesity worsens DISH. Vitamin A in large doses can cause bone spurs to form at tendon and ligament insertions into bone, but its role in DISH is uncertain.

Rheumatoid Arthritis

Although viruses are suspected as a cause of rheumatoid arthritis, there is not enough evidence to pronounce them guilty. The use of oral contraceptives protects women against the development of rheumatoid arthritis. Women who have never given birth to a baby are at greater risk for rheumatoid arthritis. Cigarette smoking increases the risk of developing rheumatoid arthritis. Emotional stress can precipitate flare-ups.

Juvenile Onset Arthritis

A viral cause is suspected here too, but proof is lacking.

Gout

Trauma to a joint in a person with gout can cause an acute attack of gout in that joint. Anything that increases the level of uric acid in the body is a risk factor for gout. Eating foods high in purines, drinking a lot of alcohol, dehydration, and starvation raise uric acid levels. Low doses of aspirin, cyclosporine, and diuretics ("water pills") also elevate the uric acid levels. Chronic lead poisoning due to drinking moonshine from lead containers or inhaling lead in contaminated work sites can cause gout. (See Chapter 11, "Diet and Nutrition.") Filipinos moving to North America have gotten gout because of a change in diet.

Pseudogout

Acute attacks can be triggered by trauma to a joint, arthroscopy, injection of hyaluronic fluid (e.g., Synvisc) into a joint, or any type of surgery (especially the removal of the parathyroid glands). Low levels of magnesium, treatment with intravenous pamidronate, and serious medical illnesses (such as heart attacks, strokes, and pneumonia) can also cause acute attacks of pseudogout.

Ankylosing Spondylitis

Klebsiella pneumoniae, a bacterium that can sometimes be found in the intestine, might interact with the HLA-B27 receptor to cause ankylosing spondylitis. This theory has yet to be proven.

Psoriatic Arthritis

Trauma to the skin in a person with psoriasis can cause a patch of psoriasis to develop at the injured site. Trauma to a joint in a person with psoriatic arthritis might cause that joint to develop psoriatic arthritis.

Infection with HIV can worsen both the skin psoriasis and the psoriatic arthritis. The skin psoriasis may be aggravated by skin infection with bacteria such as streptococcus and staphylococcus or with yeasts such as Candida and Pitysporum.

Reactive Arthritis

The HLA-B27 receptor interacts with certain infections of the bowel, cervix, and urethra. Diarrhea is the symptom of the bowel infections and the guilty bacteria are salmonella, shigella, yersinia, and campylobacter, which are found in contaminated water or food. The urethral and cervical infections implicated are due to Chlamydia trachomatis, which is transmitted by sexual contact. The urethral infection (urethritis) in men causes burning on urination and a discharge from the penis, but the infection of the cervix (cervicitis) usually has no symptoms.

Rheumatic Fever

Again, the inherited immune system of the susceptible person reacts with bacteria. The bacteria in this case are group A beta-hemolytic streptococcus, which cause a sore throat (pharyngitis or "strep throat"). This condition is more common in economically deprived inner city youngsters.

Lyme Disease

Atypical bacteria called Borrelia burgdorferi cause Lyme disease. It is spread by deer ticks found in forests, woods, brush, and grassy areas in the northeast, north central and west coast of the United States, Europe, western Russia, and Asia. Lyme disease is uncommon in Canada. It is most commonly seen in adolescents and young adults. Flying insects, transfusions, or contact with the Lyme disease patients do not spread the Borrelia.

Systemic Lupus Erythematosus

An infectious agent may cause systemic lupus erythematosus, but so far there is no proof. Infections such as the flu can worsen systemic lupus erythematosus in some people.

The onset of systemic lupus erythematosus was associated with exposure to sunlight in 30–40 percent of cases. The culprit is the ultraviolet ray: up to 70 percent of persons with systemic lupus erythematosus have had flares following ultraviolet light exposure. Other sources of ultraviolet light include fluorescent lighting.

Cigarette smoking is associated with the occurrence of leg ulcers, discoid lupus rash, lung disease and heart attacks in patients with systemic lupus erythematosus.

There are many drugs than can cause a lupus-like condition that subsides after the medication is stopped. They do not worsen pre-existing systemic lupus erythematosus, nor do they cause true systemic lupus erythematosus. Such drugs include hydralazine, procainamide, quinidine, isoniazid (INH), chlorpromazine, minocycline, d-penicillamine, interferon-alpha, and anti-tumour necrosis factor (infliximab and etanercept).

Systemic lupus erythematosus patients are more likely to be allergic to sulfa antibiotics (e.g., Bactrim and Septra). They can also cause a flare-up of systemic lupus erythematosus.

Oral contraceptives and female hormones should be used with caution. Systemic lupus erythematosus may flare with estrogen but may improve with progesterone-only oral contraceptive pills.

Hair dyes and permanent-wave solutions did not cause or aggravate systemic lupus erythematosus in studies that followed an initial study, which had suggested that they did.

Alfalfa sprouts have induced systemic lupus erythematosus in macaque monkeys. This phenomenon has been attributed to the content of l-canavanine in these sprouts. There was a report of one person with systemic lupus erythematosus worsening after eating alfalfa sprouts. Eating a diet high in saturated fats may worsen systemic lupus erythematosus.

Scleroderma

Long-term use of vibrating tools such as chainsaws or jackhammers and exposure to frostbite have sometimes resulted in Raynaud's phenomenon. Some medications are associated with Raynaud's phenomenon.

They include ergot, which may be found in some medications used to treat migraines, and beta(-adrenergic) blockers such as propranalol, which are used to treat heart disease and high blood pressure. Strenuous exercise has been associated with an uncommon scleroderma-like syndrome called eosinophilic fasciitis.

Some occupations with exposure to certain chemicals have been linked to scleroderma, although the incidence of scleroderma is still low in these occupations. A form of scleroderma has been described in factory workers exposed to the fumes of vinyl chloride. Scleroderma has been seen with exposure to silica in miners, sand-blasters, grinders, sandstone sculptors, and foundry workers. Exposure to organic solvents such as benzene, dieseline, heptane, and trichlorethane, and to epoxy resins, may be risk factors.

Several years ago in Spain, several people ate a contaminated batch of rapeseed (canola) oil, and developed a scleroderma-like syndrome referred to as toxic oil syndrome. A batch of the health food product l-tryptophan that originated from Japan caused another scleroderma-like syndrome called eosinophilia–myalgia syndrome. Bleomycin and pentazocine (Talwin) can cause some scleroderma-like effects.

Sometimes "graft versus host disease" can complicate bone marrow transplants. It resembles scleroderma.

Polymyositis and Dermatomyositis

Viruses have been implicated as causes of these inflammatory muscle disorders but there is no definitive proof so far. Some drugs, such as the cholesterol-lowering agent Lipitor, can mimic these muscle disorders.

Fibromyalgia

Many cases of fibromyalgia begin following viral illnesses, injuries, acute or chronic emotional distress, and medical events such as surgery, drug reactions, systemic lupus erythematosus, or low thyroid levels. However, many cases start just out of the blue. A disturbed sleep pattern accompanies fibromyalgia, and many different factors can be responsible for the sleep disorder. The rate of mood disorders such as depression in persons with fibromyalgia is high. There are so many possible triggers to which one can be exposed that it is difficult to pinpoint any one single environmental stressor that is responsible for fibromyalgia.

Hemochromatosis

Frequent transfusions given for years can lead to the accumulation of iron in the body; it deposits in cartilage, damaging it gradually.

Arthritis Due to Joint Infections

An infection can enter a joint from the bloodstream or by penetrating the joint externally. Bacteria, viruses, and fungi can infect the joints.

Injuries that puncture the joint, joint surgery, and joint injections can introduce infection into a joint. Human bites and bites from animals (such as dogs, cats, and rats) can cause infectious arthritis. Illicit drug users who repeatedly inject their veins and patients requiring long-term catheters in their veins for medication or feeding are at risk for introducing infections into their bloodstream. The bloodstream carries these infectious agents to the joints. Joints with foreign material in them (such as joint replacements) or joints that have some abnormality from previous injury or arthritis are more likely to be infected than normal joints. Suppression of the immune system by medications or by diseases such as AIDS, chronic liver disease, diabetes mellitus, and cancer make the patient more susceptible to infections, including those involving joints. Tuberculosis can infect joints. Bacteria called Brucella can cause an infectious arthritis. It is contracted from eating unpasteurized milk and cheese, and farmers and meat packers may also be exposed to it, although it is rare in North America.

Several viral illnesses can cause arthritis. Multiple joints are usually involved, and the arthritis eventually disappears without damaging the joints. In North America, viruses that might do this include rubella and rubella vaccinations (German measles), parvovirus B19 (Fifth disease), Hepatitis B and C, HIV, infectious mononucleosis, adenovirus, coxsackie, and echovirus. Because many people travel, infections can be picked up elsewhere in the world. There are viruses in Australia, Africa, and Asia that cause arthritis: they have such exotic names as Chikungunya, O'nyong-nyong, and Ross River virus.

There are more than a hundred types of arthritis, and ongoing research is making great strides in trying to find their causes. It is becoming clear that they have different causes, but most are associated with a combination of inherited and environmental factors. Inherited factors are studied by looking at genes and their protein products and by examining the prevalence of the arthritis in twins, families, populations, and genders. Environmental factors are studied by looking at the association of possible physical, chemical and drug, climatic, infectious, dietary, and psychological causes with the different types of arthritis. Some factors play a role in causing the arthritis, while others are involved just in modifying the arthritis.

Appendix II: further information

Organizations

You might wish to contact some of the following organizations for further information.

The Arthritis Society (Canada)
Suite 1700, 393 University Avenue
Toronto, ON M5G 1E6
Telephone: (416) 979-7228
Toll free: 1-800-321-1433
E-mail: info@arthritis.ca
Website: www.arthritis.ca

The Arthritis Society, provincial contacts

To reach your provincial office, phone: 1-800-321-1433

Other organizations

The Arthritis Foundation (USA)
P.O. Box 7669
Atlanta, GA 30357-0669
Telephone: (404) 872-7100
Toll free: 1-800-283-7800
E-mail: help@arthritis.org

The American Juvenile Arthritis Organization (AJAO)
A Council of the Arthritis Foundation
1330 West Peachtree Street
Atlanta, GA 30309
Telephone: (404) 965-7538
Toll free: 1-800-283-7800

Canadian Arthritis Patient Alliance
393 University Avenue, Suite 1700
Toronto, ON M5G 1E6
Telephone: (416) 979-3353, ext. 347
E-mail: capa@arthritis.ca
Website: www.arthritis.ca/capa

Human Resources Development Canada
Persons with disabilities including Canada Pension Plan Disability Benefits
Telephone: 1-800-277-9914 (English); 1-800-277-9915 (French)
Website: www.hrdc-drhc.gc.ca/isp/cpp/disabi_e.shtml

Books and Publications

The Arthritis Foundation's Guide to Good Living with Fibromyalgia. Atlanta: Arthritis Foundation, 2001.

The Arthritis Foundation's Guide to Good Living with Osteoarthritis. Atlanta: Arthritis Foundation, 2000.

Blumenthal, M., W. R. Busse, A. Goldberg, et al. *The Complete German Commission E Monographs: Therapeutic Guide to Herbal Medicines.* Austin, TX: American Botanical Council, 1998.

Canadian Arthritis Bill of Rights. Toronto: The Arthritis Society, 2001.

Cassileth, Barrie R. *The Alternative Medicine Handbook.* New York: W. W. Norton, 1998.

Corey, David, and S. Solomon. *Pain—Learning to Live without It.* Toronto: MacMillan Canada, 1993.

Drum, David. *The Chronic Pain Management Sourcebook*. Los Angeles: Lowell House, 1999.

Horstman, Judith. *The Arthritis Foundation's Guide to Alternate Therapies*. Atlanta: Arthritis Foundation, 1999.

Koehn, Cheryl, Taysha Palmer, and John Esdaile M.D. *Rheumatoid Arthritis: Plan to Win*. New York: Oxford University Press, 2002.

Lorig, Kate, RN, Dr.Ph., and James F. Fries M.D. *The Arthritis Helpbook: A Tested Self-Management Program for Coping with Arthritis and Fibromyalgia*. Cambridge, MA: Perseus Books, 2000.

Mayes, Maureen D., M.D. *The Scleroderma Book: A Guide for Patients and Families*. New York: Oxford University Press, 1999.

Murray, Michael, and Joseph Pizzorno. *Encyclopedia of Natural Medicine,* second edition. Rocklin, CA: Prima Publishing, 1998.

Nelson, Miriam E., Ph.D., Kristin R. Baker Ph.D., Ronenn Roubenoff M.D. M.H.S., with Lawrence Lindner M.A. *Strong Women and Men Beat Arthritis*. New York: G.P. Putnam's Sons, 2002.

Panush, Richard S., M.D., ed. *Rheumatic Disease Clinics of North America: Complementary and Alternate Therapies for Rheumatic Diseases,* volumes 1 (Nov. 1999) and 2 (Feb. 2000). Philadelphia: W. B. Saunders Company, 1999, 2000.

PDR for Herbal Medicines. Montvale, NJ: Medical Economics Co., 1998.

Petri, Michelle, ed. *Rheumatic Disease Clinics of North America: Pregnancy and Rheumatic Disease* (Feb. 1997). Philadelphia: W. B. Saunders Company, 1997.

Raising a Child with Arthritis: A Parent's Guide. Atlanta: Arthritis Foundation, 1998.

Senecal, Jean-Luc, M.D. *Lupus: The Disease with 1000 Faces*. Calgary: Lupus Canada, 1991.

Tucker, Lori B., Bethany A. DeNardo, Judith A. Stebulis, Jane G. Schaller. *Your Child with Arthritis: A Family Guide for Caregiving*. Baltimore: The John Hopkins University Press, 1996.

Tyler, Varro E., and Steven Foster. *Tyler's Honest Herbal: A Sensible Guide to the Use of Herbs and Related Remedies,* fourth edition. New York: The Haworth Press, Inc., 1999.

Walk with Ease:Your Guide to Walking for Better Health, Improved Fitness and Less Pain, second edition. Atlanta: Arthritis Foundation, 2002.

Wallace, Daniel J., M.D. *The Lupus Book: A Guide for Patients and Their Families,* revised and expanded edition. New York: Oxford University Press, 2000.

Weinblatt, Michael E., M.D. *The Arthritis Action Program: An Integrated Plan of Traditional and Complementary Therapies*. New York: Simon & Schuster, 2000.

West, Sterling G. *Rheumatology Secrets*. Philadelphia: Hanley and Belfus, Inc., 1997.

Woolaver, Lance. *The Illuminated Life of Maud Lewis*. Halifax, NS: Nimbus Publishing Limited, 1996.

Magazines

Arthritis News, published quarterly for the Arthritis Society (Canada)
Circulation Dept.
Rogers Media Healthcare
P.O. Box 80054, Station BRM B
Toronto, ON M7Y 5C8
Toll-free: 1-800-217-0591
Website: www.arthritis.ca

Arthritis Today, published by the Arthritis Foundation (USA)
P.O. Box 4284
Pittsfield, MA 01202-4284
Toll-free: 1-800-207-8633
Website: www.arthritis.org

HerbalGram, published by the American Botanical Council
P.O. Box 144345
Austin, TX 78714-4345

Websites

Alliance for a Canadian Arthritis Program: www.arthritisalliance.com
The Alternative Medicine Homepage:
www.pitt.edu/~cbw/altm.html
American Academy of Orthopaedic Surgeons: www.aaos.org
American Botanical Council: www.herbalgram.org
American College of Rheumatology: www.rheumatology.org
American Juvenile Arthritis Organization:
www.arthritis.org/communities/about_AJAO.asp
The American Pain Foundation:
www.painfoundation.org/default.asp
Arthritis Consumer Experts: www.arthritisconsumerexperts.com
The Arthritis Foundation (USA): www.arthritis.org
The Arthritis Society (Canada): www.arthritis.ca
Ask Dr. Weil: www.drweil.com/app/cds/drw_cda.php
Better Business Bureau: www.bbb.org
Canadian Rheumatology Association: www.cra-scr.ca
The Cochrane Muscularskeletal Review Group of the Cochrane Collaboration: www.cochranemsk.org
The Consumer Network of the Cochrane Collaboration:
www.cochraneconsumer.com
Eckerd Health Source for Osteoarthritis:
http://eckerd.healthcite.com/HealthReview/p3605.html
Eckerd Health Source for Osteoporosis:
http://eckerd.healthcite.com/HealthReview/p1628.html
Fibromyalgia Network: www.fmnetnews.com/index.html
Health Canada: www.hc-sc.gc.ca

Health World Online: www.healthy.net
The Herb Research Foundation: www.herbs.org/index.html
Lupus Canada: www.lupuscanada.org/
National Ankylosing Spondylitis Society (UK): www.nass.co.uk/
National Center for Complementary and Alternative Medicine (NIH): http://nccam.nih.gov/
National Institute of Arthritis and Musculoskeletal and Skin Diseases, National Institutes of Health (USA): www.nih.gov/niams
National Psoriasis Foundation (USA): www.psoriasis.org
Office of Alternative Medicine (NIH, USA): www.altmed.od.nih.gov
Pain.Com: A World of Information on Pain: www.pain.com/default.cfm
Raynaud's & Scleroderma Association: www.raynauds.demon.co.uk/
Rheumatoid Arthritis Information Network: www.healthtalk.com/rain/index.html
Rheumatology Resources: www.rheuminfo.com
Scleroderma Foundation: www.scleroderma.org/
Scleroderma Society of Ontario: www.sarnia.com/groups/sso
Sjogren's Syndrome Foundation: www.sjogrens.com
Spondylitis Association of America, Inc.: www.spondylitis.org/
US Food and Drug Administration: www.fda.gov/cder/da/da.htm

Glossary

Abortifacient A drug or other agent that causes abortion.

Acupoints Points along the meridians of the body where acupuncture is applied.

Acupressure Pressure applied to acupuncture points manually.

Acupuncture Use of thin needles inserted at designated points along the body's meridians to correct the flow of "energy" as a therapy for illness.

Adrenaline A hormone secreted by the adrenal glands in response to stress (also known as epinephrine); stimulates autonomic nerve action and makes nerve cells more responsive to pain impulses.

Aerobic exercise Exercise that increases the need for oxygen.

Afferent nerves Nerves that carry the electrical impulses of sensations from the skin, muscles, joints, etc., to the spinal cord and brain.

Alexander technique A type of movement therapy that reduces muscular tension, stress, fatigue, and neck and back pain.

Alternative therapies Non-mainstream treatments used instead of mainstream medicine.

Analgesics Drugs that reduce pain.

Anaphylaxis An allergic reaction that results in shortness of breath, wheezing, rash, and drop in blood pressure.

Androgens Male sex hormones.

Anemia A deficiency of red blood cells in the bloodstream resulting in an insufficient amount of oxygen being delivered to the tissues and organs.

Anesthesia Local or general insensibility to pain with or without the loss of consciousness, induced by a drug.

Antibody A Y-shaped protein (immunoglobulin) secreted into the blood or lymph by B-lymphocytes and plasma cells in response to a foreign stimulus (antigen) such as a bacterium or virus, in order to neutralize and remove the antigen by binding to it.

Anticoagulant A substance that reduces the ability of the blood to clot ("blood thinner").

Antigen A substance recognized by the body as being foreign to it and, when introduced into the body, elicits an antibody response. Antigens can be toxins, bacteria, foreign blood cells, viruses, and the cells of transplanted organs.

Antimicrobial An agent that can destroy disease-causing micro-organisms such as bacteria (e.g., antibiotics).

Antinuclear antibody An antibody directed against antigens that reside in the nucleus of a cell. Detection of these antinuclear antibodies in the blood is used as a diagnostic test for connective tissue diseases.

Antioxidants A substance such as Vitamin E that prevents or delays the oxidation process in cells or tissues. Used to clear unstable molecules with an odd number of electrons produced by oxidation that may be harmful to the body.

Antiphospholipid antibody An autoantibody directed against a group of phosphate-containing lipids or fats that are normal constituents of the body. Antiphospholipid antibodies are associated with a syndrome that features clots in the arteries and veins and recurrent miscarriages. It can occur with systemic lupus erythematosus.

Aromatherapy The use of pleasant odours from plant oils for healing.

Arthrodesis A surgical procedure that obliterates a joint by fusing or uniting the ends of the bones that make up the joint. The ability of the joint to move is lost.

Arthroplasty The damaged ends of the bones that make up a joint are surgically removed. If no artificial implant is inserted, it is referred to as an excision arthroplasty. If an artificial implant is inserted, it is referred to as a replacement arthroplasty.

Arthroscopy A surgical procedure that involves the insertion of a tube with a light source and camera through a small hole into a joint to look around it.

Arthrotomy The making of a surgical incision to gain access to a joint for further surgical procedures.

Art therapy Using art for therapeutic purposes.

Assistive devices Aids for protecting joints and making tasks easier. Also known as adaptive devices.

Autoantibody An antibody directed against an antigen that is not foreign to the body. The immune system is tricked into making an antibody against a chemical component of itself (e.g., an A or B antigen that is a normal component of the red blood cells).

Autoimmunity The process by which the body develops an immune response against one of its own tissues, cells, or molecules.

Ayurvedic medicine Traditional system of medicine that originated from the Hindu philosophy of ancient India.

Biofeedback The use of electrical instruments to recognize changes in body functions like heart rate, temperature, and sweating, in order to relax or contract muscle.

Botanical medicine The use of plants for medicinal purposes.

Bouchard's nodes The bony enlargement of the PIP joints of the fingers caused by osteoarthritis.

Bradykinin A biologically active 9-amino acid molecule that mediates inflammation, increases pain sensation, dilates blood vessels, and contracts smooth muscle.

Bursa A sac-like body cavity containing thick lubricating fluid, which is located between a tendon and bone or skin and bone to reduce the friction between the moving structures.

Bursitis Inflammation or irritation of a bursa.

Calcaneus The heel bone.

Cardiomyopathy A disease or disorder of the heart muscle.

Cartilage Dense, flexible connective tissue or "gristle" found at the ends of some bones where they form joints, or located in areas such as the nose, ears, and trachea. It has no nerve or blood supply.

Central nervous system (CNS) The brain and the spinal cord.

Chiropractic The use of manipulation to reposition "subluxed" or misaligned vertebrae in the spine to restore health.

Chondrocyte A cell located in the cartilage that produces the collagen and proteoglycans that constitute cartilage.

Chondroitin sulfate A chain of about 25 to 30 repeating double sugars (disaccharides) that bind to a core protein to help make up the proteoglycans of cartilage. It is also marketed as a treatment for osteoarthritis.

Chromosome A threadlike body of DNA in the cell nucleus, which carries genes in a linear order and transports them during cell division to the newly divided cells' nuclei.

CMC joints The carpometacarpal joints, located between the farthest row of carpal bones in the wrist and the bases of the metacarpals in the hand.

Collagen A group of fibrous proteins that are the supporting skeleton of skin, tendon, bone, cartilage, and other connective tissues and organs.

Co-morbid diseases Other diseases that coexist with the primary disease, such as infections, osteoporosis, and heart disease with rheumatoid arthritis.

Complement Several plasma proteins of the immune system that interact in a cascading sequence to destroy bacteria and cells and contribute to inflammation in the process.

Complementary medicine Non-mainstream treatments used together with mainstream medicine.

Contracture An often permanent shortening of a muscle or scar tissue that results in a flexion or bent-up deformity of a joint.

Cortisone A naturally occurring corticosteroid secreted by the adrenal gland that has many metabolic effects; can be used as a medication to reduce inflammation and the immune response.

Crohn's disease A chronic inflammatory disease of the intestines.

CRP C-reactive protein; a globulin-type of protein that appears in the blood during certain inflammatory conditions, such as rheumatoid arthritis, bacterial infections, and cancer. Its concentration in the blood can be measured and used to assess how active the inflammation is.

Cuboid A bone shaped like a cube located on the outer aspect of the midfoot in front of the calcaneus and behind the fourth and fifth metatarsals.

Cupping Placing on selected areas of the skin heated cups, which then adhere to the skin by the suction created as they cool.

Cytokines A group of proteins released by cells of the immune system that regulates the immune response by stimulating or inhibiting other cells to behave in a specified manner. Examples include the interleukins, interferons, and tumour necrosis factor.

Debridement Surgical excision of debris, devitalized, inflamed, or infected tissue, and foreign matter from a wound or cavity like a joint.

Deep vein thrombosis Clot formation in a deep vein as opposed to a visible superficial vein.

DHEA Dehydroepiandrosterone; a hormone secreted by the adrenal gland that is metabolized to androgens and estrogens. It is available for therapeutic use.

Diathermy A method of physical therapy that involves generating local heat in body tissues by high-frequency electromagnetic currents.

Dietary therapy The use of diet and food for health and healing.

DIP joints The distal interphalangeal joints; the joints closest to the tips of the fingers and toes.

Disc The fibrous cartilaginous cushions that lie between the vertebrae.

Dislocation The displacement or "putting out of joint" of the end of a bone from its normal position in the joint.

Diuretic Any substance that increases the production and flow of urine from the body.

DMARD Disease modifying anti-rheumatic drug. Hydroxychloroquine, gold, sulfasalazine, methotrexate, etanercept, and infliximab are DMARDs. They work slowly to inhibit joint inflammation, damage, and sometimes extra-articular features of inflammatory types of arthritis like rheumatoid arthritis.

DMSO Dimethylsulfoxide; a chemical by-product of the pulp and paper industry. It is a solvent that may have some therapeutic value.

Docosahexaenoic acid (DHA) An omega-3 fatty acid found in oils from cold-water fish.

Ductus arteriosum A heart shunt in the fetus that connects the pulmonary artery to the aorta. It should close at birth. If it does not close, it is called a patent (open) ductus arteriosum.

Efferent nerves Nerves that carry messages from the brain back to muscles and glands to initiate an active response such as muscle contraction.

Eicosapentaenoic acid (EPA) An omega-3 fatty acid found in oils from cold-water fish.

Electromagnetic therapy A type of energy therapy that uses electromagnetic waves for healing.

Embolus A mass (such as an air bubble, piece of fat, or detached blood clot) that travels through the bloodstream and lodges to obstruct or occlude a blood vessel.

Endorphins Chemical neurotransmitters found in the brain and spinal cord that act by binding to opiate receptors to reduce the perception of pain.

Endotracheal tube A breathing tube inserted through the nose or mouth into the trachea to assist in ventilating the lungs.

Enthesis The junction where a tendon or ligament inserts into bone.

Enthesitis The inflammation of an enthesis.

Enzyme A protein that controls the rate at which a chemical reaction takes place without itself being destroyed or altered during the reaction.

Epidural anesthesia The injection of an anesthetic into the space outside the dura that surrounds the spinal cord.

Ergonomics The design and arrangement of the equipment and environment in the workplace to maximize the health, comfort, and productivity of the worker.

ESR Erythrocyte sedimentation rate (also called sed. rate); a lab test done to measure how fast the red blood cells drop in a small glass tube.

The faster they fall, the more inflammation there is. The test can be used to assess how active one's inflammatory arthritis is.

Estrogens Female sex hormones that promote the shedding of an egg from the ovary for fertilization, and that are responsible for the secondary female sex characteristics.

Extra-articular features Manifestations of an arthritic disease that are not located in a joint, such as in rheumatoid nodules or a large spleen.

Feldenkrais method The use of gravity to correct physical habits of movement that unduly strain muscles and joints.

Femur The thighbone.

Fibroblast A cell that produces collagen in the soft tissues and organs for supporting their structure and for healing damaged and diseased areas.

Fibula The narrow long bone that runs along the outside of the tibia (shinbone) from the knee to the ankle.

First-degree relatives Parents, siblings, and children.

Fish oils Oils extracted from cold-water fish. They contain omega-3 fatty acids that appear to reduce inflammation.

Flexion contracture See contracture.

Foraminotomy A surgical procedure that enlarges a foramen, the bony tunnel made up of two adjacent vertebrae through which a nerve root exits from the spinal cord to the periphery, in order to relieve any pressure on a nerve as it exits through the foramen.

Gamma linolenic acid (GLA) An omega-6 fatty acid found in the seeds of plants such as evening primrose.

Gene A segment of DNA transmitted from parent to offspring that codes for one specific protein.

Gerovital Procaine hydrochloride ("Novocain"), promoted in Romania as a rejuvenating and anti-arthritis remedy.

Glucosamine This amine of glucose is a normal constituent of the proteoglycans that make up cartilage. It is available as a supplement for the treatment of osteoarthritis.

Glycosaminoglycans Long chains of repeating double sugars (disaccharides) that make up the proteoglycan molecules of cartilage. Examples include chondroitin 4-sulfate, chondroitin 6-sulfate, and keratan sulfate.

Heberden's nodes The bony enlargement of the DIP joints of the fingers by osteoarthritis.

Heparin A drug used to treat and prevent blood clots (thrombosis).

Herb, medicinal A plant or part of a plant used for health and healing.

HLA (human leukocyte antigens) Inherited protein receptors on the surface of cells that recognize foreign antigens for the start of the body's immune response to them. They are used to match organ transplants to a recipient and to study the genetic basis of disease by their greater incidence in different diseases, such as the association of HLA-B27 to ankylosing spondylitis.

Holistic Refers to therapy directed at the person as a whole: spiritual, mental, emotional, and physical with consideration of the family, friends, and environment.

Homeopathy A system of medicine that treats symptoms with minute amounts of substances that can produce the same symptoms when used in larger quantities.

Humerus The bone of the upper arm.

Hyaluronic acid The gel-like glycosaminoglycan found in joint fluid that acts as a binding, lubricating, and protective agent.

Hydrotherapy The use of hot or cold water, ice, and steam for therapeutic purposes, including pool therapy, hot and cold compresses, whirlpools, saunas, and mineral waters.

Hypermobility The ability of a joint to move beyond its normal range of movement (i.e., unusually flexible joints as in "loose-jointed" or "double-jointed").

Idiopathic Having no known cause.

Infection The invasion of the body or a part of the body by a microorganism that multiplies and causes illness.

Inflammation A protective response of the body to injury, tissue damage, or infection. The cardinal signs are pain and tenderness, heat, redness, swelling, and impaired functioning of the inflamed area.

Integrative medicine A mixture of Western and complementary medicine.

Intubation The process by which a breathing tube is inserted through the mouth or nose into the trachea.

Isometric exercise Exercise that strengthens muscle by contracting the muscle against resistance without moving the joint. The force exerted increases without any change in the length of the muscle fibres.

Isotonic exercise Exercise that strengthens muscle by using a steady resistance (like weights or elastic fitness bands) while moving the joint. The resistance is constant but the length of the muscle fibres varies during the exercise.

Juvenile onset arthritis Arthritis that begins before the age of 16 years.

Kyphosis An abnormal backward curvature of the spine that results in a humpback or hunchback of the upper back.

La antibody An autoantibody associated with systemic lupus erythematosus and Sjogren's syndrome. Also known as SS-B antibody.

Laminectomy Surgical removal of the posterior arch of a vertebra (lamina and spinous process) to decompress the nerve tissue.

Laser A device that emits highly amplified light of one or more specific frequencies that give the light different properties and uses. In medicine, a laser can provide intense light or heat. In surgery, the intense heat can be used to vaporize damaged or cancerous cells.

Leukotrienes A family of 20 carbon atom compounds derived from the fatty acid, arachidonic acid. They are related to prostaglandins and mediate inflammation.

Liefcort A mixture of prednisone, estradiol, and testosterone promoted to treat arthritis but with much controversy surrounding its use.

Ligament A band of fibrous tissue that connects bones together and supports and stabilizes joints.

Light therapy The use of light and colour to treat health problems.

Manipulation The use of hands to apply high-velocity thrusts to joints or vertebrae to improve their range of movement or alignment.

Massage The manipulation or working of tissues and muscles by hand to relieve soft- tissue pain and muscle tension.

MCP joints Metacarpophalangeal joints; the large knuckles of the hand. Each MCP joint is made up of the far end of the metacarpal and near end of the closest phalanx of each finger and thumb.

Meditation The process of focusing one's thoughts or engaging in deep contemplation or reflection. Can be used to relieve pain, stress, and fatigue.

Melatonin A hormone secreted by the pineal gland; it is marketed as a remedy for improving sleep.

Meniscus A fibrous cartilage disc that acts as a cushion between the ends of bones that meet in a joint (e.g., the "cartilage" in a knee).

Minerals Inorganic substances that are neither animal nor vegetable. They are required for the normal functioning of the body, which extracts them from food. Examples are sodium, potassium, calcium, magnesium, sulfur, iron, and copper.

Mini-incision surgery Surgery that can be done through much smaller incisions using advanced instruments, even for hip and knee replacements.

Monoarthritis Arthritis that affects only one joint.

Mood disorders (or affective disorders) These represent extremes in moods, such as depression, mania, anger, and euphoria.

Moxibustion The burning of the herb mugwort over acupuncture points to increase circulation and promote healing.

MSM Methylsulfonylmethane; a derivative of DMSO, as well as a natural food substance that is being promoted for the treatment of arthritis and other musculoskeletal ailments.

MTP joints Metatarsophalangeal joints; the balls of the forefoot. Each MTP joint is made up of the far end of the metatarsal and the near end of the closest phalanx of each toe.

Myofascial pain Pain and tenderness in a large area of soft tissue with trigger points.

Naturopathy A system of health that uses nutrition, natural substances, and lifestyle changes to reinforce the body's ability to heal itself and prevent disease.

Navicular A concave bone on the inner aspect of the midfoot and in front of the talus.

Nerve root At the level of each vertebra, from the right and left sides, a nerve root sprouts from the spinal cord to exit through an opening in the spine to join other nerve roots to form peripheral nerves that spread throughout the body. Protruding discs or bone spurs can pinch them.

Neurotransmitters Chemicals that modulate the electric current that leaps from one nerve ending to another in order to assist or impede the transmission of an electrical message (e.g., endorphins impeding pain transmission and substance P assisting it).

Nightshades Plants from the genus Solanum, such as potatoes, tomatoes, eggplant, and bell peppers.

Nociceptor A receptor on a sensory nerve ending that responds to painful stimuli.

NSAID Non-steroidal anti-inflammatory drug, such as aspirin or naproxen; reduces inflammation but does not contain corticosteroids.

Nutraceuticals Foods or food ingredients considered to have medical or health benefits.

Obstructive sleep apnea Sleep apnea is a disorder in which a person stops breathing for 10 seconds or longer up to hundreds of times during sleep. It is usually accompanied by snoring and results in daytime drowsiness. If it occurs when the tissues in the upper airway collapse at intervals during sleep to block the passage of air, it is termed obstructive sleep apnea.

Oligoarthritis Arthritis that affects four joints or fewer.

Omega fatty acids Omega-3 and omega-6 are unsaturated fatty acids. The unsaturated double carbon bond is at the third carbon from the end of the long molecule in omega-3, and at the sixth carbon from the end of the long molecule in omega-6. The omega-3 fatty acids and the omega-6 fatty acid gamma linolenic acid (GLA) shift the production of prostaglandins from inflammatory to non-inflammatory types. The other omega-6 fatty acids shift the production of prostaglandins to the inflammatory types. Omega-3 fatty acids come from cold-water fish and flax seed; omega-6 fatty acids come from plant seeds.

Orthotics Insoles made to fit inside footwear to support, position, alter pressure, and control the movement of the joints and bones of the feet for therapeutic and preventative purposes.

Osteoblast The cell found in bone, which produces the bone matrix.

Osteolysis Dissolution or absorption of bone tissue because of disease.

Osteopathy The practice of mainstream medicine with an emphasis on joint manipulation, postural re-education, and physical therapy to correct structural problems.

Osteotomy A surgical procedure that removes a wedge of bone in order to realign the bone.

Patella The kneecap.

Peripheral nervous system (PNS) The nerves that link the central nervous system with the rest of the body. It includes the afferent and efferent nerves.

Phlebitis Inflammation of a vein that is often associated with a blood clot in the vein.

PIP joints Proximal interphalangeal joints; the middle joints or knuckles in the fingers and toes.

Placebo A treatment that is not supposed to improve an illness, yet it may through the patient's belief that the intervention will work.

Plant seed oils Oils obtained from the seeds of plants like flax, evening primrose, and borage. They contain omega fatty acids that can alter the chemical structure and effects of prostaglandins, such as their pro- and anti-inflammatory effects.

Plexus A network of nerves or blood vessels.

Polarity therapy Gentle manipulative therapy used to promote health and relaxation by unblocking and rebalancing "the life energy that circulates within and around the body."

Polyarthritis Arthritis affecting more than four joints.

Progesterone A female sex hormone that prepares the uterus for reception and development of fertilized eggs.

Prostaglandins A family of chemicals containing 20 carbon atoms derived from arachidonic acid that have an array of physiological functions and mediate inflammation.

Protein A molecule made of amino acids that is an essential and primary constituent of life forms.

Proteoglycans Large molecule constituents of cartilage that hold the water in cartilage. They allow cartilage to flex and absorb physical shock. They have a core protein with numerous glycosaminoglycan chains attached to it at right angles by link proteins.

Protrusio The head of the femur migrating centrally to protrude through the acetabulum (socket) into the pelvis as a result of hip diseases like arthritis.

Psoriasis A chronic disease of the skin and nails featuring elevated red patches covered by silvery scales. Often found on the scalp, ears, genitalia, and over bony prominences. It can be associated with a type of arthritis called psoriatic arthritis.

Pulsed electromagnetic therapy The use of a circular magnetic coil through which a low level of electrical current is sent in pulses to promote healing.

Purines Organic bases like adenine and guanine that are key components of DNA. Their metabolic end product is uric acid, which is responsible for gout.

Quackery The promotion of a medical scheme or remedy known to be false for personal gain; health fraud.

Raynaud's phenomenon A condition in which the blood vessels in the extremities (fingers, toes, earlobes, nose, and lips) reversibly constrict with cold temperatures and emotional stress. The extremities will become cold, uncomfortable, and white, purple, and red.

Referred pain Pain that is felt in a location other than where the actual cause of the pain is.

Reflexology Massaging specific points on the feet, which represent different parts of the body, in order to eliminate "energy blockages that cause illness."

Reiki A Japanese therapy in which the practitioner channels "universal life energy" into a patient with little or no contact with the patient's body.

Remission A period during which the symptoms of a disease have diminished or disappeared.

Rheumatoid factor An antibody against one's own IgG immunoglobulin. It is present in the blood of 85 percent of persons with rheumatoid arthritis. Its detection in the blood is used as a diagnostic test but it is found in other conditions besides rheumatoid arthritis.

Ro antibody An autoantibody found in systemic lupus erythematosus and Sjogren's syndrome. Also known as SS-A.

Rolfing Deep massage designed to strengthen and realign the body by stretching and lengthening the fascias or connective tissues of the body.

SAD Seasonal affective disorder; a type of depression associated with reduced light that occurs in the winter.

SAMe S-adenosylmethionine; an amino acid being promoted for the treatment of osteoarthritis and depression.

Scoliosis An abnormal side-to-side curvature of the spine.

Sed. rate Another term for ESR. See ESR.

Serotonin A natural chemical found in the brain as a neurotransmitter that leads to reduced pain perception, relaxation, sleepiness, and antidepression. It also narrows blood vessels throughout the body.

Shiatsu A Japanese form of acupressure.

Soft tissues The tissues of the body other than bone, cartilage, or teeth. They include muscle, tendon, ligament, bursa, and skin.

Sound therapy The use of sound and vibration for health and healing.

Spa therapy A health system that is centred on the use of hot mineral waters and mud as therapeutic agents.

Spinal anesthesia The injection of anesthetic into the space between the spinal cord and the dura.

Spinal cord The thick cord of nerve tissue that extends from the base of the brain down through the spinal column, carrying sensory and motor nerve impulses to and from the brain. The spinal nerves branch off to various parts of the body from the spinal cord.

Spine The backbone or spinal column of connected vertebral bones that extends from the skull to the pelvis. The cervical spine is in the neck and contains seven vertebrae. The thoracic spine is in the upper back and contains 12 vertebrae. The lumbar spine is in the lower back and contains five vertebrae. The sacrum is the spine contained in the pelvis and the coccyx is the tailbone.

Spiritual healing The transfer of a healing energy or life force from a healer to a patient by the laying on of hands, prayers, incantations, etc.

Sprain A stretching injury to a ligament.

Steroids A number of hormones with a common sterol chemical structure produced in the adrenal gland and gonads. They include the androgens, estrogens, and cortisone or corticosteroids. The corticosteroids (e.g., prednisone) are used to treat inflammation.

Strain A stretching injury to a muscle or tendon.

Stress fracture A fracture resulting from excessive activity or physical stress rather than a specific injury.

Subcutaneous Under the skin; particularly in the fat layer under the skin.

Subluxation Partial dislocation of a joint. Also the term used by chiropractors to refer to misalignments of the vertebrae.

Substance P A neurotransmitter that transmits pain impulses from the peripheral nerve receptors to the spinal cord and brain, intensifying the sensation of pain.

Synovectomy The removal or reduction of the amount of inflamed synovium from a joint or tendon sheath.

Synovitis Inflammation of the synovium. A major feature of most types of arthritis.

Synovium The lining of most joints and tendon sheaths; it secretes the joint fluid and engulfs foreign material to keep the joint clean.

Systemic Relating to or affecting the body generally, for example, fever.

Tai chi An ancient Chinese system of gentle exercises, precision movements, and controlled breathing.

Talus The anklebone, situated between the shinbone (tibia) and heel bone (calcaneus).

Tender point A painful and tender area that does not refer pain elsewhere. There are many of them in specific locations in fibromyalgia.

Tendon The fibrous cord or band connecting a muscle to a bone.

Tendonitis Inflammation or irritation of a tendon.

TENS Transcutaneous electrical nerve stimulation; the application of a mild electrical current by an electrical device to nerves in a painful area in order to reduce pain.

Testimonial Statement of one person's experience.

Testosterone One type of male hormone or androgen.

Therapeutic touch A method of healing whereby a therapist's hands move in a wave-like motion from the head to the toes of a patient with no actual physical contact, in order to restore the "energy field" around the patient.

Tibia The shinbone.

Traction A sustained pull applied mechanically to the neck, back, or a limb to correct a fracture or dislocation, to overcome muscle spasm, and to relieve pressure.

Traditional Chinese medicine A system of health and healing based on ancient Chinese philosophy.

Trager approach A system of movement re-education in which gentle, rhythmic touch combined with movement exercises is applied by a therapist to release tension in posture and movement.

Trigger point A painful and very tender area in muscle and fascia. It may feel like a knot in the muscle. When it is pressed, there is a local twitch response and a referral of the pain in a predictable pattern.

Ultrasound High-frequency sound waves used to visualize organs and tissues in the body for diagnostic purposes. The waves are also used to treat painful areas of the body by causing heat in the deep structures to which they are directed.

Uric acid The end product of the breakdown of purines in the body. Its accumulation in the body by a combination of over-production and under-excretion leads to gout.

Vertebrae The 33 bones that make up the spinal column.

Vertebral artery The artery that runs through the cervical vertebrae to supply blood from the heart to the back half of the brain. There is one on the right side and one on the left side.

Visualization The formation of meaningful mental images in order to achieve relaxation, pain control, and health.

Vital force or energy A hypothetical force or power that gives life to the physical body; perhaps the soul or spirit.

Vitamins Organic chemicals that in minute quantities are vital to nutrition, good health, and normal metabolism.

Yoga An ancient Indian system of exercises, poses, deep breathing, and meditation that can be used for health reasons.

Index

Italicized numerals refer to illustrations and charts.